D0193268

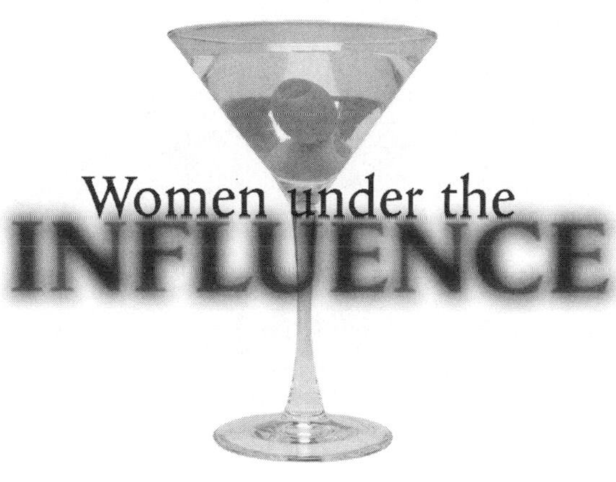
Women under the
INFLUENCE

FOREWORD BY JOSEPH A. CALIFANO, JR.

Women under the INFLUENCE

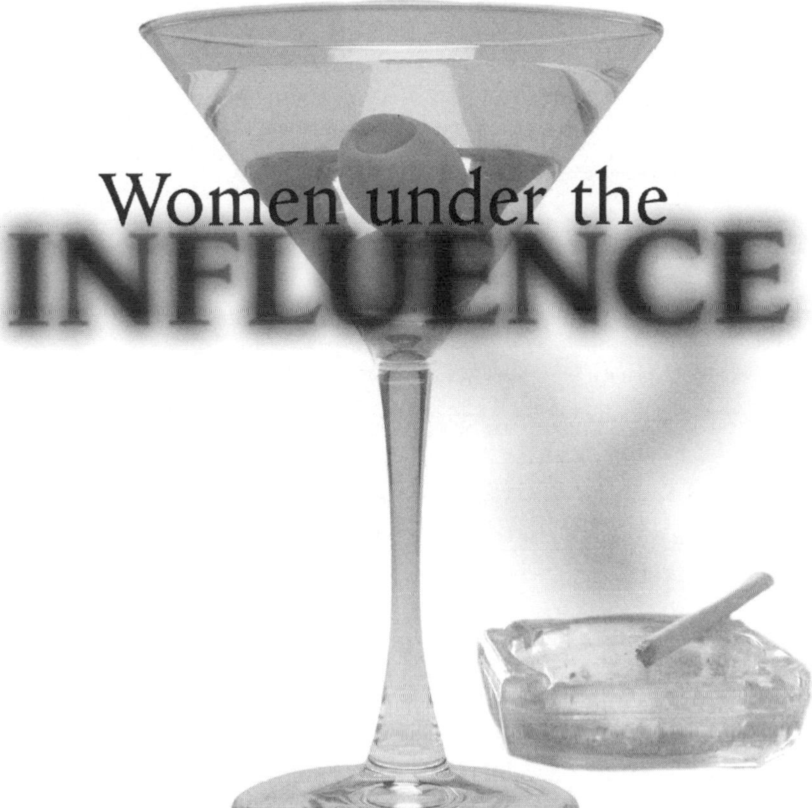

The National Center on Addiction
and Substance Abuse at Columbia University
New York, New York

The Johns Hopkins University Press
Baltimore

Printed in the United States of America on acid-free paper
9 8 7 6 5 4 3 2 1

The Johns Hopkins University Press
2715 North Charles Street
Baltimore, Maryland 21218-4363
www.press.jhu.edu

Library of Congress Cataloging-in-Publication Data

Women under the influence / the National Center on Addiction and Substance Abuse at Columbia University.
p. ; cm.
Includes bibliographical references and index.
ISBN 0-8018-8227-3 (hardcover : alk. paper) —
ISBN 0-8018-8228-1 (pbk. : alk. paper)
1. Women—Substance use—United States. 2. Women—Drug use—United States. 3. Women—Alcohol use—United States. 4. Women—Tobacco use—United States. 5. Women—Mental health—United States.
[DNLM: 1. Substance-Related Disorders—psychology. 2. Substance-Related Disorders—complications. 3. Substance-Related Disorders—prevention & control. 4. Women—psychology. WM 270 W8725 2006]
I. Columbia University. National Center on Addiction and Substance Abuse.
RC564.5. W65W66 2006
616.86′0082—dc22 2005006474

A catalog record for this book is available from the British Library.

ntents contents contents contents contents

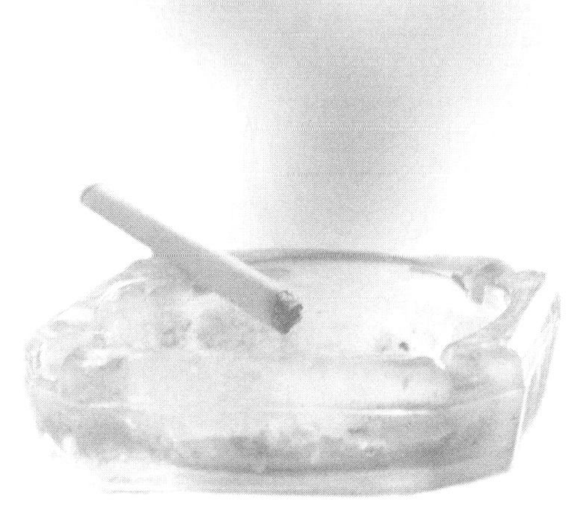

foreword

The result of more than a decade of research by the National Center on Addiction and Substance Abuse (CASA*) at Columbia University, *Women under the Influence* is the first CASA book and represents the most penetrating and comprehensive examination ever undertaken of substance abuse among American women of all ages.

The volume reveals that, compared to boys and men, girls and women become addicted to alcohol, nicotine, and illegal and prescription drugs at lower levels of use and in shorter periods of time, develop substance-related diseases like lung cancer more quickly, suffer more severe brain damage from alcohol and drugs like Ecstasy, and often pay the ultimate price sooner. Yet 92 percent of women in need of treatment for alcohol and drug problems do not receive it. Stigma, shame, and ignorance hide the scope of the problem and the severity of the consequences.

Women under the Influence demonstrates how significant a problem substance abuse has become for American women. Each year scores of thousands die from heart disease, stroke, and cancer—substance abuse is the number one preventable factor in each of these killing and crippling ailments. Some 6 million girls and women abuse or are addicted to alcohol, 15 million use illicit drugs and misuse prescription drugs, and nearly 32 million smoke cigarettes.

This book shines a light into the dark corners of this problem, removes the stigma, and suggests how women and girls with substance abuse and addiction problems can get the help they need to regain control of their lives. Doctors, nurses, teachers, social

*The National Center on Addiction and Substance Abuse at Columbia University is neither affiliated with, nor sponsored by, the National Court Appointed Special Advocate Association (also known as "CASA") or any of its member organizations or any other organization with the name of "CASA."

workers, and drug and alcohol counselors will find this book invaluable, as will policy makers and researchers in education, health care, public health, social services, corrections, and welfare. Any serious effort to improve the quality of health care, contain health care costs, and prevent disease must address this costly problem. Parents will learn here about the special characteristics that put their daughters at risk of substance abuse, and find a host of ideas to protect their daughters, detect the problem when it is taking root, find effective help, and, we hope, avoid the heartache and tragedy that so many families have suffered. Corporate executives and employee-assistance program directors will find more effective ways to tackle this problem among their female employees.

This book has special meaning for women. Substance abuse and addiction are intensely personal and isolating problems for women and young girls; many struggling with it are so paralyzed by shame, embarrassment, and denial that they don't seek the help they need. *Women under the Influence* reveals that substance abuse affects all kinds of women—rich and poor, young and old, black, brown and white, urban and rural, professional and homemaker—and that all kinds of women can confront and deal with the problem. It also uncovers situations and characteristics that increase the risk for girls and women in the conviction that such knowledge will help keep women from becoming substance abusers.

Because each stage of a woman's life harbors unique risks and great opportunities for intervention, this book takes a life-span approach. It highlights key issues for girls and teens, young adult women, adult women, and older women to help explain how the problem develops and changes as women age. Girls and young women may drink to deal with depression or with school and peer pressures, or because they believe drinking will make them more sociable and sexually uninhibited. They may also cope with stress and depression by using drugs. Drug use and heavy drinking among girls and young women can lead to everything from brain damage and serious accidents to rape, unwanted pregnancy, and suicide. As women age, their physical tolerance for alcohol and drugs decreases. At the same time, the death of loved ones, financial difficulties, serious illness, or added responsibilities as caretakers for parents or grandchildren may produce stress that increases the likelihood of alcohol and drug abuse.

Finding and gaining access to effective prevention and treatment programs for girls and women is infuriatingly difficult. Few programs are designed specifically for them, and research on prevention strategies for girls is hard to come by.

Although primary care physicians are in a position to intervene in the substance use of their female patients, physician screening for the problem is uncommon and a failure to recognize the symptoms is too common. Even when physicians screen for substance use, many fail to detect it, and those who do detect it often fail to provide adequate guidance to their patients.

Whether a woman is on welfare or Wall Street, in Manhattan, New York, or Manhattan, Kansas, substance abuse typically is accompanied by other issues that must be addressed in order to achieve recovery: co-occurring mental illness such as depression (which women are likelier to experience), low self-esteem, poor body image, high levels of stress. Women who have been physically or sexually abused are at far greater risk of becoming alcohol and drug abusers and addicts. Troubled family relations, poverty, and job-related stress increase the likelihood of smoking, drinking, and drug use.

CASA was founded in 1992 with the goal of bringing under one roof the skills needed to address all forms of substance abuse in all corners of society. CASA has five missions: to inform Americans of the economic and social costs of substance abuse and its impact on their lives; to assess what works in prevention, treatment, and law enforcement; to encourage every individual and institution to take responsibility to combat substance abuse and addiction; to provide those on the front lines with the tools they need to succeed; and to remove the stigma of abuse and replace the shame and despair with hope.

Soon after we opened our doors, we discovered the appalling lack of research on women and substance abuse. We set to work and in 1996 published *Substance Abuse and the American Woman,* the first comprehensive assessment of how women are affected by all forms of substance use. That groundbreaking report found that many women were not aware of the dangers they faced, that prevention programs failed to meet their needs, that health professionals were misdiagnosing or failing to diagnose, and that the void in research on women and substance abuse was enormous for older women. CASA then probed the hidden problem of addiction among older women. In 1998, CASA released another report, *Under the Rug: Substance Abuse and the Mature Woman.* It was so significant that then American Medical Association president Nancy Dickey, M.D., issued a special alert to physicians and called for diagnosis and treatment of alcohol and substance abuse in older women. In 2003, CASA released *The Formative Years: Pathways to Substance Abuse Among Girls and Young Women Ages 8–22,* an unprecedented analysis of the factors influencing girls and young women to smoke, drink, and use drugs and the unique risks they face. This report elicited wide attention and spurred work in the field to design prevention and treatment efforts that take into account the special needs of girls and young women.

In addition to these three reports and an extensive review of the substance abuse literature, *Women under the Influence* draws from a wealth of CASA research, including studies of eating disorders, underage drinking, diversion and abuse of prescription drugs, substance abuse and America's families, substance abuse and sex, and substance abuse in America's schools and in child welfare and criminal justice systems. This book includes data from several national surveys conducted by CASA, including its annual survey of teen and parental attitudes toward substance abuse, surveys of teens and adults on underage drinking, and surveys of primary care physicians and their patients with substance abuse problems.

The work that led to this book has influenced the development of CASA's own programs. CASAWORKS for Families[sm] was launched in June 1998 with the mission of helping drug- and alcohol-addicted mothers on welfare achieve self-sufficiency. CASAWORKS for Families[sm] combines in a single, concentrated course drug and alcohol treatment, literacy and job training, parenting and social skills, violence prevention, health care, family services, and a gradual move to work. Because of the research results from the earlier women's reports, the program included treatment specially designed for women.

Addiction is a complex and vexing health and social problem that millions of girls and women battle every day. CASA has written *Women under the Influence* to awaken health professionals, educators, parents, policy makers, and clergy to appreciate the scope and special characteristics of the substance abuse problem for girls and women, the key points of intervention for prevention and treatment, and the roads to recovery. Although research on this topic is continuing, nearly a decade after the release of CASA's *Substance Abuse and The American Woman,* there remain few studies, treatment programs, or prevention initiatives that address the unique risks, needs, and consequences of substance abuse for girls and women.

If years ago we had instituted prevention and treatment programs tailored to the needs of girls and young women, the numbers now suffering could have been significantly reduced. A 25 percent reduction—a modest estimate—would have saved almost eight million girls and women from smoking, one and a half million from abusing or becoming addicted to alcohol, and nearly four million from abusing drugs. Just think of the human wreckage, the family tragedies, that could have been prevented! And the benefits would not have ended there: one generation's burden passes on to the next—a family history of tobacco, alcohol, or drug abuse puts children at greater risk of such abuse.

Preventing and reducing substance abuse among women is crucial to improving the future of our nation and the health of our families. This is a fight worth fighting and worth fighting now. That's why CASA is publishing *Women under the Influence.*

The acknowledgments at the end of the text recognize many of the individuals who worked on this project over the past decade. I want to single out here Susan Foster, M.S.W., CASA's vice president and director of policy research and analysis, who has spearheaded, directed, and supervised this effort. Her intelligence, commitment, sensitivity, judgment, and high standard of scholarship have been critical to the research over the past decade and have shaped every chapter of this extraordinary book. She has become a national resource on women and substance abuse. I also want to recognize Peter Dolan, chief executive officer of Bristol-Myers Squibb, and John Damonti, president of the company's foundation. They provided the resources over many years to make this undertaking possible; throughout they have provided Sue Foster and all the CASA researchers complete freedom. It is a testament to their commitment to women's health.

Joseph A. Califano, Jr.
Chairman and President, The National Center on Addiction
and Substance Abuse at Columbia University
Secretary, U.S. Department of Health, Education, and Welfare, 1977–1979

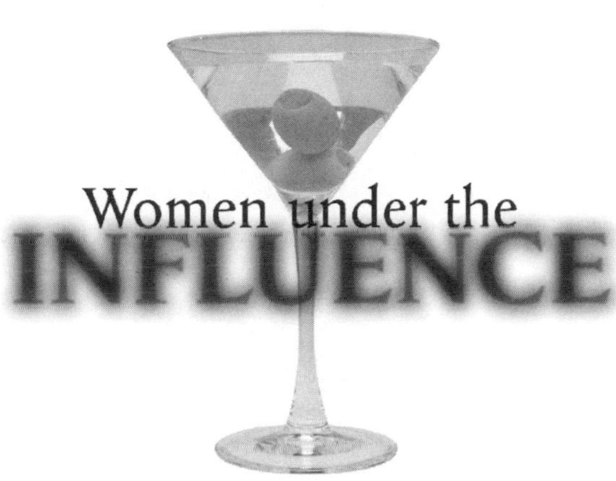
Women under the
INFLUENCE

chapter 1

Pathways to Substance Abuse among Girls and Women

There is no single point in a woman's life when a discussion of substance use or abuse is not relevant. Each stage of life offers unique challenges that can lead to addiction. And each stage poses unique risks to the health and well-being of women who abuse substances. Smoking, drinking, and drug use can interfere with girls' academic performance and family and peer relations; it can lead to other high-risk behaviors, such as getting into fights or engaging in risky sex; it can precipitate the emergence of eating disorders, depression, or anxiety; and it can hike the risk of accidents, homicide, and suicide. Women who smoke, abuse alcohol, or use drugs also are at increased risk of cancer, heart disease, and liver disease. The negative consequences of substance abuse in women often are compounded by the added responsibilities of adulthood, including marriage, pregnancy, childcare, employment, and caring for aging parents. The aging process makes older women even more susceptible to the physical and psychological effects of substance abuse, often at a time when many are losing their social support systems and facing financial limitations and other life difficulties.

Understanding how substance abuse affects women of all ages and the unique pathways to addiction that originate in childhood and progress through adulthood is essential if we are successfully to improve the quality of life for millions of women and their families.

The Experiences and Challenges of Girls and Young Women

As girls grow and develop, the transitions into adolescence and early adulthood—entering middle or junior high school, entering and graduating from high school or college, or entering the workforce—frequently involve many changes in the social and physical environment that influence their risk of unhealthy behavior.[1] Some aspects of these transitions appear to affect girls and young women differently than boys and young men as they form attitudes, beliefs, and habits that can influence their use of cigarettes, alcohol, and drugs.

Adolescence

Early adolescence often is an unstable and fragile time for girls.[2] They begin to struggle with physical and emotional maturity as they simultaneously try to define their identities and move successfully from childhood to young adulthood.[3]

The transition to middle or junior high school typically is accompanied by visible signs of puberty among girls—including rapid growth, weight gain, and development of sex characteristics.[4] Puberty is a time of higher risk for girls than boys, in part because overt pubertal changes for boys tend to emerge once they have had time to adjust to the middle school transition.[5] At this stage, girls experience an increased emphasis by peers and family on physical appearance, self-presentation, and popularity. They are likelier than boys to compare themselves physically and academically to their new peers,[6] increasing their self-doubts.[7] They also begin to shift their focus from their parents and other adults, looking instead to peers and popular culture for self-evaluation and self-critique.[8]

Perhaps as a means of managing these emerging physical, familial, and social challenges of early adolescence, girls begin to become more sensitive to others' feelings and impressions, gauging their personalities, predicting their reactions, and attempting to respond accordingly.[9] Thus begins a pattern in which girls and women suppress their own thoughts and desires in favor of those of others,[10] opening them up to peer influences to engage in substance use and other unhealthy behaviors.

During middle adolescence, girls and boys make yet another transition, from middle school to high school.[11] Girls strive to develop a unique identity but also feel the need to conform to their peer group.[12] Pressure on girls of this age to project a more feminine image sometimes is associated with less satisfaction with their physical appearance, increased depression, lower self-esteem, and decreased academic success[13]—any of which can increase their risk of substance use. Substance abuse at this time may stunt girls' emotional growth, lower their self-esteem, increase their risk of depression, hinder their ability to plan ahead, and contribute to truancy or school dropout.[14]

Later adolescence also is a period of tremendous change.[15] Girls at this stage struggle to achieve independence yet remain connected.[16] They seek greater autonomy from parents and begin to form visions of their own goals.[17] Older adolescent girls who abuse substances may lack self-confidence and be highly self-critical while pro-

COMING OF AGE IN TODAY'S WORLD

Girls today . . . are coming of age in a more dangerous, sexualized and media-saturated culture. They face incredible pressures to be beautiful and sophisticated, which in junior high means using chemicals and being sexual. As they navigate a more dangerous world, girls are less protected.

—Mary Pipher, Ph.D., author, *Reviving Ophelia: Saving the Selves of Adolescent Girls*

Source: Pipher, M. B. (1994). *Reviving Ophelia: Saving the selves of adolescent girls.* New York: Putnam. P. 12.

claiming their independence.[18] Upon entering college, young women may use their newfound independence to engage in risky behaviors that they were unable to pursue under the watchful eyes of their parents and high school teachers.[19]

Early Adulthood

After college or upon entry into the workforce, young adults are faced with the stress of pursuing their careers. Although tremendous progress has been made in ridding the work environment of gender-based discrimination, young women in certain careers still face such biases, albeit typically in more subtle forms than in the past. Many young women also begin to face the pressures of balancing career goals with their families and relationships. How a young woman copes with these adulthood pressures will influence whether or not she turns to substance use.

The Unique Challenges of Adult Women

Most adult women today grew up in a time of tremendous social and political upheaval, in which their redefined roles provided them with more autonomy and opportunities than ever before, yet still called for adherence to the traditional responsibilities of marriage and motherhood. Whereas earlier generations of women certainly faced stressful life circumstances, today's woman faces considerable demands on her time, energy, and resources as she struggles to balance career and family responsibilities. Women today often are burdened by the financial responsibilities of single-parenthood, by the need to provide continued care and support to their children long after they have passed into adulthood themselves, or by the tremendous economic and emotional costs of caring for aging parents.

Despite their enormous sacrifices and contributions to society, adult women are virtually invisible in popular culture, which fixates on youth and devalues the normal aging process. Women straining to keep up with the youth-oriented culture may become depressed by the inevitable gray hairs, emerging wrinkles, or extra pounds and the sense of "invisibility" or "disappearance" that many begin to feel in their surrounding environment.[20]

Unfortunately, the social, political, and economic equality that women have begun to achieve has been accompanied by their equality in the realm of substance abuse and addiction. Women experiencing the stresses of adulthood—including pregnancy and child rearing, maintaining steady and rewarding employment, managing a household, fostering a healthy marriage, coping with the empty nest (or the unanticipated and prolonged full nest), dealing with divorce and its consequent financial pressures, and facing family illness or parental death—may turn to alcohol or drugs for escape or solace.

Challenges of Older Adulthood

The challenges of middle adulthood—of family changes, financial stress, and moving farther away from the cultural ideal of youthfulness—often are compounded as women age. Many older women struggle with retirement, an empty nest, sudden or chronic illness, the loss of independent living, financial woes, or the deaths of spouses, relatives, or friends.[21] Some older women take care of their own aging parents;[22] others become primary caretakers for grandchildren, sometimes because their own children work long hours, are divorced, abuse substances, or are unable to be responsible parents.[23] Some less burdened older women report taking up heavy alcohol use out of boredom or having "more time to drink" once they have shed the responsibilities of earlier years.[24]

For some older women, increasing physical ailments, such as arthritis or other forms of chronic pain, can bring them into more encounters with abusable prescription drugs which, if not appropriately prescribed and monitored by their physicians, can result in misuse of these drugs and ultimately in addiction.[25] The depression and anxiety that accompanies these physical ailments can further increase the risk that older women will abuse alcohol or prescription drugs to alleviate their distress. Indeed, alcohol and prescription drug abuse are the two leading substance-related problems older women face.[26]

Pathways to Substance Abuse

Regardless of the particular life stage, no formula exists for identifying who will engage in substance use or if that use will lead to dependence or addiction. Risk and protective factors for substance use are linked to an individual's personality, family, peers, community, and culture. Successful intervention begins by recognizing who is most at risk and why. Although some risk pathways* are unique to particular substances, there are pathways that are common to all abusable substances, including tobacco, alcohol, illicit drugs, and certain psychoactive prescription drugs.

The Genetic and Biological Pathway

Whether girls and young women smoke, drink, or use drugs is determined more by their environment than by their genetics or biology.[27] However, genetic and biological factors appear to play a larger role than environmental factors in determining whether substance use will develop into abuse and addiction.[28] Therefore, understanding the role of genetics and biology is critical to informing prevention and treatment.

Twin and adoption studies† confirm a genetic role in the transmission of tobacco, alcohol, and illicit drug use behaviors from parent to child.[29] Indicators of gender differences in biological tendencies toward substance abuse also can be found in studies of physical reactions to certain substances.[30] For example, daughters of alcoholics tend to have a greater physiological tolerance for alcohol,[31] increasing their risk of heavy drinking and the development of subsequent alcohol problems. Young women with a family history of alcoholism also produce more saliva when exposed to alcohol than women without such a history, suggesting a potential risk for more intense alcohol craving and future alcohol problems.[32]

---

* CASA has conducted extensive research on the pathways leading to substance use and abuse among girls and young women, and much of that research is included here. Of note is a two-part national survey of 1,220 girls and young women making key life transitions from elementary to middle school, middle to high school, high school to college, and college into the world beyond, referred to as the *Formative Years* survey. CASA also conducted focus groups with preadolescent girls ages 8 to 12 and with their parents to better understand the perspectives and risks of younger girls with regard to substance use.

† These studies help researchers differentiate between the roles of genetics versus environment in the propensity to develop a substance use disorder. Studies of adopted children allow researchers to compare the adopted child both to her biological parents, with whom she shares genetic features but no environmental experiences, and to her adopted parents, with whom she shares environmental experiences but no genetic features. Similarly, studies of identical (monozygotic) and fraternal (dizygotic) twins allow researchers to isolate genetic similarities from environmental similarities. Identical twins are genetically identical and fraternal twins share an average of 50 percent of their genes, but both types of twins typically experience a shared environment if reared together. Some research suggests, however, that the social environment of fraternal twins actually may be less similar to that of identical twins (e.g., less overlap in friendship networks); therefore, some twin studies may overstate the strength of genetic influence on substance use disorders.

Puberty

The timing of the biological changes associated with puberty is related to a girl's risk for substance use and other problem behaviors. Girls whose physical and sexual maturation proceed faster than average are at increased risk for a spectrum of negative outcomes, including substance use and abuse.[33] Girls who experience early puberty are at increased risk of engaging in substance use earlier, more often, and in greater quantities than their peers whose physical maturity occurs later.[34]

Like the risk for substance use, there are biological and environmental influences on the timing of puberty.[35] One biological explanation for the relationship between early puberty and an increased risk for substance use points to the role of testosterone in substance use and the timing of puberty onset. Higher testosterone levels in young adult females have been associated with current smoking and smoking during adolescence as well as with the earlier onset of puberty.[36] The link also may be explained by the greater tendency of early-maturing girls to associate with older, more risk-taking peers,[37] particularly boys, and to use substances to cope with the physiological and emotional stresses associated with puberty.[38]

Falling Tolerance as Women Age

Biological changes that affect the potential for substance abuse do not end with puberty. Women of any age react differently than men to alcohol and, preliminary research suggests, psychoactive prescription drugs. They get addicted faster and after consuming smaller amounts. Particularly among older women, physical tolerance for alcohol and drugs declines with age because the amount of lean body mass (muscle and bone) and water in women's bodies decrease with age as the amount of fat increases.[39] Metabolism also slows down so that alcohol or drugs remain in the body longer and less is needed to achieve the same effect.[40] Given the same quantity of alcohol, older adults experience a higher concentration of it in the blood than younger people.[41] Reduced liver and kidney function also may slow down the metabolism and the elimination of alcohol from the body.[42]

These changes can surprise older women. What appeared to be safe and moderate drinking in their thirties and forties can be dangerous, abusive, and addicting in their sixties and seventies.[43]

Co-Occurring Disorders and Addiction

In many cases, common biological or genetic factors can account for the co-occurrence of substance abuse and psychiatric disorders. Certain mental health disorders in a biological parent relate to similar disorders in children, and these mental health disorders tend to co-occur with substance abuse.[44] Childhood conduct disorder and alcoholism, for example, appear to be genetically linked in women.[45] In one study, the increased risk of substance use among 17-year-old girls with conduct disorder (symptoms include aggression to people and animals, destruction of property, deceitfulness or theft, and serious violations of rules) was more than four times that of girls without conduct disorder; the risk for boys was two-and-a-half times greater for those with versus without conduct disorder.[46] In addition, the co-occurrence of frequent smoking and alcoholism with major depressive disorder appears to result primarily from genetics that predispose women to both conditions.[47] One study of female twins found that women with major depressive disorder were approximately three to six times more likely than those without to suffer from alcoholism.[48]

Mental Health and Addiction

Mental illness and substance use disorders are closely linked in women. Nearly two million adult women in the United States (approximately 2%) are estimated to have both a serious mental illness and substance use disorder—the rate is similar among adult men.[49]

Signs of mental-health related risk for future substance abuse often can be detected in children at a very early age.[50] Although only a few studies have examined gender differences in this regard, the general findings show that young girls and boys with difficult temperaments—who demonstrate poor adaptability, hyperactivity, insecurity, or chronic negative moods—may have more problems coping with the interpersonal demands of adolescence and young adulthood, putting them at greater risk for substance use and abuse as they age.[51] Among females and males, a tendency toward rebelliousness, risk taking, and sensation seeking is a key risk factor for substance use.[52]

Self-Esteem

Self-esteem—self-confidence or self-image—plays an important role in the use of tobacco, alcohol, and drugs. Self-esteem declines for girls and boys upon entering middle school; however, the decline among girls typically is more dramatic.[53] A national survey of girls found that 14 percent of high-school-aged girls have low self-confidence compared to 9 percent of younger girls.[54] Teenage girls with low self-confidence are twice as likely as those with higher self-confidence to report smoking (smoking several cigarettes to a pack or more in the last week), drinking (drinking alcohol at least once a month), or using drugs (using illegal drugs in the last month).[55] On the other hand, girls with high self-esteem generally are less likely to engage in delinquency and substance use.[56]

Body Image

For girls, dissatisfaction with and attempts to control body weight play an important role in promoting eating disorders and substance use. The effect of weight concerns on substance use can be seen over a wide spectrum of weight-related attitudes and behaviors, ranging from mere appearance concerns to full-blown eating disorders. CASA's *Formative Years* survey found that as girls get older, they are significantly more likely to try to control their weight, often in quite unhealthy ways (Fig. 1.1).[57]

The greatest change in the tendency to diet occurs during middle school (between the fifth and eighth grades), when most girls are going through puberty and putting on weight—a natural phenomenon that conflicts with fashion's beauty ideal. Younger girls tend to associate weight loss with being prettier and with greater popularity, whereas older girls are more likely to associate it specifically with being more attractive.[58] Although increases in dieting behaviors can be seen as early as middle school, the teen years are when girls usually begin to show symptoms of eating disorders.[59] These are precisely the same years when girls are at greatest risk for engaging in substance use.[60] Girls with eating disorders may use tobacco, alcohol, or other drugs to self-medicate negative feelings or to further help in their efforts to lose weight.[61]

The link between eating disorders and substance abuse does not end in adolescence. Women continue to feel the pressure to conform to the thin ideal throughout their lives, and many turn to smoking and drug use to help them maintain an unhealthy low weight. Indeed, increasing numbers of middle-aged women are struggling with eating disorders.[62]

Stress

Females and males tend to react differently to stressful life events, with females internalizing reactions by becoming depressed or anxious, and males externalizing stress by becoming aggressive and engaging in delinquent behaviors.[63] Girls are more likely than boys to respond to stress with substance use, particularly smoking.[64] For girls, the combination of low self-esteem and stressful life events makes depressive symptoms more

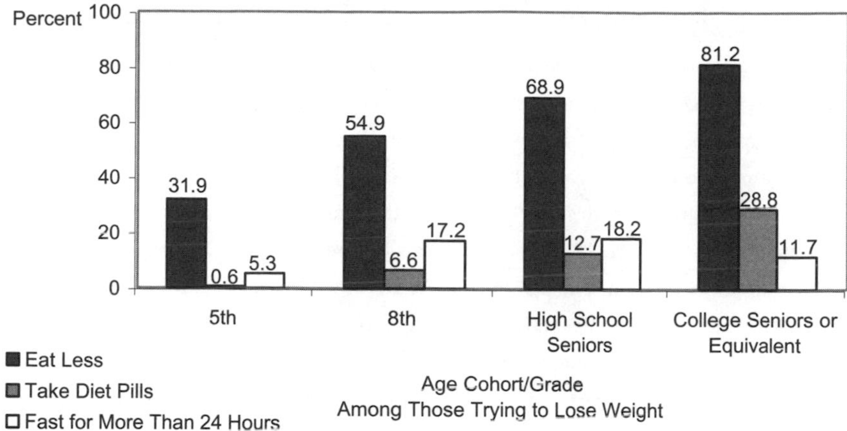

Fig. 1.1. Dieting behaviors in the formative years. *Source:* The National Center on Addiction and Substance Abuse (CASA) at Columbia University. (2003). *The formative years: Pathways to substance abuse among girls and young women ages 8–22*. New York: CASA. P. 42.

likely,[65] thereby increasing their risk of substance use.[66] In fact, one of the most common reasons given by girls in grades 5 through 12 for engaging in substance use is stress relief, and this is particularly true of those who are depressed or who have been abused.[67]

Stress is a common precursor for substance use in women of all ages. Not only do females tend to experience specific forms of life stress—such as sexual abuse, the pressures of caring for relatives, and certain forms of illness—more often than males, but also they seem to react to stress less adaptively than males.[68] One means of coping with stress is to turn to substances of abuse.

Depression

Depression is a significant risk factor for substance use, and females are likelier than males to experience depression.[69] CASA's *Formative Years* survey found that girls who reported depressive symptoms at an initial interview were significantly likelier than those with fewer depressive symptoms to report greater alcohol use, binge drinking, and more frequent marijuana use at the second interview, even after taking into consideration their earlier alcohol or marijuana use.[70] These relationships were particularly true for recent college graduates.[71]

This research supports other findings that girls who are susceptible to depression and anxiety are at particularly high risk of developing substance use disorders.[72] Depression and anxiety during preadolescence increase the risk of initiating alcohol use in adolescence and developing a drug disorder in early adulthood.[73]

Older women are twice as likely as older men to report feeling depressed; about four million women over age 65 are depressed, compared to about two million elderly men.[74] Depression after age 60 is most common among women who are unmarried, lack close friends, participate in few activities, frequently visit physicians, are in declining health or are disabled, and take several prescribed medications.[75] They may be struggling with an empty nest and the loss of their primary role as mother.[76] But perhaps the biggest factor during older adulthood is bereavement.[77] Lingering depression is common after the death of a spouse.[78] At any age, female alcoholics are twice as likely as nonalcoholic females to be depressed and almost four times more likely than male alcoholics to be depressed.[79] Smoking also is more common among women suffering from depression, which in turn makes it more difficult for women to quit.[80]

Physical and Sexual Abuse

The more adverse experiences a child has with abuse (recurrent physical, emotional, or sexual abuse) and household dysfunction (having lost a parent during childhood or growing up in a household with a family member who is in prison, or who is an alcohol or drug abuser, a victim of violence, and/or chronically mentally ill), the higher that child's risk of smoking, drinking, and using drugs in adulthood.[81] More than one in five high school girls report having experienced sexual or physical abuse.[82] These girls are twice as likely to smoke, drink, or use drugs as those who were not abused (Fig. 1.2).[83]

Substance use is one type of coping strategy that can provide escape from painful childhood experiences and serve as a means of self-medicating feelings of isolation and loneliness.[84] Sexually abused teens report significantly more anxiety, loneliness, and depression than nonabused teens,[85] all of which are significant risk factors for substance use and abuse.

Studies of teenage girls find earlier initiation of substance use and more excessive use among those who have been sexually victimized.[86] More than twice as many girls as boys in treatment for drug abuse report current physical and sexual abuse.[87] Nearly twice as many girls in drug treatment who have a history of sexual abuse began using alcohol before the age of 11 compared to those with no history of abuse. In addition, sexually abused girls were approximately three-and-a-half times likelier to use sedatives, tranquilizers, painkillers, and opiates regularly (at least once a month in the past year) than girls who were not abused.[88]

The long reach of childhood victimization can be seen in adults as well. Women who were sexually or physically abused in childhood are significantly more likely than nonabused women to drink, get intoxicated, experience alcohol-related problems and alcohol dependence symptoms, and to abuse psychoactive prescription and illicit drugs.[89]

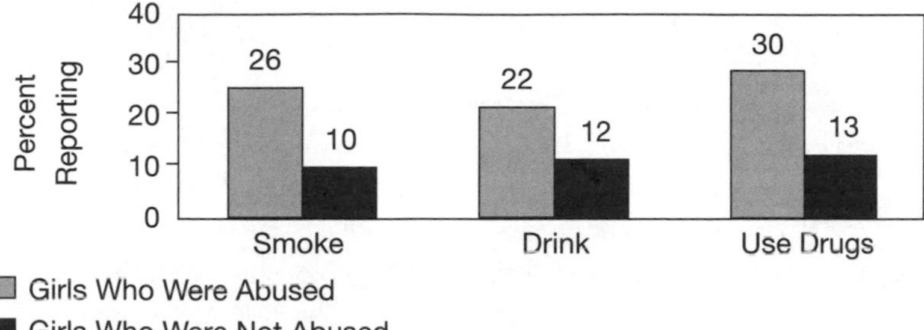

Fig. 1.2. Smoking, drinking, or using drugs, by physical or sexual abuse. *Source:* Data from Schoen, C., Davis, K., Collins, K. S., Greenberg, L., Des Roches, C., and Abrams, M. (1997). *The Commonwealth Fund survey of the health of adolescent girls.* New York: Commonwealth Fund. P. 27.

The Family and Addiction

Abundant research demonstrates that parents hold one of the most important keys to children's decisions of whether or not to smoke, drink, or use drugs.[90] And research suggests that girls appear to be more responsive than boys to parental influences on substance use.[91]

The worse a girl's relationship with her parents, the earlier her initiation of alcohol use and the greater her likelihood of drug use. In contrast, girls who communicate openly with their parents about the dangers of substance use are significantly less likely to be substance users.[92] The majority of girls (61.6%) in CASA's *Formative Years* survey who reported talking with their parents about substance use said that their conversations made them less likely to smoke, drink, or use drugs.[93]

The link between consistent messages of parental disapproval of substance use and lower rates of children's substance use is strong.[94] Five times as many teens (47%) who say their parents wouldn't particularly disapprove of their smoking one or more packs of cigarettes a day are current smokers compared to teens who say their parents would strongly disapprove (9%). Nearly three times as many teens (43%) who say their parents wouldn't particularly disapprove of their having one or two alcoholic drinks nearly every day currently use alcohol compared to teens who say their parents would strongly disapprove (15%). Five times as many teens (29%) who say their parents wouldn't particularly disapprove of their trying marijuana once or twice are current marijuana users compared to teens who say their parents would strongly disapprove (6%).[95] Girls who perceive parents as highly disapproving of substance use or who be-

LEADING BY EXAMPLE

More important than anything parents say is what they do . . . It won't work for parents to start talking to their kids about drinking "responsibly" when they themselves cannot go to a party without coming home drunk, or come home and not have a "drink before dinner." We have to be honest with ourselves if we are to be honest with our children.

—Ralph I. López, M.D., Clinical Associate Professor of Pediatrics and Associate Attending Physician, Weill Cornell Medical Center; author, *The Teen Health Book: A Parents' Guide to Adolescent Health and Well-Being*

Source: López, R. I. (2002). *The teen health book: A parents' guide to adolescent health and well-being.* New York: W. W. Norton. P. 262.

lieve there would be disciplinary consequences should they use substances experiment with fewer drugs and get high less frequently than other girls.[96]

Parents who smoke, use drugs, abuse alcohol, or demonstrate permissive attitudes about substance use put their children—girls and boys—at risk for similar behavior.[97]

Uninvolved and Disengaged Parents Increase Risk

Parents who do not monitor their children's activities or do not remain consistently involved in their lives put their children at risk for substance use.[98] Parents are likelier with daughters than with sons to make sure that they know where their daughters are and whom they are with, to make family rules clear, to discuss instances of misbehavior, to praise achievements, and to refrain from disparaging them.[99] Parents generally are less likely to allow their daughters to get away with misbehaving.[100]

Religion

Religion appears to be strongly linked to less substance use and abuse, particularly in girls.[101] Among girls, more frequent attendance at religious services is associated with less smoking, drinking, binge drinking, and drug use. Likewise, the greater importance girls attach to religion or spirituality, the less substance use they report.[102]

Not only do girls tend to be more religious than boys and to hold more favorable attitudes toward religion,[103] but also being involved in religion is more strongly associated with reduced risk for substance use among girls than among boys.[104] Among female college students, religiosity is related to less alcohol consumption and fewer drinking-related problems.[105]

Religion is a valuable protective factor throughout a woman's life. Spiritual values and social support that mature women share in religious communities may help prevent substance use and abuse. In these settings, individuals who do not use or abuse substances also may serve as role models. Mature women who are not religious are more likely to drink and smoke than those who hold religious beliefs.[106] Mature women who describe themselves as not religious are much more likely to drink (90.8%) and be current smokers (44.8%) than those who identify themselves as Catholic (64% drink, 24.8% smoke) or Protestant (52.3% drink, 20.7% smoke).[107]*

The School and Community Environment

Risk factors for youth substance use can be found within the neighborhood, school, and larger community.[108] Neighborhoods and communities that are caring and supportive, provide positive role models, hold high expectations for achievement, and encourage youth participation in events have been found to protect against substance use.[109] Neighborhoods and communities with higher rates of poverty, norms that encourage substance use, and high levels of drug availability have been found to increase the risk for substance use.[110] Girls living in more troubled neighborhoods are likelier to smoke, drink, and use drugs than those living in safer neighborhoods.[111]

School

Academic difficulty is a strong risk factor for substance use among teens. Girls who use substances of abuse in the teen years are likelier to have had academic problems.[112] Poor school performance in preadolescence and adolescence increases the risk for alcohol abuse in early adulthood as well.[113]

---

*The survey sample was too small to determine rates for other religious affiliations. Small sample size makes it impossible to determine that the difference between smoking rates among those who are not religious and those who are Protestant is statistically significant. Because the National Household Survey on Drug Abuse (NHSDA, now called the National Survey on Drug Use and Health [NSDUH]) does not contain data on religious affiliation, this data comes from the 1995 Health and Retirement Survey (HRS). The HRS does not ask about use of alcohol during the past month; those who "drink" represents those who answered "yes" to the question, "Do you ever drink any alcoholic beverages?" Overall, the reported prevalence of current drinking and smoking are higher in the HRS than in the NHSDA.

Extracurricular Activities

Teenage girls who do not participate in any extracurricular activities are twice as likely to report current smoking as those who participate in multiple (three or more) activities (25.5% vs. 12.4%). Girls not engaged in activities also are likelier than those engaged in multiple activities to drink alcohol (19.2% vs. 14.9%) and use marijuana (10% vs. 4.8%).[114]

Socioeconomic Status

Although it may be commonly believed that low-income children are at higher risk for substance use and abuse than their wealthier counterparts, the relationship between wealth and substance use risk is not clear-cut. For example, whereas low-income teens may smoke and use certain illicit drugs more than those who are more affluent, their rates of alcohol use are somewhat lower.[115] Other research finds that affluent suburban youth report higher levels of substance use than inner-city youth.[116] A study of tenth-grade girls found that those from affluent, suburban families had higher levels of tobacco, alcohol, and marijuana use than those from inner-city families (35% vs. 15% reported using these substances at least once).[117] Affluent seventh-grade girls in another study exhibited higher rates of depression and anxiety symptoms than those typically found in less affluent populations. The affluent girls at highest risk for substance use and other problems tended to lack adult after-school supervision and to feel low levels of closeness with their mothers.[118]

Frequent Moving

Frequent moving from one home or neighborhood to another is strongly related to increased risk for substance use, particularly among girls. Teenage girls who move frequently (six or more times) over the course of a five-year period are much more likely to report smoking, drinking, and drug use than those who do not move at all during that time or than boys who move frequently.[119]

Peers

Peers may influence substance use by showing approval of smoking, drinking, or drug use, by serving as role models for these behaviors, or by applying pressure to engage in these behaviors.[120] Generally, girls are more susceptible to peer influences to smoke and drink than boys, perhaps because girls tend to spend more time with friends and to be more involved in their peers' lives than boys.[121] Social relationships among girls tend to be more intimate and exclusive than those of boys.[122] Girls experiencing problems or feeling stress are more likely than boys to seek social support outside of the family, particularly from a same-sex friend.[123] Girls are likelier than boys to perceive friends as helpful in providing social support, whereas boys tend to see formal supports, such as counselors and teachers as more helpful.[124]

Peer substance use is an important predictor of smoking, drinking, and drug use.[125] The more friends a girl has who smoke cigarettes, drink regularly, and use marijuana or other illegal drugs, the likelier she is to do these things herself.[126]

Peer Pressure

Peer pressure to smoke, drink, or use drugs may occur in the form of encouragement, dares, or actual offers from peers of cigarettes, alcohol, or drugs.[127] Teens who are susceptible to peer pressure (e.g., their "friends could push them into doing just about anything") or who report experiencing peer pressure (e.g., they "often feel pressured to do things they wouldn't normally do") consume more tobacco, alcohol, and illicit drugs than those who experience less peer pressure.[128] Girls' perception of pressure by other people their age to smoke, drink, and use drugs increases as they progress through middle and high school, with the greatest increase in the perception of peer pressure to drink or use drugs occurring during this time.[129]

The extent to which girls experience peer pressure to smoke, drink, or use drugs also is strongly related to the number of friends they have who engage in those behaviors. Girls who report having been pressured to smoke, drink, or use drugs are significantly likelier to have more substance-using friends than girls who report not experiencing such pressure.[130]

Another study of teen girls found that many initiated smoking at the urging of their friends and chose to continue to smoke to fit in with their peers. Among those who wanted to quit smoking, fear of peer rejection or at least an expectation that peers would not be supportive of an attempt to quit led some girls to sustain their smoking behavior.[131]

A study of 11- and 13-year-old girls found that those at the top of the social pecking order—the most popular girls—believe they are under more pressure to smoke than less popular girls, suggesting that peer pressure sometimes is due less to active influencing by peers and more to pressure to maintain a certain image.[132] Popular girls may use smoking as a means of bolstering an image of one who is rebellious, sophisticated, and stands out from a crowd.[133]

Peer pressure may be associated more strongly with drinking for girls than it is for boys.[134] One study found that when several of a girl's closest friends smoke or drink, she is more than seven times likelier to drink alcohol; boys who have several close friends who smoke or drink are almost three times likelier to drink.[135]

Availability

Boys generally have an easier time than girls obtaining tobacco, alcohol, and drugs and are likelier than girls to receive offers to smoke, drink, or use drugs.[136] Although males generally have more opportunities than females to use drugs like marijuana, cocaine, hallucinogens, and heroin, once presented with the opportunity, equal numbers of males and females eventually will engage in drug use.[137]

One national study found that 13.8 percent of teenage girls (compared to 24.2% of teenage boys) under the age of 18 who smoke report that they obtained their own cigarettes by purchasing them in a store or gas station in the past 30 days.[138] An earlier version of this study found that among teens who purchased their own cigarettes from these venues in the past month, more girls than boys (72.9% vs. 64%) were not asked to show proof that they were of the legal age of 18 to purchase cigarettes.[139] While teenage girls are less likely to obtain their cigarettes by purchasing them, they are 58% more likely than teenage boys to acquire cigarettes through noncommercial sources (e.g., getting them from friends or by getting someone else to buy them).[140] With regard to illicit drugs, teenage girls are likelier than teenage boys to report that marijuana (55.8% vs. 51.6%), cocaine (30.1% vs. 20.5%), crack (31.8% vs. 20.5%), LSD (21.3% vs. 13.9%), and heroin (18.6% vs. 12.4%) are fairly or very easy to obtain.[141]

Thirteen percent of teen girls and 18.9 percent of teen boys reported being approached in the previous month by someone selling drugs.[142] Girls are more likely to be offered drugs by a female acquaintance, a young female relative (i.e., sister, cousin), or a boyfriend, whereas boys are more likely to be offered drugs by a male acquaintance, a young male relative (i.e., brother, cousin), a parent, or a male stranger. Girls are likelier than boys to receive a simple offer (e.g., "Do you want some?") or offers that minimize the negative effects of the drug. Boys are likelier to receive offers that play up the social image aspects of drug use. Finally, girls are likelier to receive the offers in private places such as friends' homes; boys are likelier to receive the offers in public settings (e.g., park, street).[143]

Advertising and the Entertainment Media

Tobacco and alcohol manufacturers spend billions of dollars each year on advertising and promotions, sponsorships of events, and product placements in movies and television shows. The tobacco industry has a long history of marketing to young women, exploiting their desire for independence and sophistication and appealing to perennial female concerns about weight and appearance. Alcohol industry advertising makes drinking—and by association women who drink—appear fun and sexy.

Because the media is such an important part of the lives of many young people, they are natural targets for tobacco and alcohol marketing. Cigarette- or beer-related cartoon logos, promotional materials handed out at concerts and sporting events, and the portrayal of attractive models and celebrities enjoying cigarettes and alcohol are among the many marketing strategies tobacco and alcohol industries use to make their products attractive to young people.[144] Children under the age of 21 see more magazine advertisements for alcoholic beverages—particularly beer, alcopops (fruit-flavored, malt-based alcoholic drinks), and distilled spirits—than adults. Almost one-quarter of alcohol advertising on television is more likely to be seen by youth than adults.[145] Because of this widespread marketing of alcohol to youth and the abundance of research findings on the detrimental effects of drinking for young people, the American Medical Association has called on networks and cable television to stop airing alcohol commercials that are appealing to youth or that appear on programs seen by underage viewers.[146]

More recently, the National Research Council and the Institute of Medicine have gone even further, recommending that the alcohol industry strengthen its advertising codes to prohibit advertising in venues where a large proportion of the audience is underage and that it take part in creating and funding an independent nonprofit foundation aimed at preventing and reducing underage drinking—an idea initially proposed by CASA. They also called on advertisers to refrain from marketing alcohol products in a way that appeals to young people, and they called on the entertainment media to use rating systems to warn of messages that portray alcohol consumption in a favorable light.[147]

Summary

Accurately predicting which girls or women will engage in substance use or be at risk for addiction is a difficult task. Numerous factors contribute to an individual's susceptibility to substance abuse, and there is no clear formula for determining the exact confluence of factors that will increase this susceptibility or protect against it. What is known is that the presence of multiple risk factors in a person's personality, family, or surrounding environment—rather than just a few—hikes the likelihood that an individual will develop substance use problems.

Girls and women of all ages use substances for reasons different than boys and men, the signals and situations of higher risk are different, and women tend to get hooked faster and suffer the consequences sooner than men. To help girls and women steer clear of tobacco and illicit drug use and the abuse of alcohol and prescription drugs, we need to address these differences in the prevention and treatment of substance abuse. Women in the United States thus far have paid a fearful price for our failure to do so.

chapter 2chapter 2chapter 2chapter 2chapter 2

Women and Smoking

Women who smoke like men, die like men who smoke.
—Joseph A. Califano, Jr., 1979

- Approximately one in five women in the United States smokes.[1]
- Nearly one-quarter of high school senior girls smoke.[2]
- Teenage girls are closing the gender gap by smoking at almost the same rate as boys.[3]
- Approximately 3,000 children and teens become regular tobacco users *each day;* almost half of them are girls.[4]
- 6.3 million women over age 49 are regular smokers.[5]
- Each year, approximately 178,000 women die from a smoking-related disease.[6]
- More women die each year in the United States from lung cancer than from breast, uterine, and ovarian cancers *combined.*[7]
- While the rate of lung cancer deaths has been declining among men, the rate has soared by 600 percent among women.[8]
- On average, a smoking woman loses 15 years of her life, while a smoking man loses 13 years.[9]

Cigarette smoking is the number-one preventable cause of death in the United States. Indeed, tobacco kills more people in the United States each year than alcohol, cocaine, crack, heroin, AIDS, suicide, automobile accidents, and fires *combined.*[10] Women now smoke almost as much as men (23% of women and 28% of men ages 12 and older are current smokers, that is, have smoked in the past 30 days[11]), and they have caught up with, and in some cases even surpassed, men in terms of smoking-related diseases. Each year 178,000 women die from tobacco-related maladies.[12] Heart disease, for example, once considered a man's ailment, now kills more women than men each year.[13] A woman who smokes is up to four times more likely to get heart disease than a nonsmoking woman.[14] Although lung cancer still kills more men than women, the gender gap for this disease is rapidly closing as well. While deaths related to lung cancer have been declining steadily among men since the early 1980s, there has been a 600 percent increase in lung cancer mortality among women over the past seven decades.[15] In 1987, lung cancer surpassed breast cancer as the leading cause of cancer deaths among women in the United States[16] and accounted for one-quarter of all cancer deaths among women in the past year.[17] Cigarette smoking is the main cause of lung cancer, with up to 90 percent of all lung cancer patients having smoked cigarettes in their lifetime.[18]

The Early Days

Until the twentieth century, smoking tobacco for pleasure was predominately a male habit. Women who enjoyed smoking tobacco generally were regarded as unsavory, dishonorable, and sexually promiscuous.[19] Smoking was considered fit only for "sporting girls" and professional performers.[20] Some defiant women, however, notably the wives of presidents Andrew Jackson and Zachary Taylor, openly smoked pipes for pleasure.[21] And in the nineteenth and early twentieth centuries, rebellious, artistic women—including George Sand, Colette, Gertrude Stein, and Virginia Woolf—openly smoked cigars.[22] Smoking corncob pipes was popular among women in the Appalachian Mountains.[23]

The Introduction of Cigarettes

During the French Revolution, the French began smoking tobacco rolled in paper, which they called cigarettes.[24] These cigarettes were cheap and crudely made[25] and provided an alternative to snuff, which had become associated with the hated aristocracy.[26] Improved manufacturing techniques, resulting in a higher quality cigarette paper and lower prices, contributed to their growing popularity among men in the United States in the nineteenth century.[27]

At the turn of the twentieth century, cigarette smoking in the United States was still not acceptable behavior. It was "low class," "un-American," and suitable only for "dudes and college misfits." However, many found that, compared to cigarettes, cigars and pipes were even more offensive because of the large amount of smoke and strong

A NECESSARY EVIL

King James I of England wanted to ban tobacco because he believed it caused syphilis. However, the tax revenues—which went directly to his coffers—were too tempting to turn down. He also realized that tobacco planting and exporting were essential for the colonies to prosper economically. Indeed, Jamestown, Virginia, his namesake, owed its economic flourishing to tobacco. The conflict between the need to ban or control a dangerous substance and the desire for revenues from that substance has been an unfortunate aspect of tobacco's history that continues to this day.

Source: Community Outreach Health Information System (COHIS). (2002). *COHIS: The ashtray: Smoking and tobacco abuse: The history of tobacco.* www.bu.edu (accessed December 28, 2001).

odors they emitted. By contrast, cigarettes had a mild aroma and produced less smoke. They also were easier to carry and consume, and cigarette smoking soon became the preferred method of tobacco consumption by rich and poor alike.[28]

The Narrowing of the Gender Gap

In the early 1900s, men who smoked in public were tolerated, but American women were still condemned for such conduct. For them, it had to remain a hidden vice. New York City actually banned public smoking by women,[29] and in 1904 a woman was even arrested for smoking in an automobile.[30]

In 1920, women were officially declared politically equal to men when the Nineteenth Amendment gave them the right to vote. Cigarettes quickly became the symbol of their equality and liberation, a way to challenge proprieties that still deemed women smokers to be disreputable and unladylike.[31] Cigarettes became their flaming torches of freedom.

Tobacco Companies Target Women

Not all women were suffragettes, happily flaunting convention by openly smoking cigarettes. The tobacco companies realized that these other women—the more traditional ones—were a ripe, untapped market and began targeting them as early as 1919.

The Lorillard Company developed an advertisement specifically aimed at women in the early 1920s but quickly withdrew it because of public outcry.[32] In the mid-1920s, Philip Morris promoted Marlboros to women by declaring them "Mild as May."[33] In the mid-1920s, Liggett & Myers launched an ad campaign for Chesterfield cigarettes featuring a woman with the message "Blow Some My Way." This highly successful

SINGING CIGARETTES' PRAISES

Some attribute the popularity of cigarettes among nineteenth-century women to the enormous success of Bizet's *Carmen,* an opera about a girl who worked in a tobacco factory. In a few scenes, Carmen and her fellow female factory workers smoked cigarettes on stage. Because these women were uneducated and poor, they were seen as disreputable in the eyes of the upper classes. So, while helping to popularize cigarette smoking, Carmen also reinforced the negative image of women who smoke.

Source: Cantoni, L. (1999). *Carmen.* www.reginaopera.org (accessed February 19, 2004).

campaign was well accepted by the public. Sales of the cigarette increased by 40 percent in just two years.[34] The biggest success story, however, was the American Tobacco Company's campaign in the late 1920s, which cleverly pitched Lucky Strikes as a route to thinness. "Reach for a Lucky instead of a sweet," said one ad. Two others, "You can't hide fat clumsy ankles. When tempted to over-indulge, reach for a Lucky instead" and "Avoid that future shadow. When tempted, reach for a Lucky," juxtaposed pictures of thin women over women with fat legs and double chins.[35] The American Tobacco Company described the female market as "a new gold mine right in our front yard," which indeed it was. Sales of Lucky Strikes, which increased more than 300 percent during the first year of its advertising campaign,[36] went from almost 14 billion cigarettes in 1925 to more than 40 billion in 1930, making Lucky the leading brand nationwide. While actual data do not exist on smoking prevalence before 1935,[37] the 1980 Surgeon General's Report estimated that the female smoking rate rose from about 6 percent in 1924 to 16 percent in 1929.[38]

SUFFRAGETTES AND CIGARETTES

In 1929, smoking by women in public was illegal in New York and other cities. The American Tobacco Company wanted to do something about it as well as boost the image of smoking. They pulled off a major public relations coup, with the help of public relations pioneer Edward Bernays. They held a "Torches of Freedom" march, promoting women's right to smoke in public. About a dozen society women dressed as suffragettes marched in the Fifth Avenue Easter Parade, openly smoking cigarettes and carrying placards depicting cigarettes as "torches of liberty."

Source: Bernays, E. L. (1965). *Biography of an idea: Memoirs of public relations counsel Edward L. Bernays.* New York: Simon and Schuster.

In 1935, *Fortune* magazine conducted the first national survey of smoking and found that 18 percent of women (and 52% of men) smoked.[39] While only 9 percent of women over 40 in this survey were smokers, more than 26 percent of those under 40 smoked.[40] By World War II, women almost succeeded in equaling men in their smoking habits.[41] In 1944, 36 percent of women were smoking, and by the late 1940s, an astounding 45 percent smoked. Although women's smoking rates continued to increase through the 1950s, peaking in the mid-1960s, men's smoking rates consistently were higher than those of women throughout this time.[42]

Sensing the potential for big market growth, tobacco companies again began targeting women in the 1960s. And again, they exploited the feminist movement by suggesting that smoking was the ultimate symbol of liberation.[43] At the same time, their ads and promotions were becoming increasingly sexist. In 1968, Virginia Slims was launched with its infamous slogan, "You've come a long way, baby!" But the sexism inherent in the slogan seemed to be lost on the girls and women who flocked to buy Virginia Slims, and the campaign was an enormous success. Indeed, a direct relationship can be found between the launching of Virginia Slims in the 1960s and the subsequent dramatic increase in smoking among adolescent girls.[44] Eve cigarettes, introduced in 1970, were packaged to appeal to a woman's feminine side, with an elegant, pastel-colored package.[45] Other exploitative ads followed. Winston cigarette ads featured an attractive woman saying, "My buns may not be made of steel, but my butts are all tobacco."

The tobacco industry's targeting of women was so successful that by the time the link between smoking and lung cancer and other diseases became widely known, it was too late for many of the millions of women who already were hooked on tobacco.

Emergence of the Truth

In 1950, a landmark study linking smoking to lung cancer was published in the prestigious *Journal of the American Medical Association.*[46] Over the next decade, more than 7,000 articles were published linking smoking with lung cancer and other life-threatening diseases.[47] As a result of all the scientific evidence about the negative consequences of smoking, the advisory committee of the U.S. Surgeon General convened in 1964 and produced the first Surgeon General's Report on Smoking and Health.[48] The report concluded that smoking was hazardous to the health of men and women and that immediate action was warranted.[49] It spurred a major, highly successful public health effort to reduce smoking and other tobacco use. Articles began to appear in newspapers and magazines, as did antismoking ads. The truth about the dangers of smoking finally reached the public, and smoking rates began to decline significantly.

CLOSING THE GAP

The Virginia Slims Woman is catching up to the Marlboro Man.
—Antonia C. Novella, M.D., M.P.H., former U.S. Surgeon General

Source: American Heart Association. (2004). *Tobacco industry's targeting of youth, minorities and women.* www.americanheart.org (accessed April 13, 2004).

Further Narrowing of the Gender Gap

The impact of the Surgeon General's report and the associated public health campaigns were particularly profound for men. Since its release, rates of smoking among men declined steadily—by 50 percent, according to some estimates. At the same time, the decline in smoking among women was less steep—approximately 38 percent,[50] accounting, to some extent, for the apparent narrowing of the gender gap in smoking.

Despite fluctuation in rates of smoking among women and men over the past century, by the beginning of the twenty-first century, approximately 23 percent of women and 27 percent of men were smokers.[51]

Smoking among Older Women

In general, smoking rates are lower among older adults than among younger adults. This is primarily because some older adults manage successfully to quit smoking while others die early from smoking-related illnesses.[52] However, while smoking rates have declined in the adult population since the 1960s, the rate among older women has barely changed.[53] In fact, the gender gap in smoking that once existed in this age group has narrowed considerably. In 2003, 16 percent of women ages 50 and over smoked compared to 22 percent of same-aged men.[54]

One reason older women may be catching up to their male peers is that more male smokers than female smokers die before age 60.[55] Because men tend to smoke for more years and more heavily than women, they are at higher risk of dying from smoking-related diseases at younger ages than women smokers. However, fewer women than men in this age group successfully quit smoking.[56] This may be due to the fact that women experience higher rates of nicotine dependence than men, even at the same levels of use.[57]

Teen Trends

From the mid-1940s to the mid-1960s smoking rates among adolescent girls either remained stable or increased slightly. Once the tobacco industry began targeting their advertising campaigns to girls and women in 1967, smoking rates among teenage girls, but not boys, began to increase rapidly.[58] Indeed, in the 1970s, the smoking rates of high school senior girls equaled and then surpassed those of boys their age.[59]

After a significant decrease from the late 1970s to the early 1990s, smoking rates among high school girls increased again in the late 1990s. Today, teenage girls are smoking at virtually the same rate as boys.[60] For example, middle school girls now smoke cigarettes at nearly identical rates as middle school boys (9% vs. 10%),[61] and high school girls and boys smoke at identical rates (22% each).[62] Although between the ninth and twelfth grades, there is a significant increase in smoking among girls (from 19 to 23%), boys smoke at slightly higher rates than girls in the twelfth grade.[63]

There are considerable racial/ethnic differences in the smoking rates of girls. The majority of available data on racial/ethnic differences focus on whites, blacks, and Hispanics, with less data on Asian Americans, Native Americans, and other groups. Whereas small studies show that Native American teenage girls have high rates of smoking and Asian American girls have relatively low rates,[64] large national studies show that smoking rates are highest among whites, followed by Hispanics, and blacks.[65] Black girls also start smoking significantly later than girls of other racial/ethnic backgrounds.[66] While 18 percent of white and 16 percent of Hispanic female high school students report smoking a full cigarette before the age of 13, only 12 percent of black female high school students report doing so.[67]

College Students

Historically, college students of both sexes have had lower smoking rates than their noncollege peers. While that's still the case, college students appear to be catching up. According to the 2002 *Monitoring the Future* survey, there was almost a 40 percent increase in daily cigarette smoking on college campuses between 1991 and 1999. While smoking among college students declined in 2000 and 2001, it rose again in 2002.[68]

Male and female college students smoke at virtually the same rate (about 28%). Yet, because male college students smoke cigars and use smokeless tobacco in addition to cigarettes, their tobacco use rates are slightly higher than female college students who primarily smoke cigarettes.[69] Male students also tend to be heavier smokers than female students.[70]

The overwhelming majority (over 80%) of women who smoke began before the age of 18,[71] which is consistent with a body of research that has shown that if smoking is not initiated by age 18, chances are that the person will never smoke. However, that now appears to be changing.[72] Sixteen percent of young women today are having their first cigarette between the ages of 18 and 24.[73] Eighteen is also the youngest age group that can be legally targeted for cigarette promotion,[74] making it a natural mark for the tobacco industry. The industry is taking full advantage of this and pouring money into reaching this age group[75] through cigarette and smokeless tobacco promotions at fraternity parties, bars, and clubs, and it appears to be getting its money's worth.[76] CASA's *Formative Years* survey found that the greatest increase in smoking among girls takes place during the transition from high school to college, when many girls turn 18. On average, girls in the study reported smoking six more days per month in their freshman year of college than they did in their senior year of high school.[77] Another study found that 28 percent of college smokers had begun smoking regularly at age 19 or older, when most were in college, not high school.[78]

Nicotine Addiction

The addictive powers of smoking have been known for centuries. In 1623, Sir Francis Bacon warned, "The use of tobacco is growing greatly and conquers men with a certain secret pleasure, so that those who have once become accustomed thereto can later hardly be restrained therefrom."[79]

Nicotine is one of the most addictive drugs known to man . . . and woman. It is an alkaloid, a class of compounds that includes morphine and cocaine. In fact, some experts consider nicotine more addictive than heroin or alcohol.[80] Nicotine stimulates nicotine receptors in the spinal cord and parts of the brain. This, in turn, activates the sympathetic nervous system and increases heart rate and blood pressure.[81] Nicotine affects the same brain mechanism as other drugs of abuse by increasing brain levels of the neurotransmitter dopamine, producing nicotine-induced feelings of pleasure and reward and, over time, addiction and vulnerability to withdrawal symptoms.[82] Even a brief exposure to low levels of nicotine can cause lasting changes in the brain's reward areas, amplifying the pleasing effects and boosting the desire to repeat the exposure.[83] When a person quits smoking, the presence of pleasure-inducing brain chemicals is reduced, altering mood and making smoking cessation more difficult.[84] Indeed, physical addiction to nicotine is the main barrier to smoking cessation for women and men.[85] Yet, women who smoke a half a pack of cigarettes a day have higher rates of nicotine addiction than men who smoke comparable amounts.[86]

Although adults tend to smoke more than teens, teens experience higher rates of nicotine dependence than adults at the same levels of cigarette use.[87] A longitudinal study of 12- to 13-year-old smokers found that 40 percent developed symptoms of tobacco dependence after just trying smoking and 53 percent after inhaling. Of those who reported symptoms, fully half developed them by the time they were smoking only two cigarettes one day a week, and two-thirds had symptoms by the time they were smoking one cigarette a day. Girls in this study reported having more symptoms of tobacco dependence than the boys. They also became dependent more rapidly than the boys; it took the girls an average of only three weeks to develop symptoms of tobacco dependence while it took boys an average of 26 weeks.[88]

Girls who begin smoking in their teens are likely to have greater difficulty quitting, to smoke for a greater number of years, and to smoke more heavily than those who start smoking as adults.[89] This puts teenage girls who smoke at especially high risk of dying prematurely from smoking-related diseases.

The Deadly Consequences of Smoking

Because smoking among women was not widespread until the 1940s, the full spectrum of illness and death wrought by tobacco on women did not become apparent until several decades later when this first generation of women to have smoked heavily began reaching age 60.[90] In 1980, U.S. Surgeon General Julius Richmond warned the public, "The first signs of an epidemic of smoking-related disease among women are now appearing."[91]

His prophesy of an epidemic among smoking women unfortunately came true. Women now account for 39 percent of all smoking-related deaths in the United States.[92] This is more than double the rate it was in the 1960s. During 1995–1999, the smoking-attributable death rate for men declined for cancer and cardiovascular disease and remained stable for respiratory diseases. During this time period, there was an increase in the number of women smokers who died of cancer and respiratory diseases, while the number of cardiovascular deaths among smoking women decreased by almost 10 percent. However, smoking does appear to take a greater toll on women than men; on average, a man who smokes will lose 13 years of life, while a woman who smokes will lose 15 years of life.[93]

Mortality from smoking-related illnesses is even higher among black women than white women.[94] While the exact reasons for this are unclear, it may be because black women retain nicotine in their bodies longer than do white women.[95] In addition, compared to white women, black women are more likely to smoke menthol cigarettes, which have a higher tar and nicotine content than other cigarettes and are easier to inhale deeply.[96] The higher rates of poverty and limited access to health care among black

MISCONCEPTION ABOUT SMOKING

A previous belief that smoking was less hazardous for women "is an illusion reflecting the fact that women lagged one-quarter century behind men in their widespread use of cigarettes."

Source: Office of the Surgeon General. (1980). *The health consequences of smoking for women: A report of the surgeon general.* Washington, DC: U.S. Department of Health and Human Services, Public Health Service, Office of Assistant Secretary for Health, Office on Smoking and Health. P. v.

women also are likely significant in the relationship between race, smoking, and illness or death.[97] Smoking, however, is an equal opportunity killer, and smoking women of all races are dying in unprecedented numbers. Almost half the women who smoke (47%) will ultimately die from smoking-related diseases.[98] (See chapter 6 for a discussion of smoking cessation.)

Cancer

Tobacco accounts for almost one in three cancer deaths in the United States.[99] Smoking causes cancer of the lung, larynx, oral cavity, and esophagus. The carcinogenic effects from a single cigarette smoked by a woman are equal to nearly two cigarettes smoked by a man.[100] At the same level of exposure to tobacco smoke, women have a greater risk of developing lung cancer than men.[101] Indeed, female smokers are up to three times more likely than male smokers to develop lung cancer.[102]

Lung cancer in women was virtually nonexistent in the 1950s. However, in the mid-1950s, the rate began rising and has not stopped since.[103] From the early 1960s to the mid-1980s, the death rate from lung cancer among female smokers soared 496 percent (from 26 to 155 per 100,000), six times the rate of increase among male smokers (from 187 to 341 per 100,000).[104] In 1987, for the first time, more women died of lung cancer than of breast cancer. In the year 2000, more women died from lung cancer than from breast, uterine, and ovarian cancers *combined.* In fact, the United States has one of the highest lung cancer death rates among women in the industrialized world.[105] Although the rate of lung cancer cases has been declining among men, it continues to rise among women.[106] Cigarette smoking is responsible for 80 percent of cases of lung cancer in women.[107]

In addition to lung cancer, a woman who smokes more than doubles her risk of getting bladder or pancreatic cancer.[108] Smoking also increases a woman's risk of stomach and cervical cancer by at least 50 percent and can double her risk of ovarian cysts.[109]

SMOKING-RELATED CANCERS AMONG WOMEN

Lung	Stomach	Laryngeal
Pancreatic	Nasal cavities	Myeloid leukemia
Bladder	Oral/Pharyngeal	Cervical
Kidney	Esophageal	Uterine
Liver		

Sources: National Cancer Institute. (2003). *Cigarette smoking and cancer: Questions and answers.* http://cis.nci.nih.gov/ (accessed March 22, 2004); American Cancer Society. (2003). *Cancer facts and figures, 2003.* Atlanta: American Cancer Society.

Women who smoke also are at increased risk for developing breast cancer. One study found that women who smoked for 40 years or longer had a 60 percent higher risk of breast cancer than women who never smoked, and those women who smoked over 20 cigarettes a day for at least 40 years were at 83 percent greater risk of breast cancer than nonsmoking women.[110]

Unfortunately, smoking and drinking often go hand in hand. And because alcohol also contributes to oral, pharyngeal, laryngeal, and esophageal cancer, the combination of tobacco and alcohol considerably heightens a woman's risk of developing such cancers.[111]

Cardiovascular Disease

Since 1984, heart attack, stroke, and other cardiovascular diseases have killed more women than men; cardiovascular diseases account for 33.5 percent of smoking-related deaths.[112] Cardiovascular disease is the number one killer of women in later adulthood, and smoking is a leading preventable cause of cardiovascular problems.[113] Women in later adulthood who smoke are about twice as likely to develop heart disease as nonsmokers.[114] A smoker has twice the risk of having a heart attack as a nonsmoker.[115] Smoking increases a woman's chance of having a heart attack as well as of dying from one.[116] In fact, cigarette smoking is the biggest risk factor for sudden cardiac death; smokers who have heart attacks are more likely than nonsmokers not only to die from the attack but also to die within an hour of it.[117]

Women who are heavy smokers (smoke 20 or more cigarettes a day) are up to four times more likely to get heart disease than nonsmoking women.[118] Also, women who smoke 25 or more cigarettes a day are 5.5 times likelier to get fatal heart disease than nonsmokers.[119] Women who smoke and use oral contraceptives increase their risk of a heart attack by 1,000 percent.[120] Among women, smoking doubles the risk of having a stroke.[121]

THE SADDEST JOURNEY OF MY LIFE

At age 16, Trudy Grover moved out of her parents' house. "I loved the feeling of taking care of myself. I had my own apartment, worked as a waitress and always had a pack of Marlboros in my pocket. One day when I was 35, I was running back and forth between tables and suddenly couldn't catch my breath. It was like somebody was holding me underwater. I told myself I was just getting older. At age 42, I was diagnosed with emphysema . . . The doctor put me on an oxygen tank, an ugly thing with green rubber tubes running into my nose . . . In the struggle to breathe, you can lose control of your bladder . . . I cried in shame . . . In 1993, I had a lung transplant—my only option, said the doctor . . . Now a year and a half later, I take 23 pills a day . . . To pay bills, I was forced to sell my home and possessions. And I made the saddest journey of my life: back to my mother's house. 'Mom,' I said, averting my eyes, 'I'm broke. Will you take me in?' . . . I was begging my 73-year-old mother to take care of me again. I couldn't help crying."

Source: Ecenbarger, W. (2004). *So you think you want to smoke! The stories of four who did.* www.svcc.cc.il.us (accessed March 31, 2004).

Respiratory Diseases

In addition to cancer and heart disease, smoking causes chronic obstructive pulmonary diseases (COPD) such as chronic bronchitis and emphysema. Smoking increases the risk of death from these diseases tenfold and is responsible for approximately 90 percent of COPD deaths in women.[122] Smokers have more respiratory problems than nonsmokers, and women who smoke have more respiratory disorders than men who smoke.[123] These disorders include persistent coughing, wheezing, breathlessness, and asthma.[124]

Cosmetic Considerations

Smoking is linked to a whole host of cosmetic and aesthetic problems. These include skin conditions such as finger and fingernail discoloration and psoriasis. By reducing blood flow to the skin, smoking increases facial wrinkling, particularly crow's feet around the eyes. Over time, "smoker's face"—lines or wrinkles, gaunt facial features, grayish skin, and a red florid complexion—can be found among 46 percent of smokers.[125] In addition, smoking causes halitosis, tooth discoloration, and tooth loss.[126] Indeed, smoking is one of the most significant contributors to the development and progression of periodontal disease.[127]

Dangers of Secondhand Smoke

Secondhand smoke is a major public health concern for both adults and children. Whether it is referred to as secondhand smoke, sidestream smoke, passive smoking, or environmental tobacco smoke (ETS), exposure to other people's tobacco use contributes to approximately 35,000 heart-disease deaths and 3,000 lung cancer deaths in nonsmokers each year in the United States alone.[128]

Approximately 7,000 more women die each year from secondhand smoke than men.[129] Women living with a spouse who smokes have a 30 percent higher risk of lung cancer than women who are not chronically exposed to passive smoke.[130] Furthermore, being around others who smoke makes it harder to quit and multiplies the effects of secondhand smoke for everyone in the household.[131] Having a smoke-free home and a smoke-free workplace are essential to the health and well-being of people of all ages.[132]

The Risks to Older Women

Even if smoking doesn't kill her, it can sabotage an older woman's ability to live independently. Smoking has been linked to weak muscles, poor balance, and impaired neuromuscular function among women over age 65.[133] One study found the decrease in muscle function comparable to five years of aging.[134] Smoking also causes macular degeneration, the leading cause of blindness among elderly Americans. Women who smoke 25 or more cigarettes a day are more than twice as likely to suffer this eye disease, compared with women who have never smoked.[135]

Smoking increases a woman's risk of osteoporosis.[136] Women who smoke a pack a day throughout adulthood cut their bone density up to 10 percent by the time they reach menopause.[137] One or more factors may be at work: smoking may inhibit calcium absorption or reduce a woman's estrogen levels, which in turn leads to bone loss and fragility.[138] Osteoporosis also may be more common among smokers because smokers tend to weigh less than nonsmokers and low weight tends to decrease estrogen levels and increase the risk of hip fracture.[139] Women between the ages of 44 and 54 who smoke are twice as likely to experience menopause one to two years earlier than those who have never smoked[140] and may experience more menopausal symptoms such as hot flashes.[141] Early menopause, in turn, contributes to osteoporosis.[142]

More research is needed to assess the precise impact of smoking on a woman's endocrine system. What we do know is that because of the damage to women's bones, the risk of suffering a fracture of the spine, hip, and other sites is more than double among smokers.[143] Estrogen replacement, the most effective therapy known to preserve bone mass, appears to be less effective in women who smoke.[144]

Between the ages of 65 and 74, women who smoke are more than twice as likely to die of smoking-related cardiovascular problems and cancers as women who do not smoke.[145] This increase in the risk of death is highest for those who have been heavy smokers for many years.[146] As more women who are heavy smokers pass into later adulthood, the personal tragedies and health care costs incurred by these heavy smokers in the years before death will increase significantly.

The Risks to Youth

A smoker doesn't have to wait until adulthood to experience the negative consequences of smoking. Teen smokers are at risk for a whole host of physical problems during adolescence. Compared with nonsmokers, teens who smoke are less physically fit, and have retarded lung growth and diminished lung function. Young smokers frequently report such symptoms as wheezing, shortness of breath, coughing, and an increase in phlegm production. In general, teen smokers have a greater susceptibility to respiratory diseases than nonsmokers. And because they are less physically fit, teen smokers suffer in terms of physical performance and endurance.[147]

Relatively few studies have examined the effects of smoking specifically on girls and young women. One study that has examined this population found that smoking slows the growth of lung function in boys and girls but that the deficits may be greater in girls. In support of this, the study found that rates of wheezing are higher among girls than boys at all levels of smoking.[148]

A recent study found that 30 percent of girls who were daily smokers reported poor health compared with only 8 percent of nonsmoking girls. Smoking girls tend to complain more of respiratory symptoms, asthma, headache, neck and shoulder pain, stomachache, nausea, nervousness, restlessness, and sleep problems than do nonsmoking girls. Daily smokers also report using more medications and health services.[149]

In addition to reporting actual health problems, girls tend to perceive their own general health as worse than males, particularly if they smoke frequently and in large quantities. While boys generally give higher ratings of their own health compared to girls, this gender gap in self-perceived health widens at increasing levels of tobacco-use frequency and intensity, with girls' self-ratings becoming progressively worse than boys' self-ratings.[150]

Smoking also poses some unique threats to young women. Nearly 40 percent of teenage girls who use oral contraceptives also smoke cigarettes,[151] putting them at increased risk of heart disease. Cigarette smoking also may affect menstrual function, increasing the risks for dysmenorrhea (painful menstruation) and menstrual irregularity.[152]

In addition to the physical consequences, girls and young women are at risk for certain mental health effects of smoking. Teen smokers have been found to be three times more likely to have consulted a doctor or mental health professional because of emotional or psychological problems[153] and almost twice as likely as nonsmokers to develop symptoms of depression.[154]

Teen smoking appears to precede depression rather than the other way around.[155] CASA's *Formative Years* survey, a two-part survey with a six-month interval between interviews, found that girls who reported smoking at the time of the first interview were more likely to report being depressed six months later than girls who did not smoke. This relationship remained statistically significant even after taking into consideration the girls' earlier levels of depression.[156] Another study found that teens who were not depressed when they started smoking were four times more likely to develop depressive symptoms during the course of one year than their nonsmoking peers. Furthermore, 12 percent of pack-a-day smokers developed symptoms of depression compared with 5 percent of nonsmoking teens.[157]

In addition to depression, frequent smoking is related to an increased risk of panic attacks and panic disorder in young adults. Like depression, there is little evidence that panic attacks or panic disorder increase the risk for smoking; rather, smoking appears to precede these symptoms. One possible explanation for this relationship is that smoking can affect breathing and cause lung problems, which can give the false sensation of suffocation, leading to panic attacks.[158]

Other Problems for Teens

Students who smoke are more likely to do poorly in school than nonsmoking students. One study of middle schoolers found that *D* and *F* students were almost six times as likely to smoke cigarettes as those students who received *A*s and *B*s.[159] Smoking status also is linked to academic plans; high school senior girls who do not plan to go to college are more likely to smoke cigarettes than those with college plans.[160] CASA's *Formative Years* survey found that 85 percent of nonsmoking high school senior girls wanted to go to college compared with 15 percent of those who smoked.[161]

Smoking often precedes the use of alcohol, marijuana, and other illicit drugs.[162] In general, teens who smoke are significantly more likely than their nonsmoking peers to use alcohol and drugs, and the more they smoke, the greater the likelihood of other substance use. Indeed, a recent study found that only about 5 percent of nonsmoking teens reported using illicit drugs, while 26 percent of those who smoke up to five cigarettes a day and 47 percent of those who smoke about 10 cigarettes a day did so.[163]

The Road to Tobacco Use

Although the majority of teenage girls have tried smoking at some point, only one-third to one-half go on to become regular smokers.[164] Most girls choose *not* to smoke, most (65%) would rather date a nonsmoker than a smoker, and 42 percent strongly dislike being around smokers.[165] Yet some girls do choose to smoke. What motivates or predisposes them to become regular smokers while others avoid it at all costs?

Parents, personality characteristics, peers, personal concerns, and the larger social environment are key factors in influencing a young person's health-related attitudes and behavior. They are especially important in determining which girls choose to smoke and which ones decide not to.

Parental Smoking

Parental smoking is perhaps one of the most important determinants of children's smoking.[166] Research consistently indicates that parents who smoke, compared to non-smoking parents, are significantly more likely to have children who smoke or plan to smoke.[167] Girls appear to be more influenced than boys by their parents' smoking behavior.[168] In addition, daughters of smoking mothers are more likely to smoke than sons.[169] Parental attitudes also have been shown to be strong determining factors for children's smoking.[170] Again, this appears to be especially true for daughters of smoking mothers.[171]

Maternal smoking, even prenatally, can influence a daughter's risk of smoking. Girls whose mothers smoked during pregnancy are four times likelier to smoke during adolescence and into young adulthood than girls whose mothers did not smoke during pregnancy. The relationship between prenatal exposure to maternal tobacco use and smoking during adolescence is stronger for daughters than for sons and exists regardless of the amount the mother smoked during pregnancy.[172] Although the reason for this link between prenatal exposure to mothers' smoking and daughters' later smoking is not well understood, researchers speculate that during brain development, nicotine or other substances released by maternal smoking may impact the developing brain and modify its threshold of tolerance to nicotine, predisposing the child to smoke.[173]

Smoking mothers also may be passing on genes that put their children at risk of becoming smokers. Estimates for the heritability of tobacco use and dependence in women range considerably from 37 to 84 percent. (For men, the range is from 28 to 84%.)[174] Although it is difficult to sort out the genetic contributions and the environmental influences on smoking, both appear to be important.[175] Even if genetics play a role in smoking, screening for genetic susceptibility to smoking initiation and nicotine dependence can backfire; those not at genetic risk may be inclined to try smoking because they feel immune to nicotine addiction.[176]

Personality and Self-Image

An individual's personality is a result of a combination of biological, family, and social factors. Therefore, it is difficult to ascertain whether or not certain personality factors themselves are related causally to smoking and other substance use and abuse. There are, however, some common personality traits that often are found in teens who smoke and use other drugs.

Research consistently indicates that one of the key risk factors for smoking is a tendency toward rebelliousness, risk taking, and sensation seeking. One study of fifth graders found that girls who exhibited high levels of risk-taking behavior were twice as likely to smoke in the twelfth grade.[177] Girls who initiate smoking early in adolescence tend to have extroverted and sociable personalities; however, if these girls continue to smoke and increase their levels of tobacco use in later adolescence and young adulthood, they tend to become depressed and have poor social relationships.[178]

Young smokers also appear to be concerned with sexuality and body image, while older girls seem to define their self-image more through style and fashion. One study found that 12- and 13-year-old smoking girls wanted to be more sexy, slim, and attractive than nonsmokers of the same age and tended to rate themselves as sexy and or seductive. On the other hand, the 15- and 16-year-old smoking girls focused more on being trendy and fashionable rather than on being sexy and seductive. The self-image of older girls who smoke is more similar to that of smoking teenage boys and more reflective of cigarette advertising campaigns. The study found that 18- and 19-year-old female smokers rated themselves as being more wild, cool, tough, and arrogant than nonsmoking girls of this age.[179]

In addition to smoking as a means of enhancing their image, fitting in, or appearing mature or cool,[180] girls also smoke as a way of being sociable, to connect with others, or to break the ice in potentially uncomfortable social situations.[181] A study of 11- and 13-year-old girls found that girls at the top of the social pecking order—the most popular girls—are under more pressure to smoke than less popular girls, suggesting that peer pressure sometimes is due less to active influencing by peers and more to pressure to maintain a certain image. Popular girls may use smoking as a means of bolstering their image of being rebellious, sophisticated, and standing out from a crowd. The popular boys in this study felt less pressure than the girls did to smoke in order to be "cool" because smoking interfered with their main "cool" activity of participating in sports.[182]

Peer Influences

While parents and personality characteristics have a lot to do with whether or not a girl smokes, peer influence is often the deciding factor. Indeed, teens with friends who smoke cigarettes are nine times more likely to smoke than their classmates with non-smoking friends.[183] Friends' smoking is more strongly related to girls' smoking than it is to boys' smoking. In general, girls are more susceptible than boys to social influences to smoke. This may be because girls tend to be more peer-oriented than boys and also tend to spend more time with their friends.[184]

Girls who believe that their friends approve of smoking are more likely to become regular smokers than those who think their friends disapprove of smoking.[185] In addition, the smoking behavior of a girl's best friend, especially if the best friend is female, is a strong risk factor for her own tobacco use.[186] Girls may be influenced to smoke by their peers because they are modeling their behavior, seeking their approval, or being pressured by them to smoke.[187]

CASA's *Formative Years* survey found that girls' perception of pressure to smoke by other people their age increases as they progress through middle and high school: 4.1 percent of fifth graders, 29.5 percent of eighth graders, and 40.5 percent of high school seniors report pressure to smoke.[188]

One study of teen girls found that many initiated smoking at the urging of their friends and chose to continue to smoke to fit in with their peers. Among those who wanted to quit smoking, fear of peer rejection or at least an expectation that peers would not be supportive of a quit attempt led some girls to sustain their smoking behavior.[189]

Stress Relief

The belief that smoking will be beneficial in some way—such as improving a depressed mood,[190] relieving stress or anxiety, or otherwise helping women to cope with stressful personal problems[191]—increases the risk of smoking. Stress reduction is one of the most frequently cited reasons girls and women smoke.[192] Indeed, focus groups with girls as young as eight years old reveal that stress is seen as the key motivating factor in smoking among girls.[193]

In general, girls report experiencing more stress, particularly school-related stress, than boys. They also are more likely to respond to this stress with substance use, particularly smoking.[194] One survey found that 68 percent of 10- to 17-year-old girls and 76 percent of 18- to 22-year-old women smoked because it made them feel calmer or more relaxed.[195] In another, more recent survey, 66 percent of the girls reported stress relief as their main reason for smoking.[196]

A study of black teenage girls found that those who reported having smoked in their lifetime experienced significantly more daily life "hassles" or stress than girls who reported never smoking—particularly with regard to academics and family or economic troubles. Furthermore, black girls who reported more daily life hassles also began smoking at a younger age.[197] Other research suggests that racial discrimination, which increases life stress, may be related to the smoking habits of black girls. The experience of discrimination also may lead to depression and low self-esteem, both of which are related to smoking among girls.[198]

Contrary to popular belief, however, using cigarettes for stress reduction can backfire. Smoking actually increases the risk for panic attacks and other stress- or anxiety-related disorders.[199]

Obsession with Weight

Stress can increase not only a woman's desire to smoke but also her desire to eat. Men, on the other hand, tend to eat less when stressed. Women also tend to be more obsessed with thinness and losing weight than men.[200] Between 33 and 40 percent of women are on diets compared with only 20 to 24 percent of men. A recent survey of college freshmen found that 89 percent of the freshman women versus 53 percent of the freshman men who were of normal weight wanted to be thinner.[201]

Adolescent girls are especially concerned about their weight, and many, if not most, are on diets at some point during middle or high school.[202] Research indicates that 42 percent of girls in grades one through three want to be thinner, 81 percent of 10 year olds report that they are afraid of being fat, and the number one wish of girls ages 11 to 17 is to lose weight.[203]

A national survey of high school students found that 59 percent of high school girls reported that they were trying to lose weight.[204] The concern about weight and the desire for thinness is one of the major reasons girls not only start smoking[205] but also continue to smoke into adulthood and beyond.[206] They believe that they look sophisticated and glamorous while smoking and that smoking will help them ward off hunger and keep their weight down.[207] Unfortunately, women of all ages have discovered one of the few benefits of smoking—that nicotine is an appetite suppressant.[208] Smoking, especially in women, is associated with a decreased consumption of sweets and carbohydrates.[209] And nicotine does appear to increase metabolism and suppress appetite.[210] This is not a recent discovery. The effect of tobacco on appetite and weight has been known for hundreds of years. A French monk in the sixteenth century wrote that "[Tobacco] keepeth the parties from hu[n]ger and thirst for a time."[211]

The tobacco industry has cashed in on the connection between smoking and weight for decades. A Silva Thins ad from 1967 exclaimed, "Cigarettes are like girls; the best ones are thin and rich." The tobacco industry continues to exploit young girls' and women's obsessions with thinness by promoting thin cigarettes, using thin models, and using references to thinness in their advertising copy. Misty cigarette's slogan is "Slim 'n Sassy"[212] and Capri, described as "super slim," advertises that there is "no slimmer way to smoke."[213] Not surprisingly, Virginia Slims is still one of the more popular brands designed for women.[214]

Availability

The legal age to buy tobacco in most states is 18 (19 in Alaska, Alabama, and Utah).[215] So how do younger smokers get their Virginia Slims and Marlboros? Surveys of school children confirm that teens and even preteens have no trouble obtaining cigarettes. For example, 6 out of 10 (60%) eighth graders and 8 out of 10 (81%) tenth graders report little if any trouble obtaining cigarettes.[216] Cigarettes are widely available from friends and illegally from stores.[217] In spite of fines and other penalties, many newsstands and drug, grocery, and convenience stores sell cigarettes to children without checking their identifications. Children who try to buy cigarettes are able to do so 25 percent of the time.[218] Underage girls tend to have an easier time buying cigarettes than underage boys.[219] Among teens who purchased their own cigarettes from stores or gas stations, more girls than boys (72.9% vs. 64%) reported that they were *not* asked to show proof that they were of legal age to purchase cigarettes.[220] This may be because it is easier for girls than for boys to make themselves look older than they really are.

Teen Targets

Advertising has a tremendous impact on smoking initiation in the United States, not just among women but among teenage girls as well.[221] In fact, the tobacco industry is pumping more money than ever into advertising. In 1998, the Master Settlement Agreement (MSA) banned the tobacco industry from marketing their products to minors. Despite this, since the MSA, the tobacco industry increased spending on cigarette ads by 26 percent,[222] and increasing numbers of teens report seeing tobacco ads in magazines.[223] A recent study found that while the tobacco industry did reduce ads in maga-

IN THEIR OWN WORDS

The base of our business is the high school student.[a]
—Lorillard, 1978
It is important to know as much as possible about teenage smoking patterns and attitudes. Today's teenager is tomorrow's potential regular customer.[b]
—Philip Morris, 1981
The ability to attract new smokers and develop them into a young adult franchise is key to brand development.[c]
—Philip Morris, 1999

Sources: [a]Hammond, R., and Rowell, A. Campaign for Tobacco-free Kids, and Action on Smoking and Health. (2001). *Trust us: We're the tobacco industry.* www.ash.org.uk (accessed March 18, 2004). [b]Hammond and Rowell. (2001). [c]Campaign for Tobacco-free Kids. (2002). *Tobacco company quotes on marketing to kids.* www.tobaccofreekids.org (accessed March 22, 2004).

zines with the highest teen readership, it increased ads in other magazines read by substantial numbers of teens, such as fashion magazines.[224] The majority of women's magazines accept cigarette ads, and those that do tend to be less likely to run articles about the hazards of smoking than the magazines that do not accept such ads.[225]

Cigarette-marketing strategies, regardless of their stated audience, have been successful at attracting young smokers. One study examined 1,752 California teens who were identified as having never smoked and as being nonsusceptible to smoking influences—"susceptible nonsmokers" were teens who did not rule out smoking in the future, while "nonsusceptible nonsmokers" indicated that they were very unlikely to ever smoke. Three years later, about half the boys and girls in the study had progressed toward smoking, either by showing susceptibility to or experimenting with smoking or becoming established smokers (identified as those who smoked at least 100 cigarettes). Over 62 percent of those who progressed toward smoking had high exposure to tobacco promotions or advertising.[226]

Another study examined a group of teens who indicated that they had smoked no more than one cigarette in 1993. The adolescents were reinterviewed in 1997. Those teens who, in 1993, had owned a tobacco promotional item and named a brand whose advertisements attracted their attention were twice as likely to become established smokers than those who did neither.[227] Yet another study found that 73 percent of teens ages 12 to 17 recalled seeing a tobacco advertisement in the previous two weeks, compared to only 33 percent of adults.[228]

TARGETING MINORITY WOMEN

African-Americans, Hispanics and women comprise a significant percentage of RJR's business. To ignore their business—only featuring white males in our advertising, and only manufacturing styles white males prefer—would leave us open to criticism for racism and sexism, and rightly so . . . We believe all adult Americans are capable of assessing the smoking and health controversy. To say that minorities and women are less capable than white males of deciding whether they want to smoke, or if so, what brand, is demeaning. We do not believe minorities or women should be set aside as a "protected class."
—R. J. Reynolds, public statement on marketing to minorities

Source: Action on Smoking and Health and Cancer Research Campaign. (1998). *Big tobacco and women: What the tobacco industry's confidential documents reveal.* www.ash.org.uk (accessed January 3, 2002).

The really bad news is that initiating smoking in the teen years is a virtual death sentence for millions of teens who will ultimately die prematurely because of it.[229]

Marketing to Women, Minorities, and Developing Countries

In order to sustain itself economically, the cigarette industry must replace the 400,000 smokers who either die or quit smoking each year. This has motivated them to target not only teens but also adult women and minorities. For example, in 1999, Virginia Slims launched an ad campaign, "Find Your Voice," which directly targeted minority women.[230]

Cigarette companies are increasingly targeting their products to developing countries, particularly to women in those countries.[231] In China, an estimated 20 million women began smoking in the past decade, and smoking rates among women in Japan doubled over the course of only five years (from 9% in 1986 to 18% in 1991).[232]

Smoking in the Movies

The tobacco industry targets teens and women in ways that go beyond blatant advertising; Hollywood films are major vehicles of product promotion for the tobacco industry.[233] Recent studies of smoking in movies indicate that since 1991, there has been a tremendous increase in films that show characters smoking. And the smokers in films typically are attractive, sexy, and glamorous and often are depicted smoking in sexy, romantic, adventuresome, and rebellious roles.[234]

The average teen in the United States watches three movies (or videos) a week,

TARGETING UNDERDEVELOPED COUNTRIES

Demographically, the population explosion in many underdeveloped countries ensures a large potential market for cigarettes. Culturally, demand may increase with the continuing emancipation of women and the linkage in the minds of many consumers of smoking manufactured cigarettes with modernization, sophistication, wealth and success, a connection encouraged by much of the advertising of cigarettes throughout the world.
—Philip Morris, Inc.

Source: Hammond, R., and Rowell, A. Campaign for Tobacco-free Kids, and Action on Smoking and Health. (2001). *Trust us: We're the tobacco industry.* www.ash.org.uk (accessed March 18, 2004).

and the majority of the movies they see has one or more characters in them who smokes.[235] A study evaluating the top-grossing films from 1985 to 1995 found that 98 percent of the films had references that supported tobacco use and 46 percent depicted a lead character using tobacco.[236] Another study found that 90 percent of films rated PG or PG-13 featured someone smoking. This study also found a strong positive relationship between smoking experimentation among teens and viewing films that depict tobacco use.[237]

Lead Hollywood actresses often are portrayed using tobacco products to control their emotions, to manifest power and sex appeal, to enhance their body image or self-image, or to control weight.[238] One study found that from 1990 to 1996, 27 percent of female lead characters compared to 80 percent of male lead characters smoked tobacco in a film.[239] However, a study examining a sample of movies from 1993 to 1997 that featured 1 of 10 leading Hollywood actresses found that the percentage of lead actors or supporting actors shown smoking was similar for women and men (42% and 38%, respectively). Yet this same study found that while leading female actors were equally likely to be seen smoking in PG- or PG-13-rated movies as in R-rated movies, male leading actors were 2.5 times more likely to be shown smoking in R-rated or un-

STOPPING THE SPREAD OF SMOKING

Curtailing the increase in tobacco use among women in developing countries represents one of the greatest opportunities for disease prevention in the world today.

Source: Patel, J. D., Bach, P. B., and Kris, M. G. (2004). Lung cancer in U.S. women: A contemporary epidemic. *JAMA* 291(14):1767.

SOME FEMALE STARS WHO SMOKE ON-SCREEN

Scarlett Johansson
Nicole Kidman
Gwyneth Paltrow
Julia Roberts
Meg Ryan
Winona Ryder
Sissy Spacek
Sharon Stone

rated movies than in PG or PG-13 films; furthermore, the PG or PG-13 movies were less likely to contain negative messages about smoking than the R-rated movies.[240]

Not only is smoking in movies widespread, it tends to be portrayed in an ambivalent manner. Among the 200 most popular movie rentals of 1996 and 1997, 89 percent displayed tobacco use, and only 7 percent of the adult characters who smoked experienced some consequence of their tobacco use, while none of the young characters who smoked experienced any apparent consequence. Furthermore, only 7 percent of these movies portrayed characters who refused to smoke. Less than one in four (22%) movies that depict youth cigarette use express negative statements about smoking or smokers; at the same time, positive statements about smoking and smokers are expressed rather infrequently (6%).[241]

Teenagers are not the only ones exposed to celebrity smoking in films. A study of 50 G-rated children's animated films from 1937 to 1997 found that 56 percent portrayed one or more incidences of tobacco use. Smoking frequently was used to signify inde-

Table 2.1 Women Celebrities Who Died from Smoking-Related Diseases

Celebrity	*Age at Death*	*Disease*
Susan Hayward	55	Lung cancer
Lee Remick	55	Lung cancer
Betty Grable	57	Lung cancer
Tallulah Bankhead	65	Emphysema
Sarah Vaughan	66	Lung cancer
Colleen Dewhurst	67	Lung cancer
Melina Mercouri	68	Lung cancer
Nancy Walker	69	Lung cancer
Audrey Meadows	69	Lung cancer

Source: Data from American Lung Association of Kansas. *Famous dead smokers.* www.kslung.org (accessed March 22, 2004).

CIGAR PROMOTION ON A COLLEGE CAMPUS IN 2002

It is the intent of the Cigar Society to bring together all persons who are interested in the gaining of leadership and life skills, while acquiring the knowledge and appreciation for the world of cigars. The Cigar Society intends to focus on giving back to the community by channeling the energy of its members, created by the love of cigars, towards participation in charitable events and Community Impact programs.
—From a college Web site

Source: Cigar Society. *Cigar society description.*www.columbia.edu/cu/bbb/events/moreinfo/cigar.html (accessed March 22, 2004).

pendence and sexiness in characters,[242] qualities that may have a particular appeal to girls and young women.

The MSA banned the common practice of paying the film or television industries for placing tobacco products in movies. In spite of this ban, tobacco use in the most popular PG-13, youth-oriented films has *increased* by 50 percent from two years before to two years after the passage of the MSA. In addition, the percentage of films that portrayed tobacco use in a negative manner fell after the settlement (from 31 to 17%).[243]

Hollywood primarily shows the glamorous side of smoking. Most teens never hear about the deadly toll smoking takes on the lives of many celebrities. And if they do, it's often too late. Unfortunately, many of today's teens will already have been smoking for decades by the time their idols die of smoking-related diseases.

The Cigar Campaign

In the 1990s, the tobacco industry hit upon a new item to promote: cigars. Cigar smoking among Americans had been declining for decades. Few young men and even fewer young women smoked "stogies." Indeed, 1980s market research found that women made up only one-tenth of 1 percent of the U.S. cigar market.[244] All this changed in the early 1990s when the cigar manufacturers and enthusiasts began a major promotional campaign,[245] which resulted in a 50 percent increase in cigar smoking in the United States between 1993 and 1998.[246]

The cigar campaign involved the promotion of fancy cigar dinners in expensive hotels and restaurants, and the publishing of two magazines, *Cigar Aficionado* and *Smoke.*[247] Cigar-smoking celebrities, such as Rudolph Giuliani, Mel Gibson, Raquel Welch, and Bo Derek have appeared on their covers. And ads in these and other popular magazines have depicted famous or elegant young women and men smoking cigars.

NOT JUST FOR MEN

Whoever said it was a man's tradition to enjoy a good stogie? We are working very hard to bring women cigar smokers a place they can feel comfortable and secure about smoking cigars.
—CigarWoman.com

Source: CigarWoman.com. (2002). www.cigarwoman.com (accessed January 3, 2002).

The increase in cigar smoking associated with this new campaign was especially dramatic among adolescents and young women between 18 and 24 years old.[248] In 1992, 5 percent of women had smoked cigars but in 1998 almost 10 percent had. A study in California found that while cigar use doubled among men, it increased five-fold among women from 1990 to 1996.[249]

More teenage girls in the United States currently smoke cigars than do adult women, but boys still are twice as likely to smoke cigars as girls. Cigar manufacturers continue to aggressively market their product to women through sporting and other events, magazines, the Internet, and films.[250] Although they cannot legally target adolescents, the cigar manufacturer's message is getting through to them. In 2003, 9.4 percent of high school girls admitted to having smoked cigars in the past 30 days.[251]

Cigars also have become very popular on college campuses, and an unprecedented number of college women are smoking them. Indeed, a recent survey found that one in four college women has smoked cigars, and about one-third of these women tried their first cigar while in college.[252]

It's more than just cigars and cigarettes; high school girls increasingly are smoking alternative forms of cigarettes such as *bidis* and *kreteks*. *Bidis* are small, hand-rolled, fla-

REACHING FOR THE CIGAR

We've seen a dramatic increase in women buying cigars. It seems that as women make advances in the corporate world—which was male-dominated for so long—they also experience more stress. They have more disposable income. Now, women seem to be less afraid of embracing typical male pastimes for relaxation, for instance, cigar smoking. I think it's great.
—Allan Whitlatch, owner, Lone Star Cigars, Dallas, Texas

Source: Kasper, R. (1996). *The new cigar smoker: Women aren't waiting to exhale.* www.restaurant.org (accessed March 19, 2004).

vored cigarettes imported from India and other Southern Asian countries. They come in such flavors as chocolate, cherry, and mango, and produce higher levels of nicotine, tar, and carbon monoxide than cigarettes.[253] Four percent of girls in the twelfth grade reported using *bidis* in 2002.[254] *Kreteks* are Indonesian cigarettes that contain clove extract and tobacco;[255] 6.7 percent of twelfth grade girls used them in 2002.[256] At least for the time being, very few girls and young women smoke pipes or use smokeless (chewing) tobacco.[257]

Promotion of Smoking and Drinking

The tobacco industry is finding new venues for its marketing efforts. Its latest ventures involve promotional activities in bars and nightclubs in an effort to tap the young adult market, and these promotions have been shown to be a very effective means of encouraging young people to smoke and drink.[258]

The marriage between the tobacco and alcohol industries is nothing new. Ads depicting smoking and drinking have been in magazines for decades, and ashtrays, coasters, bar towels, napkins, and, of course, matches are covered with smoking ads.[259] Alcohol and tobacco, too, often go hand in hand.

Only recently have some states, cities, and counties begun outlawing smoking in lounges and bars.[260] California, Connecticut, Delaware, Maine, Massachusetts, and New York have succeeded in banning smoking in all bars. Hundreds of cities across the United States have also banned smoking in bars.[261]

chapter 3

Women and Alcohol

(Alcoholism) is a slow, insidious, difficult and progressive problem . . . I'm really happy that my family and my friends intervened because I was personally miserable during the time that I was drinking.
—Former governor Ann Richards, recovering alcoholic, 2003

- 6 million women in the United States abuse or are dependent on alcohol.[1]
- Approximately one-third of all girls had their first alcoholic drink* before entering high school.[2]
- Nearly half of high school girls drink alcohol and more than one in four binge drink.[3] †
- Teenage girls who are heavy drinkers‡ are five times more likely to have sex—and a third less likely to use protection—than girls who don't drink.[4]

---

*More than a few sips.

† Defined as consuming five or more drinks on the same occasion at least once in the past 30 days. Some studies use "past two weeks." Still other researchers define binge drinking as four drinks in a row for women and five drinks in a row for men because of women's biological sensitivities to intoxication, including lower body weight and metabolic processing and higher fat-to-water ratios than men.

‡For women, defined as consuming more than seven drinks per week, on average, or more than one drink per day.

- Frequent binge drinking in women's colleges increased by 124 percent between 1993 and 2001.[5]
- Alcohol is involved in as many as 73 percent of all rapes and up to 70 percent of all incidents of domestic violence.[6]
- Women who drink get drunk faster, become addicted more easily, and develop alcohol-related diseases more readily than men who drink.[7]

Alcohol is the number-one drug of abuse in the United States today. The costs are staggering, and women often bear the brunt. Women get drunk faster, become addicted more quickly, and develop alcohol-related diseases—such as hypertension and liver, brain, and heart damage—more rapidly than men.[8] Women are at increased risk for alcohol-related problems such as suicide. And when either a woman or a man, or both, are drinking, the risk of sexual assault and domestic violence increases as well.[9]

Most adult women who drink are moderate drinkers, defined by the U.S. Department of Health and Human Services as consuming no more than one drink per day for women and no more than two drinks per day for men.[10]* Only 1 in every 10 women who drinks surpasses this one drink per day guideline,[11] but the numbers are still startling. Six million girls and women either abuse or are dependent on alcohol, according to the *Diagnostic and Statistical Manual of Mental Disorders* (*DSM-IV*) criteria defining abuse and dependence.[12] The consequences of their drinking can be swift, long-term, and severe.

Drinking Women Today

Almost half (47%) of American women over the legal drinking age of 21 are current drinkers (defined as having at least one drink of alcohol in the past 30 days).[13] The average woman who drinks is young, white, employed, or in school. White adult (age 21 or older) women are significantly more likely to be current drinkers (51%) than Hispanic (36%), black (33%), or Asian American women (30%).[14] Better-educated women are more likely to drink than less educated; 60 percent of women who attended college drink alcohol compared with 36 percent of women with less than a high school diploma.[15] Women employed outside the home are more likely to drink and drink more frequently than homemakers; however, underemployment and unemployment are risk factors for—and the result of—alcohol abuse.[16] Married women have the lowest rates of heavy drinking, while unmarried women who live with men have the high-

*An alcoholic drink is equivalent to one 12-ounce bottle of beer or wine cooler, one 5-ounce glass of wine, or 1.5 ounces of 80-proof distilled spirits.

est.[17] Women of all ages, ethnic backgrounds, and social and economic levels abuse alcohol; however, most of the problem drinkers (defined as persons who have physical, social, psychological, or other problems as a result of drinking) are white, under 30, and unmarried.[18]

Men generally tend to drink more than women, but women are catching up.[19] In the last quarter century, the gender gap in heavy drinking among high school seniors has been cut in half (from a 23 percentage-point difference in 1975 to a 12 percentage-point difference in 2003)[20] and, among younger teenagers, the gender gap in alcohol use and risky drinking virtually has evaporated.[21] Girls also begin to drink at a very young age; 23 percent have had their first drink before reaching their teen years.[22]

An Early Start

Today's teenagers have tried alcohol at virtually equal rates—approximately 74 percent of males and 76 percent of females in grades 9 through 12. Forty-six percent of high school girls use alcohol monthly, and 28 percent binge drink.[23] Although teenagers drink less frequently than adults, they consume more alcohol at a time.[24]

Even more troubling, girls now are starting to drink at younger ages than ever before. In the 1960s, only 7 percent of girls reported having their first drink between the ages of 10 and 14.[25] Today, nearly one-quarter of all girls report beginning to drink alcohol before age 13.[26] Those who initiate alcohol use early in life are at increased risk of becoming problem drinkers.[27]

The older girls get, the more alcohol they drink. Thirty-nine percent of ninth grade girls report current alcohol use compared to 56 percent of high school senior girls.[28]

There also are racial/ethnic differences among girls who drink and girls who don't. Compared to black girls, more teenage white and Hispanic girls report current alcohol use (37% vs. 48% and 48%) and binge drinking (13% vs. 32% and 30%).[29] Asian American girls are less likely to drink and binge drink. One reason might be that, in general, they are more likely than other teens to believe binge drinking to be very risky.[30]

The College Years

Given the lack of parental supervision, coupled with the pro-drinking culture on most campuses, it is not surprising that most college students drink—many for the first time, and many to excess. Eighty-six percent of college women (and men) have consumed alcohol in their lifetimes and more than two-thirds report past-month alcohol use.[31]

Although fewer college women than men binge drink (33% vs. 47%), they do so more than their noncollege peers (27%).[32] College women also drink more heavily and more frequently than they have in the past.[33] Freshman women are more likely to binge drink than upper-class women, while the reverse is true for college men.[34] Not surprisingly, students living in fraternities and sororities have the highest binge-drinking rates. Indeed, women who live in sorority houses are more likely to drink and binge drink than women living in other college housing.[35]

In general, women at co-ed colleges drink more than those at all-women's colleges, but that, too, is changing. Historically, women in women's colleges had fairly low rates of binge drinking. However, the rate of frequent binge drinking in all-women's colleges increased by 124 percent between 1993 and 2001.[36]

Although college males are slightly more likely to be dependent on alcohol (according to *DSM-IV* diagnostic criteria), college females are more likely to be alcohol abusers. Approximately 55 percent of college students who meet clinical criteria for alcohol abuse are women.[37]

A Hidden Problem for Adult Women

Forty-seven percent of adult women (aged 21 and over) are current drinkers, and 15 percent admit to binge drinking. Rates of clinically defined alcohol abuse or dependence among women peak between the ages of 18 and 25 (at over 12%) before dropping off.[38] Fewer than 5 percent of women aged 35 to 64 and less than 1 percent of women age 65 or older abuse or are dependent on alcohol.[39] As with other surveys of alcohol use and abuse, these data derive from women's own self-reports and therefore may underestimate rates of abuse and dependence, particularly for older women. These figures also do not take into account those women whose patterns of drinking may not reach the diagnostic level of abuse or dependence but still put them at risk for a host of negative physical, familial, and social consequences.

Some research has shown that women suffer higher rates of late-onset alcoholism than men.[40] Roughly half of all cases of alcoholism among older women begin after age 59, while among older men, only a quarter of all cases do.[41] This difference may stem from higher rates of stress, due to loss of a spouse, social isolation, or financial crises that contribute to alcohol problems in life.[42]

Drinking's History among Women

In colonial America, drinking alcohol at home and on social occasions was acceptable for women and occasionally considered acceptable even for children.[43] Drinking in taverns was seen as improper for women. Ironically, by the mid-eighteenth century, tavern keeping was considered women's work, and about half of all tavern owners were women.[44]

BAR NONE

By the nineteenth century, the sight of women drinking in a bar and getting drunk became increasingly commonplace, but no less shocking. As one nineteenth-century commentator described, "Twenty years ago I rarely ever saw a female drinking at the bar of a public house or beerhouse. Now I see numbers so engaged from an early hour in the morning, not a few of these early risers and early drinkers having had an infant at the breast, and giving the child a share of the morning dram."

Sources: Straussner, S. L. A., and Attia, P. R. (2002). Women's addiction and treatment through a historical lens. In Straussner, S. L. A., and Brown, S., *The handbook of addiction treatment for women*. San Francisco: Jossey-Bass. Pp. 3–25. Quote from Fillmore, K. M. (1984). When angels fall: Women's drinking as cultural preoccupation and as reality. In Wilsnack, S. C., and Beckman, L. J., *Alcohol problems in women: Antecedents, consequences and interventions*. New York: Guilford. P. 8.

Not only did women drink socially but also they consumed alcohol in other ways; many patent and prescription medicines and tonics used frequently by women in the eighteenth and nineteenth centuries contained up to 50 percent alcohol. By the end of the eighteenth century, Dr. Benjamin Rush—a signer of the Declaration of Independence—expressed concern about excessive drinking by women who were seeking relief from menstrual pain and other "female troubles."[45]

Excessive drinking was condemned for women and men in the nineteenth century, but it was considered especially reprehensible for women. Women who got drunk were thought to be promiscuous and considered "fallen."[46] The typical punishment for public drunkenness for both sexes was imprisonment,[47] but in some cases even more drastic measures were imposed on women.[48] In an address to the Medico-Legal Society in 1897, one doctor recommended that a woman "be desexualized . . . whether maid or matron"[49] if she could not be cured of alcoholism*—a term first coined in 1849 by Swedish physician Magnus Huss. Sterilization of alcohol-abusing women actually continued into the middle of the twentieth century.[50]

Women became the driving force behind the nineteenth-century temperance movement, but it was not women's excessive drinking that concerned them. Countless women were being abused physically and emotionally and victimized economically by men who drank too much. A woman married to a drunk had little recourse because divorce was rare. Women had to obtain the ability to vote in order to pass antidrinking

---

*There is much disagreement surrounding the use of the term *alcoholism*. Some organizations—including the World Health Organization (WHO) and the American Psychiatric Association (APA)—have replaced the term *alcoholism* with *alcohol abuse* and *alcohol dependence*.

TEMPERANCE TIMELINE

1802	First U.S. alcohol law passed, forbidding the sale of alcohol to Indians
1851	Maine passed the nation's first state alcohol prohibition law
1874	Women's Christian Temperance Union founded
1914–1918	World War I
1919	Prohibition (Volstead Act) becomes law
1920	Women granted the right to vote
1933	Prohibition repealed

laws, and so the temperance movement merged with the women's suffrage movement. Both were largely responsible for prohibition in 1919 and—the following year—securing women's right to vote.[51]

But prohibition didn't put an end to either public or private drinking; speakeasies and the illegal use and sale of alcohol flourished. During the "roaring twenties," there were women who drank openly in speakeasies and at cocktail parties, ladies' luncheons, and country club dinners. The *American Independent,* a Kentucky newspaper, declared that women who opposed prohibition in either word or deed were "drunkards" or immoral and concluded that "Most of them are no more than the scum of the earth, parading around in skirts, and possibly late at night flirting with other women's husbands."[52]

After prohibition was overturned in 1933, their hard-won right to vote spurred additional freedoms for women, especially the freedom to work. As women became socially and economically independent, they began drinking more frequently and more openly.[53] In 1939, 45 percent of women drank alcohol. After World War II, more women were working, driving, attending college, using contraceptives, smoking, and drinking than ever before. In 1945, 60 percent of American women drank alcohol. Since then, the rates have fluctuated year to year; the percentage of women who drank dropped to 45 percent in 1958 but rose to a peak of 66 percent in 1981. From 1990 to 1994, the rate increased from 51 to 61 percent and then began to decline once again;[54] the current rate is back to about 45 percent.[55] The recent decline may be due, in part, to the heightened awareness and media coverage of the problems of heavy drinking, especially among women.[56]

Why Women Drink Excessively

Many women, like men, occasionally drink alcohol. Indeed, alcohol was and still is a normal part of everyday life for many in the United States. Yet those women and girls who drink excessively often differ in key ways from their nondrinking peers. Specific biological tendencies, family life, and/or life experiences can heighten significantly the risk of alcohol use and abuse for females.

Biological Risks

Teenage girls whose mothers drank moderately to heavily (a minimum of a third of a drink, or 0.14 oz. of absolute alcohol per day to a maximum of 3.5 drinks, or 1.78 oz. of absolute alcohol per day) during pregnancy are six times likelier to report having drunk alcohol in the past year than girls whose mothers did not drink alcohol. The relationship between prenatal exposure to alcohol and drinking among girls remains strong even when taking into account other possible influential factors, such as prenatal exposure to cigarette smoking, current maternal drinking, child-rearing practices (i.e., maternal-child closeness, monitoring, and having rules against drinking), and the girl's problem behaviors in childhood. No such relationship between maternal drinking during pregnancy and teen alcohol use has been found for boys. Although the explanation for this link is not yet well understood, researchers believe that a biological or genetic explanation can best account for it.[57]

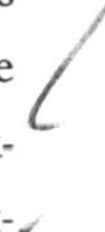

Genetics also indisputably play a role in the susceptibility to alcohol abuse and dependence in women and men, although some research indicates that the link may be stronger for men.[58] Among women, genetic factors account for up to 66 percent of the risk for alcohol dependence.[59] There is some evidence that the threshold for substance abuse and dependence in females is higher than it is for males, suggesting that greater genetic influences are necessary for females to develop a substance use disorder.[60] That is, women who end up developing alcohol- or other drug-related problems tend to have a greater genetic risk for substance dependence than do men who develop such problems.[61]

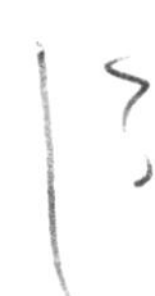

Some research has shown that daughters of alcoholics tend to have less of a physiological response to alcohol, perhaps because of a genetic predisposition, increasing the risk of heavy drinking and the development of subsequent alcohol problems.[62] Another study, however, found that young women with a family history of alcoholism produced more saliva when exposed to alcohol than women without such a history, suggesting a potential risk for more intense alcohol craving and future alcohol problems.[63]

Family Influences

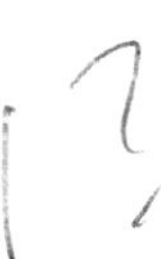

Female alcohol abusers are more likely than their male counterparts to have a family history of alcohol abuse,[64] and some research suggests that a family history of such abuse is a stronger predictor of alcohol dependence in women than in men.[65]

Many aspects of the family environment, including parents' own drinking-related attitudes and behavior, and their level of communication and involvement with their children, influence alcohol use among girls and young women. Whenever parents don't clearly communicate anti-substance-use messages to their children, they put their children at increased risk for substance use; this is especially true for drinking. Because drinking is a regular part of most adults' lives and many see it as a normal rite of passage for teens, many parents inadvertently encourage their daughters' drinking by being too lenient and permissive. For example, 18 percent of teens (25% of 15 to 17 year olds) report having attended a party in the past two years at which parents purchased alcohol for them or served alcohol to them.[66] Nearly three times as many teens (43%) who say their parents wouldn't particularly disapprove of their having one or two alcoholic drinks nearly every day report current alcohol use compared to teens who say their parents would strongly disapprove (15%).[67]

Personal Characteristics

Certain personal traits and experiences tied to the development of alcohol-related problems put girls and young women at particularly high risk. For example, women with a history of childhood conduct disorder are nearly five times likelier than those without such a history to develop alcohol dependence, whereas men with a history of conduct disorder are only twice as likely to develop alcohol dependence.[68] Because conduct problems are more unusual in girls than in boys, girls with such problems may be at greater risk of rejection by peers, attraction to groups of peers who take risks, or more punitive responses from parents, all of which increase the risk for future substance abuse.[69]

Low self-esteem also is a strong predictor of alcohol use and abuse in young women.[70] Teenage girls with low self-esteem or low self-confidence are twice as likely as those with higher self-confidence to report alcohol use.[71] One study found that girls, who at age 12 were low in self-esteem, were nearly two and a half times likelier to engage in heavy alcohol use (defined as using alcohol three or more times during the last

DRINKING HELPED ME LOOSEN UP

[Drinking] helped me deal with being able to talk to people. It helped me loosen up and lose my inhibitions in many respects. It made me feel gregarious, I didn't feel so . . . less than, or not quite good enough.

—Mary Fisher, AIDS activist and recovering alcoholic

Source: Fisher, M., personal communication, June 3, 2003.

30 days and having been intoxicated three or more times during this period) at age 15 than those higher in self-esteem. No such relationship was found in boys.[72] Self-esteem also is related to alcohol use in female college students. College-aged women with a diagnosis of an alcohol use disorder have lower self-esteem than males with the same diagnosis.[73] In comparison to female college students who do not report having a drinking problem, those who do are approximately four times likelier to report feeling worthless.[74]

Childhood Abuse

Women who were sexually or physically abused in childhood are significantly more likely than nonabused women to drink, get intoxicated, and experience alcohol-related problems and alcohol dependence symptoms.[75] In one study, 69 percent of women in treatment reported being sexually abused as children, compared to 12 percent of men. Roughly half of these women were victims of incest.[76] More than two-thirds of alcohol-abusing women seeking treatment have experienced some form of childhood sexual abuse compared to one-third of women in the general population.[77]

The more adverse experiences a child has with abuse (recurrent physical, emotional, or sexual abuse) and other forms of family dysfunction (defined as having lost a parent during childhood or growing up in a household with a family member who is in prison, an alcohol or drug abuser, a victim of violence, and/or chronically mentally ill), the higher her risk of drinking in adulthood.[78] Girls who have been sexually or physically abused are twice as likely to drink as those who were not abused. Sadly, one in five high school girls (20%) report having experienced sexual or physical abuse.[79]

Peer Pressure

Peer pressure may be more strongly associated with drinking for girls than it is for boys.[80] Middle school girls who report high levels of peer pressure to drink are twice as likely to use alcohol as those who report less peer pressure; this relationship between

A BADGE OF HONOR

You don't want to be that dumb girly girl who looks wasted and can't hold her liquor . . . To be able to drink like a guy is kind of a badge of honor.
—College senior, as quoted in *Time* magazine, 2002

Source: Morse, J., and Bower, A. (2002). Women on a binge. *Time* 159(13):57.

SPRING BREAK: EXCESSIVE DRINKING AND DANGERS

Female students—while drinking less than their male counterparts—still consume an average of 10 drinks per day while on spring break, and 78 percent of them binge drink. Forty percent of females (and more than 50% of males) drink until they are sick or pass out, and 33 percent (40% of males) report getting drunk *every* day during spring break.[a]

Not only are such high drinking levels dangerous in terms of alcohol poisoning—especially when combined with sun and potential dehydration—but also they are particularly perilous when they lead to alcohol-related disinhibition and unsafe sex. While women are less likely than men to have sex with someone they just met during spring break, they also are less likely to use a condom when having sex with someone new on spring break or to take condoms with them on spring break, putting them at risk for AIDS, other STDs, and unintended pregnancy. Women on spring break often attribute both their sexual encounters (38%) and their neglect of condom use (32%) to drinking just before having sex. Women on spring break also perceive that "everyone" drinks and that their friends all have sex.[b] As one twenty-year-old female college student on spring break put it, "We want to get drunk and naked; that's why we're down here. This is sun and alcohol 24/7."[c]

Alcohol-related accidents and arrests also are common during spring break. For example, spring break alcohol-related arrests in Florida numbered 5,220 in 2004.[d] State Department officer Glen Keiser dreads the spring break accidents he covers in Mexico: "That's what ties all of our cases together: excessive drinking. Booze, sex, and acting like idiots. The hardest thing I have to do . . . is call a parent in the United States and tell them their son or daughter has died."[e]

Sources: [a]Smeaton, G. L., Josiam, B. M., and Dietrich, U. C. (1998). College students' binge drinking at a beach-front destination during spring break. *Journal of American College Health* 46(6):247–54. [b]Apostolopoulos, Y., Sönmez, S., and Yu, C. H. (2002). HIV-risk behaviours of American spring break vacationers: A case of situational disinhibition? *International Journal of STD and AIDS* 13(11):733–43. [c]Strauss, G. (2004). "Drunk and naked" in Cancun. *USA Today,* March 31, 2004, p. 1D. [d]United Press International. (2004). *Florida spring break arrests show increase.* April 17, 2004, http://about.upi.com/ (accessed September 17, 2004). [e]Leinwand, D. (2003). Alcohol-soaked spring break lures students abroad. *USA Today,* January 6, 2003, p. 1A.

peer pressure and alcohol use is not found for boys.[81] When several of a girl's closest friends smoke or drink, they are more than seven times likelier to drink alcohol. Boys who have several close friends who smoke or drink are almost three times likelier to drink alcohol.[82]

Peers affect college women's drinking behavior as well. Young women who belong to sororities are significantly more likely to drink than those who do not;[83] 80 percent of women living in sororities binge drink compared with 35 percent of women who live elsewhere.[84] However, by the time they reach college, female students are more likely than male students to resist peer pressure to drink alcohol.[85]

Older women are not immune to the effects of their peers' drinking habits. Some older women drink heavily because their spouses, friends, or acquaintances do.[86] For example, high drinking rates are found in retirement communities that emphasize social activities involving alcohol use.[87] In fact, an increase in drinking often occurs after adults move to retirement communities.[88]

Life Transitions, Stress Relief, and Coping

Difficult life transitions increase the risk of alcohol use and abuse in girls and young women. Among young people, the greatest increases in alcohol use and binge drinking take place during the transition from high school to college. Girls drink more and on more days and report binge drinking more frequently in their freshman year of college than in their senior year of high school.[89]

Life transitions also may be an impetus for alcohol abuse in older women. Women suffer higher rates of late-onset alcohol abuse than men.[90] Indeed, roughly half of all cases of alcohol abuse among older women begin at age 60 or older, compared to a quarter of all cases among older men.[91]

Late-onset alcohol abuse appears less likely to be caused by a genetic predisposition than does earlier-onset alcohol abuse[92] and more likely to be the result of women's greater sensitivity to alcohol combined with the use of alcohol to cope with age-related stresses.[93] The problem often emerges when a person is struggling with stressful life events such as retirement; an empty nest; death of a spouse, relative, or friend; loss of independent living; sudden or chronic illness; employment problems; or financial concerns.[94] Women are more likely than men to say their heavy drinking followed a crisis, such as a miscarriage, divorce, unemployment, or the recent departure of a child from the home.[95] These dramatic changes may make days seem endless. Older alcohol abusers often say they started drinking heavily out of boredom and having "more time to drink" after shedding the responsibilities of their earlier years.[96] It is important to note, however, that it is difficult to determine how often these events precede a woman's drinking and how often drinking causes or contributes to them.

Loneliness may be a particular concern for older women. Many older women who live alone are socially isolated and receive diminished social support from family and friends. A solitary lifestyle can contribute to alcohol abuse and dependence and may prevent early detection and intervention by friends or relatives.[97] Poor social support can aggravate anxiety or depression, which in turn contributes to problem drinking. And of course, excessive drinking can drive friends and family members away, increasing the likelihood of drinking alone and perpetuating a pernicious cycle where heavy drinking leads to social isolation and social isolation leads to excessive drinking.

Poor coping skills increase the risk of alcohol use by women encountering stressful life experiences. Young women who tend to wait and hope things will get better or who report that they use alcohol or drugs to cope in the face of a serious problem are more likely to use and abuse alcohol than those with better coping skills. As with older women, this response to adversity can have a cyclical effect. Girls who report more alcohol-related trouble or problems are more likely to use more alcohol, binge drink, and get drunk than those who have fewer alcohol-related problems.[98]

High Expectations

People's expectations about how alcohol will affect them predict to some extent how frequently and how much they drink. For example, girls who believe that drinking alcohol alleviates boredom or helps them deal with sadness or depression report more alcohol use than those who do not.[99]

Girls appear to be attuned to the self-medicating powers of alcohol even before they begin to drink. As early as the sixth grade, girls are likelier than boys to believe that a positive effect of alcohol is its ability to allay bad moods or feelings.[100] Girls who drink heavily are more likely than boys who do so to attribute their alcohol use to the desire to escape their problems, anger, or frustration.[101]

Young women are likely to drink in the context of emotional pain, such as when they are depressed or concerned about personal or academic problems.[102] College women tend to believe that alcohol helps them feel sociable and assertive while decreasing their social anxiety and depression.[103] Both young women and men who drink frequently or intensely tend to drink in social settings, often with the goal of becoming less inhibited.[104] Up to 60 percent of women report that alcohol reduces sexual inhibi-

HERE'S LOOKING AT YOU

A recent study at the University of Glasgow found that alcohol makes the opposite sex appear more facially attractive, at least in the eyes of the drinker. Compared to abstainers, drinkers were more likely to rate someone of the opposite sex as attractive. Alcohol had no effect on the rating of same-sex attractiveness. This may explain why drinking in bars and at parties often leads to sex.

Source: Join Together. (2002). *Study: Booze makes opposite sex more attractive.* www.jointogether.org (accessed February 12, 2004).

tions.[105] The more women drink, the more likely they are to report that alcohol makes them feel less sexually inhibited.[106] Some women drink to provide an excuse for their sexual conduct or to relieve themselves of some responsibility for it.[107]

Women may hold higher expectations than men of alcohol's ability to enhance sexual pleasure.[108] The belief that alcohol is a disinhibitor or aphrodisiac has roots as far back as ancient Greece and Rome, and most people today still believe that alcohol facilitates sexual enjoyment.[109] Yet women's sexual arousal and ability to achieve orgasm actually decrease with increasing levels of alcohol. Alcohol's depressive effect on the central nervous system may contribute to sexual dysfunction and reduced sexual response.[110]

Availability

As is true for obtaining cigarettes, individuals under the legal drinking age of 21 have little to no trouble obtaining alcohol. The majority of teens say that alcohol is readily available to them: 67 percent of eighth graders, 83 percent of tenth graders, and 94 percent of twelfth graders say that they can get alcohol fairly or very easily.[111] Although most students who drink obtain alcohol from their friends and/or at parties,[112] children's homes and family members are common sources of alcohol, especially for younger children.[113] One study found that teens cite other people's homes as the most common setting for drinking.[114] A study of sixth, ninth, and twelfth graders found that one-third of the sixth and ninth graders were getting alcohol from their homes. Only 2 percent of teens relied solely on commercial sources for alcohol.[115] Another study found that adults over the age of 21 were the primary source of alcohol for teens in the ninth and twelfth grades and for 18 to 20 year olds.[116] At the same time, other studies suggest that it is fairly easy for teens to purchase alcohol from commercial establishments.[117] A survey found that approximately two-thirds of teenagers who drink report that they can buy their own alcohol.[118] Among college students, for whom alcohol is practically universally available, the number of alcohol outlets in the college vicinity is linked to their likelihood of drinking and binge drinking. Furthermore, having a bar on campus is associated with a slightly heightened risk that underage students will drink and binge drink.[119] Efforts to reduce availability of alcohol to young people are complicated by the fact that because alcohol is a legal drug with perceived social benefits, many adults are reluctant to abide by restrictions on its availability.

From Promotion to Exploitation

Why might women believe in the sexually enhancing properties of alcohol despite concrete evidence to the contrary? One explanation may be that the alcohol industry has

FROM DISCUS CODE OF ETHICS (OCTOBER 2003)

Beverage alcohol advertising and marketing materials should reflect generally accepted contemporary standards of good taste. Beverage alcohol advertising and marketing materials should not degrade the image, form or status of women . . . *Beverage alcohol advertising and marketing materials should not contain any lewd or indecent images* . . . Beverage alcohol advertising and marketing materials should not rely upon sexual prowess or sexual success as a selling point for the brand. Accordingly, advertising and marketing materials should not contain or depict:

- graphic or gratuitous nudity;
- overt sexual activity;
- *promiscuity; or sexually lewd* or indecent images or language.

Source: Distilled Spirits Council of the United States. (2003). *Code of responsible practices for beverage alcohol advertising and marketing.* www.discus.org (accessed February 4, 2004).

reinforced the link between sex and alcohol for years by aggressively promoting alcohol to women as a way to help them overcome sexual inhibition and a means to improve communication with men.[120]

This wasn't always the case. Before 1958, the alcohol industry's own code of ethics forbade the use of women in its ads.[121] In the 1960s, the industry realized that the women's alcohol market was primed for tapping,[122] and by later in the decade, it directly targeted women by promoting milk-based and heavily sweetened alcoholic drinks.[123] In 1975, the Distilled Spirits Council of the United States (DISCUS) finally allowed its members to put women in ads that were "dignified, modest and in good taste."[124]

In the late 1970s, an ad for the liquor Cherry Kijafa depicted a virginal-looking young woman dressed in white; the copy read, "Put a little cherry in your life." Clearly, the industry had begun to take license with their own code of ethics. Alcohol ads depicting sexy, bare-breasted women and even women in the throes of orgasm have graced the pages of virtually every popular magazine targeted to men and women.[125]

For instance, comparing a Bacardi advertisement that appeared in *Rolling Stone* magazine in 2001[126] with the industry's own stated ethical guidelines, it is evident that "sexually lewd or indecent images" certainly have not been eradicated from contemporary alcohol advertising.

Like the tobacco companies, alcohol companies recently have tried to align their image with that of the liberated woman. In addition to showing women as sex objects, alcohol ads have begun to depict independent, working women. For example, in the 1990s, a Dewar's Scotch ad showed a woman putting on her work clothes while a bare-

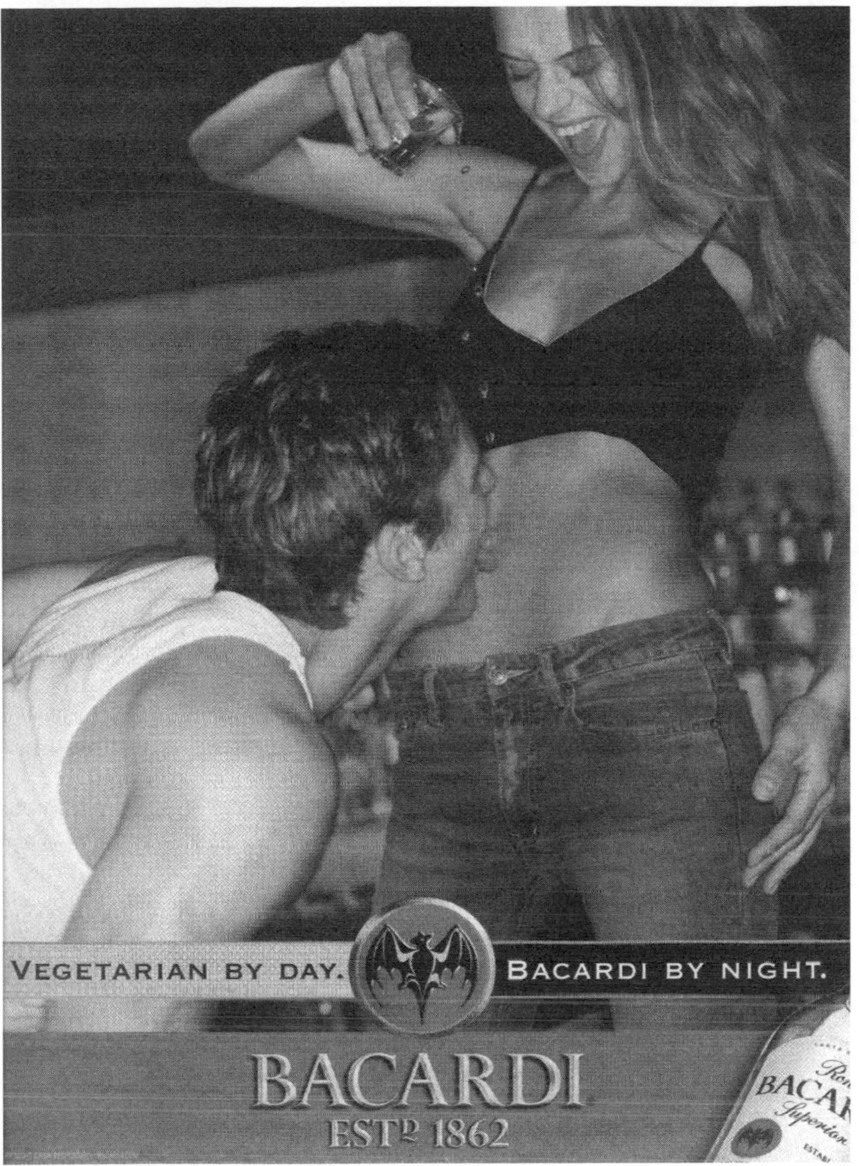

Fig. 3.1. Bacardi advertisement

PROMOTING DRINKING, SEX, AND VIOLENCE

In 2003, alcohol ads became even more sexually explicit and exploitative of women. One of the most controversial ads, a Miller Lite commercial called "Catfight," went even further by using the link of alcohol, sex, and violence to sell beer. The ad shows two sexy women by a pool arguing about why they like Miller Lite. They fall fighting into the pool and rip each other's clothes off. In the last scene, after mud wrestling in their bras and panties, one says to the other, "Want to make out?"

chested man slept in the bed beside her. The slogan: "You finally have a real job, a real place and a real boyfriend. How about a real drink?"[127]

Targeting Teens

Recent marketing efforts have turned to young drinkers by promoting sweet tasting "hard" lemonades, sodas, and other drinks—referred to as *malternatives* or *alcopops.* Drinks such as Rick's Spiked Lemonade, Tequiza, Hooper's Hooch, Smirnoff Ice, and Skyy Blue are widely advertised in magazines and billboards available to or aimed at teenagers.

These sweet-tasting alcoholic beverages are fruit-flavored and malt-based, and come in colorful, child-oriented packaging. Young teens—especially girls—often prefer alcopops to beer or mixed drinks. The sweetness and flavoring hide the taste of alcohol and may be particularly appealing to girls who prefer the sweeter taste. Most alcopops contain about 5 to 7 percent alcohol, a level that is comparable to beer. One survey found that 41 percent of 14 to 18 year olds have tried an alcopop, and more than 80 percent of these underage drinkers say that such products are easy to get.[128]

"Zippers" are another new alcoholic item on the market. Zippers are brightly colored, fruit-flavored cups of gelatin "shots" with an alcohol content of 12 percent. The packaging of these products resembles harmless cups of Jell-O. The producers of Zippers claim that they are marketed to 24- to 44-year-old women who like "entertaining, nights out with friends and fun with no regrets." However, Zippers appear to be marketed to appeal to underage drinkers. Legally sold in 26 states, in some states Zippers can be found in grocery and convenience stores as well as liquor stores and bars.[129]

The industry's gain is teens' loss, and not just in dollars. Drinking before the age of 21 more than doubles the likelihood of developing alcohol-related problems.[130] From 1990 to 2000, the number of girls who started drinking before they turned 18 doubled from one to two million—an increase equal to that among boys.[131]

THE SKINNY ON BEER

Women's (and men's) obsession with weight and the recent low-carbohydrate craze haven't been lost on the alcohol industry. While "lite" beer has been around for years, "low-carb" drinks are the latest option for dieting drinkers. One beer, Michelob Ultra, is advertised as containing only 2.6 grams of carbohydrates, compared to the usual 11 grams in a regular beer. As recently reported in the *New York Times*, the director of Michelob brands wanted to develop a beer for the "health conscious 50-plus consumer." The TV ad, however, according to the *Times* article, "shows a lithe young woman whose bare-midriff jog through downtown is rewarded with a bottle of Ultra from a scruffy young stud." Their ad campaign apparently hit the right note with women in general; while only 21 percent of beer drinkers are women, 37 percent of Ultra drinkers are women.

Source: Walker, R. (2004). The idea of a beer with a "health benefit" is debatable, but that's clearly what's resonating. *New York Times Magazine*, February 1, 2004, p. 18.

Targeting Older Women

Recently, the industry has been directing its efforts towards older female consumers as well. While wine sales have been increasing dramatically, beer sales have been declining over the past 20 years. The beer industry is now trying to lure more women—who currently account for 26 percent of beer drunk outside the home and 11 percent of beer bought in stores—to its products.[132] Interbrew, an international company that sells such beers as Rolling Rock and Lowenbrau, wants to boost sales not only to women in general, whom they consider "beer's lost drinkers," but especially to women over 50 whom they describe as a "grey opportunity."[133]

From Use to Abuse

Women metabolize alcohol differently than men; their bodies contain less water and more fatty tissue compared with men of similar sizes. Because alcohol dissolves more in water than in fat, women maintain higher concentrations of alcohol in their blood. It also is possible that women's bodies do not metabolize alcohol as well as men's due to decreased activity of the enzyme alcohol dehydrogenase (ADH), which breaks down alcohol in the liver and stomach, keeping it from entering the bloodstream.[134]* As a re-

*Further research is needed to determine whether women and men differ in initial metabolization of alcohol via ADH activity. Early research indicated gender differences, while more recent studies have found none.

DEFINING ALCOHOL ABUSE AND DEPENDENCE

Alcohol Abuse[a]

Alcohol abuse is defined as a pattern of drinking that results in one or more of the following situations within a 12-month period:

- Failure to fulfill major work, school, or home responsibilities;
- Drinking in situations that are physically dangerous, such as while driving a car or operating machinery;
- Having recurring alcohol-related legal problems, such as being arrested for driving under the influence of alcohol or for physically hurting someone while drunk; and
- Continued drinking despite having ongoing relationship problems that are caused or worsened by the drinking.

Alcohol Dependence[b]

Alcohol dependence (sometime referred to as alcoholism) is a disease that includes the following four symptoms:

- *Craving*—A strong need, or urge, to drink;
- *Loss of control*—Not being able to stop drinking once drinking has begun;
- *Physical dependence*—Withdrawal symptoms, such as nausea, sweating, shakiness, and anxiety after stopping drinking; and
- *Tolerance*—The need to drink greater amounts of alcohol to get "high."

Sources: [a]National Institute on Alcohol Abuse and Alcoholism. (2001). *Alcoholism: Getting the facts* (NIH publication no. 96-4153). U.S. Department of Health and Human Services, National Institutes of Health, National Institute on Alcohol Abuse and Alcoholism. [b]National Institute on Alcohol Abuse and Alcoholism. (2003). *FAQs on alcohol abuse and alcoholism.* www.niaaa.nih.gov (accessed February 6, 2004).

sult, women get intoxicated faster and experience worse hangovers even when drinking the same amount as men. In fact, one drink for a woman tends to have the same impact as two drinks for a man.[135]

Hormones—especially estrogen—also play a significant role in the effects of alcohol on women. Even moderate amounts of alcohol have been shown to increase estrogen levels in both women and men.[136] Researchers theorize that women might metabolize alcohol differently at different stages of their menstrual cycles, but studies examining this notion have produced conflicting findings. One review of the research found that 5 of 18 studies showed that women's physiological responsiveness to alcohol varies with stages of their menstrual cycle. The findings, however, are not clear as to which stage of the menstrual cycle is significant, and many of these studies have significant methodological limitations that make it difficult to draw firm conclusions from the findings.[137]

When a girl begins drinking is important in determining her risk for future alcohol-related problems; the younger a teen starts to drink, the greater the risk of developing a drinking problem.[138] Among teens ages 12 to 17, the average reported age of initiating drinking is 13—in the larger population, ages 12 and older, the average reported age of drinking initiation is 16 for males and 18 for females.[139] Drinking before the age of 15 quadruples the likelihood of becoming alcohol dependent.[140] Indeed, those who begin drinking between the ages of 11 and 14 have the highest incidence of lifetime alcohol abuse and dependence.[141]

Older women are at particular risk for alcohol abuse because tolerance falls as people age. As the amount of lean mass and water in the body decline, older adults experience a higher concentration of alcohol in the blood with any given drink. Reduced liver and kidney function also may slow down the metabolism and elimination of alcohol from older women's bodies. What was safe and moderate drinking in a middle-aged woman may lead to abuse or dependence in a woman in her sixties or seventies.[142] Because women get drunk faster with less alcohol and become addicted faster, they may be blindsided by its effects and become dependent before they know it. (See chapter 6 for a discussion of treatment of alcohol abuse and dependence.)

Immediate Consequences

Alcohol can have a devastating impact on girls and women. For girls under 21,* any drinking increases risk for negative health and social outcomes; for women over the legal age, consuming more than seven drinks a week (anything more than moderate drinking) is associated with increased risk.

Underage drinking is associated with risky sex, teen pregnancy, and poor academic performance and can even land a girl in juvenile hall or prison rather than in school or a good job. Drinking in early adolescence can delay puberty in girls, and alcohol abuse may cause various endocrine disorders during puberty.[143] Chronic heavy drinking can precipitate menstrual disorders such as heavy flow, painful periods, and irregular cycles.[144] Even moderate drinking can contribute to infertility in women, and the more alcohol a woman consumes, the greater her risk of infertility[145] and miscarriages.[146] (See chapter 5 for more information on the effects of alcohol on pregnancy.) Also, heavy drinking can increase the risk of premature menopause.[147]

*The National Institute on Alcohol Abuse and Alcoholism excludes individuals under 21 years of age from its definition of "moderate drinking," as it is not legal for them to drink at all.

While many of the consequences of alcohol abuse take years to show up, they also can occur suddenly, without warning, and with tragic results. Indeed, the more immediate consequences of drinking can be the deadliest; underage drinking is implicated in the three leading causes of teen death: suicide, accidents, and homicide.[148]

Suicide

Alcohol is estimated to be involved in 8 percent of teenage girls' and 12 percent of teenage boys' suicides.[149] Compared with nondrinking teens, adolescent heavy drinkers and binge drinkers are more than twice as likely to say they contemplated suicide and three times more likely to say they deliberately tried to hurt or kill themselves.[150] Teenage girls who drink frequently are almost six times more likely to attempt suicide than girls who never drink,[151] and girls who are diagnosed with alcohol use disorders are twice as likely to have attempted suicide.[152] Adult women who abuse alcohol also are much more likely to attempt suicide than other women.[153]

It is not always clear whether drinking problems precede suicidal thoughts and behavior or whether the reverse is true. For example, a study of adolescents found that for girls, suicidal thoughts and behavior tended to lead to problem drinking, while for boys, the reverse was true.[154]

Because alcohol is a central nervous system (CNS) depressant, it may increase the risk of suicide in already depressed or suicidal individuals. Drinking may reduce inhibitions and impair the judgment of someone who is contemplating suicide, making suicide attempts more likely.[155]

Accidents

Drinking is involved in a variety of often-fatal accidents including fires, car crashes, boating accidents, and drownings. Alcohol is implicated in up to 50 percent of accidental drownings among teens and adults.[156] Motor vehicle crashes are the leading cause of death in the United States for 16 to 24 year olds, and alcohol is the major factor in most of these fatal crashes.[157] The alcohol-related death rate from car crashes, which stands at 41 percent, decreased after 1991.[158] However, from 1977 to 2000 there was a 13 percent *increase* in the number of women drivers involved in alcohol-related fatal crashes, while there was a 29 percent *decrease* for male drivers.[159] This increase may be an unfortunate consequence of the "designated driver" movement; some women may drink and drive because they have had less to drink than their male companions. However, although women may drink less, they may be more intoxicated than men because

ONE FOR THE ROAD

In 2003, the American Beverage Institute (ABI) started promoting drinking and driving with their "Drink responsibly. Drive responsibly" ad campaign. While they are opposed to drunk driving, ABI claims that there's nothing wrong with having a drink or two with dinner and then driving home. Recent studies, however, prove that even a small amount of alcohol can affect judgment, perception, and impair reaction time and these effects last longer than previously believed—possibly as long as six hours.

Source: Pihl, R. O., Paylan, S. S., Gentes-Hawn, A., and Hoaken, P. N. S. (2003). Alcohol affects executive cognitive functioning differentially on the ascending versus descending limb of the blood alcohol concentration curve. *Alcoholism: Clinical and Experimental Research* 27(5):773–79.

of their greater sensitivity to the effects of alcohol.[160] If men and women have equal blood alcohol contents (BAC), women still are at higher risk of driver fatalities.[161]

Violence Toward and by Women

The link between alcohol and sexual assault, rape, marital abuse, and other violence toward women is extremely strong.[162] Alcohol is associated more closely with crimes of sexual violence than any other drug;[163] it is implicated in as many as 73 percent of all rapes and 70 percent of all incidents of domestic violence.[164] It is linked to more incidences of violence than illicit drugs, including cocaine, heroin, and PCP ("angel dust").[165] Teenage girls and young women who drink are at increased risk of being victims of dating violence such as shoving, kicking, punching, and rape.[166] Alcohol is the chief culprit in date rape on college campuses.[167] Among adult women, in more than 40 percent of alcohol-related marital assaults, both spouses have been drinking; women who abuse alcohol often have male partners who also drink heavily.[168]

Alcohol also puts young girls at risk for exhibiting violent behavior. Indeed, girls who binge drink are three times more likely than their nondrinking peers recently to have gotten into a physical fight.[169]

Unsafe Sex

Unwanted and unsafe sex are common consequences of excessive drinking.[170] Alcohol use is one of the best predictors of sexual activity and risky sexual behavior among teens.[171] Those who drink are more likely to have sexual intercourse, to have it at an

POTENT POTIONS

Passion cocktails—a combination of vodka, passion fruit, and Chinese aphrodisiacs—are hitting the British market, and there is concern they may be headed for the United States. The first of these, Roxxoff, contains 5.4 percent alcohol and horny goat weed, a sexual performance enhancer used for hundreds of years in China, India, and South America. There is now concern that these seductive new drinks may cause an increase in binge drinking, unsafe sex, teenage pregnancy, and date rape.

Source: Khan, S. (2003). *Brewers prepare to seduce young drinkers with wave of "Viagra" pops.* www.observer.co.uk (accessed May 12, 2003).

earlier age, and to have sex with more partners than teens who do not drink.[172] High school students who have drunk at least once in their lives are seven times more likely to have had sex—and twice as likely to have had sex with four or more partners—than teens who have never drunk.[173] Teenage girls who drink are more likely than girls who do not drink to have unprotected sex, which puts them at risk for unplanned pregnancies and sexually transmitted diseases, including AIDS.[174]

Adult women who use and abuse alcohol are more likely to have more sexual partners, more casual sex partners, and higher rates of sexually transmitted diseases and HIV/AIDS than nondrinking women.[175] Indeed, one study found that alcohol-abusing women in treatment are 20 times more likely than other women to be HIV-positive. Possible explanations for the high rate of infection include higher rates of unprotected sex or a general risk-taking personality that manifests in unsafe drinking and unsafe sex.[176] Other research has found that alcohol abuse weakens the body's mechanisms for destroying viruses, which increases a person's vulnerability to HIV infection and can speed up the development of AIDS-related illnesses.[177]

Longer-Term Consequences

Brain Damage

Drinking affects the brains of alcohol abusers in ways that impair learning, memory, abstract thinking, problem solving, and perceptual motor skills (such as eye-hand coordination).[178] Women, however, appear to be more susceptible than men to alcohol-induced brain impairment and damage.[179]

Alcohol appears to have a dramatic effect on adolescents' brains and ability to learn.[180] Teenagers who drink may be exposing their brains to the toxic effects of alcohol during a critical time in brain development. Preliminary research—mostly involving animal studies—suggests that because their brains are still developing, heavy drinking in teens may be more detrimental to their mental capacity than heavy drinking in adults, and the younger the drinker, the greater the risk.[181]

Women who abuse alcohol have proportionally smaller brains in early middle age after fewer years of heavy drinking than alcohol-abusing men.[182] One study found the degree of brain shrinkage in alcohol-abusing women and men to be similar even though women consumed significantly less alcohol than men.[183]

Although a recent study found that women in their seventies who drink less than one drink a day appear to have better cognitive functioning than women the same age who did not drink at all,[184] drinking at levels greater than this appears to hasten the effects of aging on the brain, a phenomenon called "premature aging."[185] This can result in mental confusion, irritability, short-term memory loss, and difficulty in problem solving.[186] While the majority of older alcohol abusers suffer from some degree of memory loss and mental deterioration, older women alcohol abusers do so after fewer years of drinking than older alcohol-abusing men.[187] These effects may be reversible in younger people who stop abusing alcohol but may be permanent in older adults.[188]

An animal study found that after several days of binge drinking, brain cells could die. This suggests that the pattern of drinking may be more important than the quantity of alcohol consumed in determining the extent of alcohol-related brain damage. Indeed, the study found that the extent of brain damage from episodes of short-term binges was similar to that which occurs after a decade of heavy drinking.[189]

Liver Disease

Women who abuse alcohol are more likely than men who do so to develop cirrhosis of the liver and other liver diseases, and to develop them sooner and at lower levels of drinking.[190] A recent study found that while men could safely drink two to three drinks a day without liver damage, more than two drinks a day for women puts them at heightened risk. The study also found that women who drank without eating and drank only on weekends were at increased risk for liver damage compared to those who primarily drank with a meal.[191]

Cardiovascular Disease

Heart disease is the number-one killer of women, and alcohol abuse can be a significant contributing factor.[192] Women of any age who drink to excess are at increased risk for cardiovascular diseases (CVD) such as coronary artery disease, arrhythmias, and cardiomyopathy (a degenerative disease of the heart muscle).[193] Women who abuse alcohol are more susceptible to developing cardiomyopathy than men who do so.[194] Binge drinking also can increase a woman's risk of dying from a heart attack.[195]

One study found that women aged 42 or younger who consume more than one drink per day appear to be at increased risk of hypertension, a major risk factor for heart disease.[196] Black women have a higher likelihood of dying from CVD than white women,[197] particularly those who drink alcohol.[198]

Falls and Fractures

Older adults who have more than one drink a day are at increased risk of injuries from falls and other accidents.[199] Falling due to alcohol abuse can have extremely serious consequences for older women, as falls are the leading cause of injury-related death among older adults.[200] Most deaths from falls are the result of hip fractures,[201] and older women who have more than one drink a day have a higher risk of hip fracture than those who drink less or abstain.[202]

The effects of alcohol on the bones of older women are both positive and negative. Because alcohol increases estrogen levels, light drinking may help counteract osteoporosis resulting from the decline in estrogen after menopause.[203] On the other hand, heavy drinking can interfere with bone growth,[204] resulting in a decrease in bone density and an increase in brittle bones[205] and bone fractures.[206] Women are especially at risk for bone disease and fractures as they age and lose estrogen during their premenopausal and menopausal years.

Breast Cancer

Alcohol appears to increase the risk of breast cancer in some women who are even moderate drinkers.[207] Another study found that women who drink two and a half to three drinks per day are at one-third greater risk for developing breast cancer than women who abstain. The study found that breast cancer risk increases by 7 percent for each additional drink consumed per day.[208] Other research suggests that women with a family history of breast cancer may be more vulnerable to the risks of alcohol consumption on breast cancer.[209]

Alcohol's effect on estrogen might be partially to blame. Women on hormone replacement therapy (HRT) for at least five years appear to be at significantly increased risk of developing breast cancer.[210] This risk appears to increase in women who drink more than two drinks on any given occasion.[211]

Coexisting Problems

Alcohol abuse does not exist in a vacuum; many women with alcohol problems have an array of other disorders. Seventy-two percent of women who abuse alcohol have had at least one episode of mental illness, compared with 57 percent of men.[212] The rates of mental illness are even higher for women diagnosed as alcohol dependent.[213]

The most commonly diagnosed mental health problems among girls and women with alcohol problems are depression, anxiety disorders, borderline personality disorder, and eating disorders. It often is difficult to discern which problem comes first; in some cases alcohol abuse precedes these disorders and in other cases the reverse is true.[214] Women who abuse alcohol also are at increased risk of smoking and abusing prescription and illicit drugs.

Depression

Depression is the most frequent of the coexisting psychological problems for women with drinking problems,[215] and women who abuse alcohol are twice as likely as other women to be depressed. They also are almost four times more likely to suffer from depression as alcohol-abusing men.[216] In the general population, women are approximately twice as likely to suffer from depression as men.[217]

Research shows that the relationship between alcohol use and depression can be found as early as adolescence. The more frequently a girl drinks or the larger the quantities of alcohol she drinks, the greater the likelihood that she is depressed or will be-

DECIDING WHETHER OR NOT TO DRINK

There is insufficient information to encourage patients who do not drink alcohol to start. The data on alcohol and cardiovascular disease are still correlative, whereas the toxic effects of alcohol are well established . . . If alcohol were a newly discovered drug . . . we can be sure that no pharmaceutical company would develop it to prevent cardiovascular disease. Nor would many physicians use a therapy that might reduce the rate of myocardial infarction by 25 to 50 percent, but that would result in thousands of additional deaths per year due to cancer, motor vehicle accidents and liver disease.
—Ira J. Goldberg, M.D., Chief, Division of Preventive Medicine and Nutrition, Columbia University College of Physicians and Surgeons

Source: Goldberg, I. J. (2003). To drink or not to drink? [Editorial]. *New England Journal of Medicine* 348(2):163.

come depressed in the near future. High school girls who drink or binge drink are approximately twice as likely to report feeling depressed, sad, or hopeless as girls who never drink alcohol. And the earlier girls initiate alcohol use, the more likely they are to report feeling sad or depressed.[218]

The link between depression and alcohol abuse may be particularly dangerous among older women, who may live alone or be socially isolated. Older people who commit suicide are nine times more likely to have consumed at least three drinks of alcohol a day than older people who die of natural causes.[219]

Eating Disorders

Alcohol abuse in teenage girls and young women is strongly linked to eating disorders such as bulimia and anorexia. Indeed, up to 50 percent of people with eating disorders abuse alcohol (and illicit drugs), compared with 9 percent of the general population, and up to 35 percent of people who abuse alcohol (and illicit drugs) have eating disorders, compared with three percent of the population.[220]

Teenage girls who engage in unhealthy dieting behavior are significantly more likely to drink alcohol than girls who eat normally. In addition, girls who consider themselves overweight or are planning to diet are at increased risk for drinking.[221] A study of incoming college freshman women found that over 70 percent of those who were bulimic or at risk for bulimia were current drinkers, compared to 44 percent of those who did not diet.[222] Bulimic women who are alcohol dependent have higher rates of other substance abuse, suicide attempts, and anxiety, personality, and conduct disorders than bulimic women who are not alcohol dependent. They also are at increased risk for multiple drug abuse.[223]

Poly-Drug Use

Alcohol use and abuse rarely occur alone; many drinkers also smoke, use illicit drugs, or abuse prescription medications.

Teens who drink are more likely to smoke regularly[224] and use illicit drugs[225] than those who do not drink. Teens who drink and smoke both cigarettes and marijuana are far more likely to get involved with such drugs as heroin and cocaine than nondrinking teens.[226]

Alcohol-abusing girls and women are likely to abuse prescription drugs as well.[227] Alcohol, tranquilizers, and sedatives all depress the central nervous system, and their combined use can cause drowsiness, confusion and delirium, fainting, and falling.[228] Combining alcohol with narcotic painkillers—such as morphine or codeine—can be extremely dangerous. Alcohol can boost the strong sedating effect of these narcotics[229] to the point of stupor and even unconsciousness. Because they are prone to life-threatening injuries from falls and accidents, the combination of drugs and alcohol is especially dangerous for older women.[230] (See chapter 4 for more information on illicit and prescription drug abuse in women.)

Weighing the Health Effects of Light to Moderate Drinking

Numerous studies have been conducted and well publicized that demonstrate the health benefits to adults of light to moderate drinking. For example, studies have found that light to moderate alcohol use may raise "good" cholesterol (HDL)[231] and lower "bad" cholesterol (LDL) and blood pressure, reducing the risk of heart disease;[232] help prevent Alzheimer's disease,[233] ischemic stroke (due to an obstruction of blood flow to an artery, but not hemorrhagic stroke),[234] type-2 diabetes,[235] and stomach ulcers;[236] and that wine in particular may reduce the risk of the common cold.[237]

Although the evidence for the beneficial effects of moderate alcohol use on coronary heart disease and ischemic stroke is substantial, the evidence for many of the other benefits cited is less conclusive.[238] Furthermore, research suggests that some of the positive effects of alcohol—particularly those touted to prevent heart disease—may be stronger for certain groups, such as men rather than women[239] and for older people[240] (primarily those with other risk factors for heart disease).[241] Still other health benefits appear to derive more from ingredients other than the alcohol itself, such as the antioxidant flavonoids found in grape seeds and skins that are fermented in making red wine.[242]

Finally, and perhaps most importantly, many studies demonstrating the health benefits of alcohol are observational; that is, health records are assessed against an individual's self-reported alcohol use. Some of these studies are methodologically flawed. For example, they do not take into account other factors that coincide both with light to moderate alcohol use and better health, such as healthy exercise and diet patterns,[243] or they include former drinkers in the abstainers group when demonstrating increased risk among abstainers.[244] In addition, some findings are overstated or inappropriately generalized to the larger population, even when studies are conducted on a particular subpopulation. More definitive evidence would involve a large, controlled, long-term study in which people of relatively equal health, age, and other demographic characteristics would be randomly assigned to one of several alcohol use conditions (e.g., various levels of alcohol use, drinking various types of alcohol) and followed over time with regular monitoring of a number of health indicators. This type of study is difficult, costly to perform, and largely unethical.

Drinking alcohol to improve one's health is a risky endeavor requiring a delicate balance, as individual women have different—and often unknown—susceptibilities to the health risks of alcohol and since even light alcohol use can have significant health risks. Improving diet and increasing physical activity often can provide a woman the same—or better—protection against heart disease and other health problems, without any of the inherent drawbacks of alcohol use.[245] Health experts agree that, given the evidence, moderate drinkers need not stop drinking but abstainers should not feel the need to drink alcohol to improve their health.

Because each woman is unique in terms of the relative healthful versus adverse consequences of light to moderate alcohol use (given her particular genetic susceptibility, physiology, age, ethnicity, family history of substance abuse and other diseases, drinking patterns, etc.), it is not possible to make a valid recommendation regarding an optimal level of alcohol consumption for women. Rather, women (and men) should consult on these matters with their personal physicians[246] and exercise common sense and healthy skepticism in wading through the barrage of media reports on research studies extolling the benefits or decrying the dangers of alcohol use.

chapter 4

Women and Prescription and Illicit Drugs

Under the influence of the drug, the woman loses control of herself . . . When she acquires the habit, she does not know what lies before her; later, she does not care. She is a young woman who is years upon years old.
—Judge Emily Murphy, 1922

- More than 7.5 million girls and women a year misuse or abuse prescription drugs.[1]
- Women are up to 48 percent more likely than men to be prescribed a narcotic, antianxiety, or other potentially abusable drug.[2]
- Women who use sedatives, antianxiety drugs, or hypnotics are almost twice as likely as men to become addicted to these drugs.[3]
- Teenage girls are more likely than teenage boys to use prescription drugs for non-medical reasons.[4]
- More than half of American women between the ages of 18 and 25 have used illicit drugs at least once in their lives.[5]
- More than 2.5 million women abuse or are dependent on illicit drugs.[6]
- Two out of three AIDS cases in American women are associated with drug abuse.[7]

The increasingly pervasive notion of a "pill for every ill" has offered women a means of self-medicating their negative thoughts and feelings and the medical profession a means of offering their patients quick and easy treatments for numerous complaints. Drugs that are now illegal and known to be highly addictive, such as morphine and cocaine, once were prescribed by doctors to ease ailments, and some were even added to beverages. Many newer and legal prescription medications, like OxyContin, Vicodin, or Valium, though tremendously beneficial when used properly, have become infamous for their addictive properties.

Women of all ages become addicted to prescription and illicit drugs more quickly than men and suffer greater physical, psychological, and social consequences.[8] Because prescription drugs are medications with known benefits and are prescribed by doctors, they often are assumed to be safe and pure. It is this perception of benefit and aid, in addition to the issues surrounding the illegality of illicit drugs, that have influenced how different types of drugs are acquired and used and how their users are perceived and treated. Yet whether one is on OxyContin or crack cocaine, the ravaging effects of addiction to drugs are equally grave.

Because prescription and illicit drug abuse have a shared history, it is difficult to discuss one without the other. The nonmedical use of prescription drugs is the fastest growing drug problem in the United States. After marijuana, prescription drugs are the most commonly abused. More than 7.5 million girls and women misused or abused prescription drugs in 2003.[9] More than 2.5 million women abuse or are dependent on illicit drugs. More than half of American women between the ages of 18 and 25 have used illicit drugs at least once in their lives.[10]

A Prescription for Addiction: A Historical Perspective

Most addicts in the nineteenth and early twentieth centuries became dependent on drugs containing opium or other narcotics that were prescribed to them by their doctors. By the end of the nineteenth century, most of the nation's approximately 250,000 opiate addicts were white, middle- or upper-class housewives or socialites.[11] In an 1871 report to the Massachusetts State Board of Health, a physician wrote: "I have talked with some of our most intelligent apothecaries, who tell me the use of opium has greatly increased, especially among women . . . The doctors are prescribing it more to their patients, and thus the habit is acquired."[12] Indeed, the prescribing and dispensing of opiates by physicians and pharmacists were the major causes of increased narcotic use and addiction.[13] Opium and morphine were believed to cure a variety of conditions including masturbation, violent hiccoughs,[14] and such "female troubles" as morning sickness, nervousness, and nymphomania.[15] Women also were widely prescribed opiates for melancholia and neurasthenia (a condition—introduced into psychiatry in 1869 and largely abandoned today—characterized by general lassitude, irritability, lack of concentration, worry, and hypochondria).[16]

DRUGS COMMONLY PRESCRIBED TO WOMEN IN THE EIGHTEENTH AND NINETEENTH CENTURIES

Opium Produced from the seeds of the Asian poppy, this drug was prescribed to women and babies for a variety of health problems, including melancholia and neurasthenia.[a]

Laudanum A mixture of alcohol and tincture of opium commonly prescribed for "women's problems" and also given to soldiers during the Civil War.

Morphine Derived from opium and first produced commercially in 1827, it was used as a pain reliever and cure for "women's problems" and alcoholism.

Codeine Derived from opium. Until the early 1980s, codeine was an active ingredient in most over-the-counter cough medicines.[b]

Cannabis Widely prescribed from 1840 to 1900 for gonorrhea, headache, labor pains, postpartum depression, and various other "women's problems."

Cocaine Introduced in the United States in 1876 and used often as a treatment for alcohol and opiate addiction as well as neurasthenia.[c] Cocaine was a major ingredient in Coca-Cola and many other drinks and tonics.

Sources: [a]Aldrich, M. R. (1994). Historical notes on women addicts. *Journal of Psychoactive Drugs* 26(1):61–64; Sandmaier, M. (1992). *The invisible alcoholics: Women and alcohol* (2nd ed.). Blue Ridge Summit, PA: TAB Books. [b]University of Buffalo, Addiction Research Unit. (2001). *Before prohibition: Images from the preprohibition era when many psychotropic substances were legally available in America and Europe.* http://wings.buffalo.edu/aru (accessed March 4, 2004). [c]Kandall, S. R. (1998). The history of drug abuse and women in the United States. In Wetherington, C. L., and Roman, A. B., *Drug addiction research and the health of women: Executive summary* (NIH publication no. 98-4289). Rockville, MD: U.S. Department of Health and Human Services, National Institutes of Health, National Institute on Drug Abuse. Pp. 8–16.

Dubbed "God's Own Medicine," morphine not only was given to injured and dying soldiers during the Civil War but also it helped, according to an observer in 1868, "anguished and hopeless wives and mothers, made so by the slaughter of those who were dearest to them."[17] With the invention of the syringe in the mid-nineteenth century, "morphinism" rapidly spread across the globe.

The pharmaceutical industry had its hand in promoting drug use among women. Manufacturers often advertised drugs containing opiates as "women's friends" or "mother's helpers" in catalogues and magazines. One such popular drug, Mrs. Winslow's Soothing Syrup, contained morphine and was widely promoted for teething and for regulating infants' bowels.[18] Mothers and doctors gave opium to pacify wailing babies and irritable children.[19]

THE INVENTION OF THE HYPODERMIC NEEDLE

Because taking opium orally often caused unpleasant gastric side effects, various other methods of delivering opium were used, including enemas, suppositories, skin patches, and crude forms of syringes. In the mid-nineteenth century, an Edinburgh physician, Dr. Alexander Wood, perfected a "hypodermic needle" that could successfully inject morphine into the bloodstream. Injected morphine was believed to be free from unpleasant side effects and not addictive. And because it worked more quickly and was more potent than oral morphine, Wood and his colleagues enthusiastically promoted its use. As a result, many of their patients became morphine addicts. Sadly, the first person recorded to have died from a drug overdose by hypodermic needle was Wood's wife.

Source: Booth, M. (1998). *Opium: A history.* New York: St. Martin's Press.

At the turn of the twentieth century, the Bayer Pharmaceutical Company was doing more than selling aspirin; it was promoting heroin as "the sedative for coughs." Cocaine was widely available in various medications, cough drops, and beverage syrups.[20] These concoctions were advertised as curing such conditions as insomnia and melancholy.[21] The drugs appeared to work because they seemed to make the original symptoms disappear.[22] Repeat customers eventually lead to addicted ones.

The use of opiates during and after the Civil War by women and men alike, the invention of the hypodermic needle, and the widespread use of opiates and cocaine in prescribed and over-the-counter medicine led to inadvertent addiction.[23] By 1900, an estimated 1 in 200 Americans were addicted to narcotics, and, as in the previous century, the majority of addicts were middle- to upper-class white women.[24]

During the early 1900s, there were approximately 50,000 opiate-containing patent medicines available in stores or by mail order in the United States,[25] and Americans were spending $100 million a year for such potions. Not all were *iatrogenically* (medically) addicted. Yet the wide availability of these drugs created a larger market for them. According to a 1921 article in the *New York Times,* "The drug and narcotic habit is ruining hundreds of young girls and women annually. Business women, it would appear, are particularly subject to the habit because of its temporary energizing effect."[26]

Vice or Victimization

At the turn of the twentieth century, there was some concern about the "moral degradation" *caused* by opiate use. However, drug addicts were not subject to legal sanctions.[27] Increased concern about the spread of opiate and cocaine addiction prompted the passage of the Pure Food and Drug Act (1906) and the Harrison Narcotics Act (1914). The Harrison Act restricted the use and distribution of narcotics. It made illegal the nonmedical use of narcotics, and doctors could only prescribe drugs in the course of their professional practice.[28] They could no longer prescribe to maintain an addict's habit, and those doctors who did were arrested.[29]

Repercussions of the Harrison Act

The repercussions of the Harrison Act were immediate and devastating. Within six weeks of its passage, an editorial in the *New York Medical Journal* noted that hoards of addicts had flocked to sanatoriums and hospitals, and out of desperation many resorted to committing crimes in order to obtain their drugs.[30]

Some female addicts were able to continue getting their drugs from their physicians.[31] A large number of the female addicts were nurses and physicians' wives, who tended to have fairly easy access to opiates. Unfortunately, many women turned to the underworld for drugs and the money to buy them. Forced into petty crime and prostitution, many wound up behind bars.[32] An editorial in *American Medicine* in 1915 sympathetically described the situation of "female habitués" after the passing of the Harrison Act: "Houses of ill fame are usually their sources of supply, and one has only to think of what repeated visitations to such places mean to countless good women and girls unblemished in most instances except for an unfortunate addiction to some narcotic drug, to appreciate the terrible menace."[33]

As a result of the Harrison Act, the percentage of female narcotic addicts fell from as high as 80 percent of the addict population near the end of the nineteenth century to around 50 percent of this population in 1918.[34]

The female addict population, once consisting of upper- and middle-class women, increasingly comprised "marginalized" women—often prostitutes and poor women living in slums.[35] They received little sympathy, concern, and help,[36] and this, too, contributed to the likelihood that they would become involved in the criminal underworld of drug dealers. By the early 1930s, instead of being iatrogenically (medically) addicted, many—if not the majority—of female addicts had become so through association with other addicts or self-medication.[37] Drug abuse and addiction among prostitutes increased tremendously after 1939. Before World War II, madams who did not want their prostitutes using drugs carefully scrutinized those who worked in their brothels. As prostitutes started working alone or having pimps, their drug addiction rates increased.[38] By the second half of the twentieth century, women made up around 25 to 30 percent of the addict population.[39] The typical addict was no longer a white middle- or upper-class woman but rather a poor, urban male who mainlined heroin.[40]

HISTORY REPEATS ITSELF

Like their nineteenth-century counterparts, who had recommended opiate-laden "soothing syrups" and related compounds for patients suffering from psychic stress, overzealous physicians began to prescribe these medications with little sense of control, once again reaching for the prescription pad to treat women's neuroses and maladjustments.
—Stephen Kandall, M.D.

Source: Kandall, S. R. (1996). *Substance and shadow: Women and addiction in the United States.* Cambridge, MA: Harvard University Press. P. 139.

Even before the Harrison Act, doctors actively promoted and heavily prescribed tranquilizers and sedatives to women suffering from everything from singlehood to motherhood to widowhood. During the next two decades, doctors—who had little awareness of these drugs' potential for abuse—increasingly prescribed them and by the end of the 1930s had written millions of prescriptions.[41]

The use of these drugs by women increased dramatically in the post–World War II period. Many women who had worked happily during the war had difficulty readapting to the role of housewife. Masses of these and other discontented housewives were prescribed tranquilizers and sedatives.[42] Indeed, white, middle-class women were four times more likely to be prescribed tranquilizers such as Miltown than any other social or economic group.[43]

Physicians and the pharmaceutical industry continued to aggressively promote the use of these drugs as safe and nonaddicting, and their use and abuse increased dramatically in the 1950s. The World Health Organization started including psychoactive drugs in its definition of drug abuse, and large numbers of women in the United States found themselves officially labeled addicts.[44] Dubbed "mother's little helpers" and "dolls," tranquilizers and sedatives were popularized in the Rolling Stones song "Mother's Little Helper" and in Jacqueline Susann's best-selling novel *Valley of the Dolls*.[45]

By the end of the 1960s, an estimated two-thirds of the users of psychoactive drugs—such as Valium and Librium—were women.[46] Valium, a tranquilizer, became the most frequently prescribed drug between 1969 and 1982.[47]

During that time, an estimated one to two million women were addicted to some degree to prescription drugs.[48] The National Commission on Marihuana and Drug Abuse—which was commissioned by President Nixon to research drug use in the United States—acknowledged in their 1973 report that large numbers of women were developing abuse problems with prescription drugs. They also noted, however, that "self-medication by a housewife . . . with amphetamines or tranquilizers . . . is gener-

OVERPRESCRIBING TO WOMEN

Women in the late 1960s accounted for:

- 53 percent of the adult population
- 59 percent of all visits to doctors
- 63 percent of all barbiturates prescribed
- 66 percent of all nonbarbiturates, sedatives, and hypnotics prescribed
- 68 percent of all antianxiety drugs prescribed
- 71 percent of all antidepressants prescribed
- 80 percent of all amphetamines prescribed

Source: Brecher, E. M., and Editors of *Consumer Reports Magazine*. (1972). *Consumers Union report on licit and illicit drugs*. www.druglibrary.org (accessed December 28, 2001).

ally viewed as a personal judgment of little concern to the larger community."[49] A year later, women accounted for three out of four Valium and Librium admissions to emergency rooms and 40 percent of drug-related deaths.[50] By 1978, an estimated 20 percent of American women were using Valium.[51]

The reputation of Valium and other prescription drugs as magic pills already had begun to fade in the wake of celebrities battling prescription drug addictions or dying from overdoses. In the 1960s, tranquilizers were involved in the deaths of Marilyn Monroe, Judy Garland, and Jimi Hendrix. Valium and other prescription drugs were reportedly involved in Elvis Presley's death in 1977,[52] and two years later TV producer Barbara Gordon vividly described her struggle with Valium addiction in the best-selling autobiography *I'm Dancing as Fast as I Can*.[53]

In the 1960s, the drug industry heavily promoted amphetamines as an appetite suppressant. Doctors prescribed them to large numbers of weight-conscious women.[54] Students of both sexes discovered another benefit of amphetamines—they helped keep them up all night to study . . . or party. By the late 1960s, women consumed 80 percent of the amphetamines in the United States,[55] with their peak usage in the summer bathing suit season. A sizable black market dealing in "speed" also had developed. As the health risks posed by amphetamine use became more apparent, the "Speed Kills" campaign was launched to emphasize just how dangerous amphetamines were. Although many young women stopped using amphetamines as a result of the "Speed Kills" campaign, they were switching to what they thought was a safer stimulant—cocaine.[56]

In the mid-1960s marijuana use increased dramatically among women.[57] As women gained rights and freedoms previously denied them, their experimentation with drug use rose as well. Everyone from hippies to housewives to female executives began to experiment with drugs. In fact, women in the 1960s had more in common with the well-bred drug-using women of the nineteenth century than with their poorer drug-abusing sisters of the 1940s and 1950s.[58] Drug users in the 1960s and 1970s had a wider range of available drugs than any generation before them—marijuana, LSD, cocaine, and heroin all were readily available, particularly in the cities where members of the counterculture lived, but also in middle America.[59] In the mid-1970s, the number of new female marijuana users peaked at 1.6 million women per year.[60]

The 1970s also brought women's unique reasons for using drugs to the attention of researchers and policy makers, often for the first time. Gender research began to uncover the specific life stresses that contribute to abuse: broken families, physical and sexual abuse, and association with drug-using men.[61] When the National Institute on Drug Abuse was founded in 1974, the Program for Women's Concerns was created to investigate and monitor the theretofore-overlooked problem of drug abuse among women.

Despite increased federal attention to the problem, the use of illicit drugs increased among women; from 1960 to the late-1970s, the percentage of female addicts doubled from 14 to 30 percent.[62] In 1970, the proportion of female heroin addicts rose from 18 to 30 percent.[63] Cocaine use surged among middle- and upper-class women during the 1970s. Popularized by athletes and musicians, women found that the drug suppressed their appetites and increased their energy, and cocaine use rose accordingly among female high school seniors.[64] The 1980s brought crack cocaine onto the scene, followed by the synthetic drugs of the rave scene in the 1990s.

Who Is at Risk Today?

The misuse and abuse of prescription drugs and the use and abuse of illicit drugs affects millions of American women (Table 4.1). Approximately 19 percent of girls and women in the United States have used prescription drugs for nonmedical reasons at some point,[65] and nearly 3 percent report using them in the past month.[66] Women account for almost half the treatment admissions for abuse of prescription opioids and stimulants and half the admissions for abuse of prescription tranquilizers and sedatives.[67] In general, those most likely to abuse or misuse prescription drugs alone (not in combination with other drugs) are adolescents, young women, and the elderly.[68] However, of all those who abuse prescription drugs, the typical abuser is a young, white, unmarried woman or man from a lower socioeconomic background. Those who live in the southern and western states also appear to be at increased risk.[69]

About 42 percent of girls and women in the United States have used illicit drugs at some point, and more than 2 percent abused or were addicted to these drugs in 2003.

Table 4.1 Females Reporting Drug Use, 2003

Drug Type	*Use during Lifetime*	*Use during Past Year*	*Use during Past Month*
Any illicit drug	41.8%	12.5%	6.6%
Marijuana	35.8	8.3	4.5
LSD	7.6	0.2	0.0
Methamphetamine	4.0	0.5	0.2
MDMA/Ecstasy	3.8	0.7	0.2
Crack	2.2	0.4	0.1
Heroin	1.0	0.1	0.0
Any prescription drug	18.9	6.1	2.7
Pain relievers	11.8	4.6	1.9
Stimulants	7.8	1.1	0.5
Tranquilizers	8.2	2.0	0.8
Sedatives	3.1	0.4	0.2

Source: The National Center on Addiction and Substance Abuse (CASA) at Columbia University. (2005). *CASA's analysis of the National Survey on Drug Use and Health (NSDUH) 2003* [Data file]. Rockville, MD: Substance Abuse and Mental Health Services Administration.

Although women of all ages, races, and social classes use and abuse drugs, as with prescription drugs, the majority of female illicit drug users are white, young (25 and under), less educated, and of lower socioeconomic status than nonusers.[70]

Poly-substance abusers also are at increased risk of prescription drug abuse;[71] girls and young women who abuse alcohol or such illicit drugs as heroin, cocaine, or Ecstasy are at increased risk of abusing prescription drugs.[72] Indeed, more than half (54 percent) of prescription drug abusers also abuse illicit drugs.[73]

A Closer Look

TEENAGE GIRLS. There has been a recent dramatic increase in the abuse of prescription drugs among 12 to 17 year olds. During the past decade, the nonmedical use of painkillers alone has increased approximately 200 percent in this age group.[74] Almost 14 percent of teenagers have used prescription medications nonmedically during their lives (14.1% of girls and 12.8% of boys). Painkillers are the most widely abused prescription drug among teenage girls (8.3% used in the past year), followed by tranquilizers (2.7%), stimulants (2.6%), and sedatives (0.5%). Teenage girls report slightly higher rates of nonmedical use of prescription drugs than boys not only in their lifetimes but also in the past year (10.1% vs. 8.6%) and past month (4.3% vs. 3.7%).[75] They are more likely than boys to use over-the-counter drugs to get high.[76] This is of serious concern since females are almost twice as likely as males to become addicted to certain forms of these drugs, such as sedatives, hypnotics, or antianxiety drugs.[77] No definitive studies have been conducted to explain these gender differences in prescription drug abuse; however, the perception of the safety and purity of these drugs relative to illicit drugs may help account for their higher rates of use among girls.

Of all prescription or illicit drugs of abuse, marijuana typically is the first one tried and the most frequently used.[78] Girls generally use illicit drugs at slightly lower rates than boys: 15.2 percent of teenage girls report using marijuana in the past year (vs. 16.3% of boys), 4.1 percent used inhalants (vs. 4.6% of boys), 3.7 percent used hallucinogens (vs. 4% of boys), 2 percent used cocaine (vs. 2.1% of boys), and 0.3 percent used heroin (vs. 0.2% of boys). Inhalants are unique in that they are used predominantly by younger teens; in fact, reports of inhalant use peak at age 14. National data indicate that while boys are more likely to have used inhalants in the past year compared to girls, boys' and girls' past-month rates of use are very similar (1.3% and 1.2%, respectively). Teenage girls' monthly use of inhalants is six times higher than the rate for all women. Trends in illicit drug use show that rates have either remained relatively stable or declined in recent years among teens.[79]

Prescription and illicit drug abuse among teens vary by race. White girls use most types of drugs at higher rates than Hispanic girls, and both use at higher rates than black or Asian girls.[80]

YOUNG WOMEN. The transition period from high school to college is when there is the greatest surge in drug initiation—especially marijuana use—for girls.[81] Approximately one-third (29%) of young women report engaging in the nonmedical use of prescription drugs or using illicit drugs during the past year (compared to 34% of young men). As with teen girls, the most widely used drug is marijuana; one quarter of young women report using marijuana in the past year. Thirty-five percent of full-time college women used illicit drugs in 2003—primarily marijuana.[82] Prescription drug abuse is the second most popular, with 13 percent of young women reporting using prescription drugs nonmedically in the past year (primarily painkillers)[83]—about 7 percent of college women used pain relievers, stimulants, or tranquilizers, and 4 percent used sedatives. With the exception of pain relievers, these rates generally are lower than for college males, and lower than for noncollege males and females (Table 4.2). The gender gap, however, has closed for some drugs; since 1989, for example, college women and men have used amphetamines at virtually the same rates, due mainly to a greater decline among males in the 1980s. Although fewer college women are daily

Table 4.2 Gender and Educational Differences in Annual Illicit Drug Use among Young Adults

	College Students		*Nonenrolled Young Adults*	
Drug Type	*Male*	*Female*	*Male*	*Female*
Any illicit drug	39.2%	34.8%	42.2%	40.0%
Marijuana	37.3	31.5	38.8	33.9
Inhalants	3.4	0.9	2.4	1.4
Hallucinogens	10.5	5.5	10.0	5.5
Cocaine/crack	6.2	5.0	10.9	7.3
Ecstasy	4.4	4.4	7.3	6.2
Heroin	0.4	0.2	0.7	0.5
Pain relievers	10.2	7.7	11.7	11.2
Stimulants	7.7	6.8	11.7	7.7
Sedatives	3.7	4.4	8.1	4.8
Tranquilizers	6.3	7.3	8.6	8.3

Source: Johnston, L.D., O'Malley, P.M., Bachman, J.G., and Schulenberg, J. E. (2004). *Monitoring the future: National survey results on drug use, 1975–2003. Volume 2: College students and adults ages 19–45* (NIH publication no. 04-5508). Bethesda, MD: U.S. Department of Health and Human Services, National Institutes of Health, National Institute on Drug Abuse.

marijuana users than college men (4% vs. 6%), daily use has risen more sharply among females since 1994.[84] The gender gap also has narrowed for cocaine and LSD use in the past decade.

ADULT WOMEN. For adults (generally over age 26), the gender gap is wider; adult men are likelier than adult women to abuse prescription or illicit drugs (13% vs. 8% in the past year). Although males and females are about equally as likely to use prescription drugs nonmedically (4.7% vs. 4.3%), males are about twice as likely as females to use marijuana (9.4% vs. 4.8%), cocaine (2.7% vs. 1.1%), and hallucinogens (0.9% vs. 0.4%).[85]

As with teens and young adults, prescription drug abuse among adult women varies by race: white women (20.4%) are more likely to have used these drugs nonmedically at some point in their lives than black (11.6%), Hispanic (12.8%), and Asian (7.5%) women. White women also are more likely to have used illicit drugs during their lifetimes than black, Hispanic, and Asian women. Rates of illicit drug abuse and dependence are higher for black women (1.8%) than for white (1.1%), Asian (0.7%), and Hispanic (0.6%) women.[86]

OLDER WOMEN. The largest substance abuse problem among older women is the misuse of prescription drugs. Pain relievers and sedatives are believed to be among the most widely abused substances among older people.[87] More than 10 percent of women over the age of 50 report using prescription drugs for nonmedical purposes in their lifetimes; the rates are somewhat higher for men ages 50 and older (12%). Females are slightly likelier than males to have misused prescription drugs in the past year (2.0% vs. 1.7%). Rates of abuse or dependence on prescription drugs are relatively low in this population (0.2% of females vs. 0.4% of males). Among those age 65 and older, the pattern shows that females are slightly likelier than males to report ever using prescription drugs nonmedically (3.9% vs. 2.9%) and to have done so in the past year (1.1% vs. 0.1%).[88]

CASA's survey of physicians found that women over the age of 59 take an average of five drugs at the same time. These physicians estimated that as many as 11 percent of their older female patients had problems with prescription drug misuse or abuse.[89] Many older women are inappropriately prescribed drugs that have a high potential for misuse and abuse, such as painkillers, tranquilizers, sedatives, and antidepressants.[90] One study found that one out of six Medicare beneficiaries—3.5 million older women—receives at least one inappropriate prescription.[91] * Many physicians mistakenly diagnose depression rather than prescription drug abuse or alcoholism in older women. As a result, they may inappropriately prescribe another psychoactive drug to treat the depression, thus exacerbating the problems and consequences.[92]

Older women become addicted faster to prescription drugs—even when using smaller amounts—than any other group of adults. The effects of aging decrease an older woman's tolerance for these drugs, making her more vulnerable to misusing and becoming addicted to them. Older women constitute the largest group of psychoactive drug users and are the demographic group most likely to be long-term users. They also tend to be the group most likely to be prescribed medication and most likely to take more than one medication at a time.[93] Older adults use prescription medications approximately three times as frequently as the rest of the population, and they have the lowest rates of compliance with physicians' directions about taking drugs.[94]

Misuse and abuse of psychoactive prescription drugs increase problems associated with aging, such as confusion, memory loss, and depression.[95] Misuse of these drugs also can cause unwanted drowsiness and sedation, resulting in falls or other accidents.[96]

---

*Prescriptions can be inappropriate for several reasons: They may be inherently ineffective or unsafe for the patient; they may be prescribed in doses that are too high or for durations that are too long, and thus ineffective or unsafe; or they may interact dangerously with alcohol or other drugs that a patient is taking.

Indeed, inappropriate prescriptions and misuse of psychoactive prescription drugs double the risk of falls and fractures among older adults[97] and increase their risk of car accidents by up to 50 percent.[98] And those older women who abuse alcohol as well as psychoactive drugs are at especially high risk for accidents and overdoses.[99]

Older women rarely use or abuse illicit drugs.[100] One possible reason is that older women (referring here to women over the age of 59) who previously used drugs "matured out." This could be due to increased wisdom and responsibilities that come with getting older,[101] illness, or other age-related factors. Another explanation is that women of an older age cohort were raised in a different, "nondrug" culture. However, the number of older illicit drugs users is predicted to increase as the baby boomers (defined as people born between 1946 and 1964)—who have grown up in an era of wider experimentation with illicit drugs—reach their sixties.[102]

Becoming Addicted

What leads girls or women to try a drug varies from individual to individual, but once they try, some go back in search of escape and the high. The high may range from feelings of euphoria, empowerment, and increased energy—as with cocaine and amphetamines—to the lassitude that can occur with marijuana or the sense of altered reality achieved with hallucinogens. The more quickly and effectively a substance enters the user's bloodstream, the greater the high and the greater the likelihood of addiction. Therefore, drugs that are taken intravenously, smoked, or snorted—such as heroin, powder cocaine, and crack—are more highly addictive. In addition, the more immediate and the shorter the duration of the high, the more likely the user will come to physically depend upon the drug.[103] Preliminary results from current research suggest that women become dependent on cocaine, heroin, or marijuana more quickly than men.[104] With some drugs, like heroin, a user can build up a physical tolerance requiring more of the drug to produce the same effects.[105]

Girls and women can become physically dependent—and potentially addicted—to prescription drugs even when taking them purely for medical purposes and as directed. This form of iatrogenic addiction may be likelier to occur among individuals with a substance abuse history or with a genetic predisposition toward addiction. Nevertheless, determining which women will become addicted to prescription drugs that are taken as intended can be difficult.

Regardless of how or why one becomes addicted to prescription or illicit drugs, quitting is not easy. Not only can a user crave a drug, but when she stops using, the negative physical and emotional results can be acute and immediate. Many drugs—including certain prescription medications and illicit drugs—result in physical dependence, even if not accompanied by symptoms of psychological addiction, where the body adapts to the drug intake. Over time, more of the drug is needed for it to have the intended effects. Withdrawal occurs when one stops using a drug upon which one has become physically dependent. The substance, dose, length of use, and the presence or absence of other conditions can all affect withdrawal symptoms, which can last anywhere from a few days to a few weeks. According to the *Diagnostic and Statistical Manual of Mental Disorders* (*DSM-IV*), stimulants (such as amphetamines or cocaine), opioids, and central nervous system (CNS) depressants (such as sedatives, hypnotics, and some antianxiety drugs) are associated with withdrawal symptoms,[106] although some research has found evidence of certain withdrawal symptoms among long-term marijuana users as well.[107] Characteristic symptoms of stimulant withdrawal include depressed mood, fatigue, vivid and unpleasant dreams, insomnia or hypersomnia, increased appetite, and either the speeding up (i.e., fidgeting) or slowing down of movement and speech. Opioid withdrawal is characterized by depressed mood, nausea and vomiting, muscle aches, excessive discharge from the eyes and nose, dilation of the pupils, goose bumps, sweating, diarrhea, yawning, fever, and insomnia. Withdrawal from CNS depressants is associated with sweating, increased pulse rate, hand tremors, insomnia, nausea or vomiting, increased motor activity, anxiety and, in some cases, hallucinations and/or seizures.[108] Marijuana withdrawal has been associated with increased aggression, irritability, anxiety, stomach pain, and decreased appetite.[109]

Poly-Substance Use

Most substance abusers use multiple drugs. Fifty-four percent of those admitted to substance abuse treatment programs report using multiple drugs. Heroin is more often a primary drug of abuse for those treated, while cocaine and marijuana are more often used in addition to a primary substance of abuse.[110] One study found that among female methamphetamine users seeking treatment, 100 percent had used alcohol, 99 percent had used marijuana, 97 percent had used tobacco, 86 percent had used cocaine, and 28 percent had used heroin—all levels much higher than among women in the general population.[111] Smoking, drinking, and use of multiple illicit substances are interrelated among teen girls.[112] One study found that 44 percent of college poly-substance users (those who binge drink and use drugs) are women, and that more college women are poly-substance users than users of one drug alone. [113] *

Poly-substance use can have more serious consequences than the use of one drug

*Although the percentages of both were very small in this study (2.98% use a single drug vs. 3.13% are poly-substance users), possibly because marijuana use was excluded due to its high level of popularity.

PRESCRIPTION DRUGS OF CHOICE

Painkillers

Commonly abused painkillers, also known as opioids, narcotics, or analgesics—such as morphine, codeine, OxyContin, Vicodin, Darvon, and Demerol—are highly addictive. A large single dose of certain painkillers can severely depress the respiratory system and even lead to death. Sudden withdrawal from these drugs can lead to violent shaking, bone and muscle pain, diarrhea, and vomiting.

Source: National Institute on Drug Abuse. (2001). *NIDA research report: Prescription drugs: Abuse and addiction* (NIH publication no. 01-4881). Bethesda, MD: U.S. Department of Health and Human Services, National Institutes of Health, National Institute on Drug Abuse.

Tranquilizers and Sedatives

Tranquilizers and sedatives fall under the heading of central nervous system (CNS) depressants. Often referred to on the street as "downers" or "chill pills," these drugs commonly are prescribed to relieve anxiety, quell panic attacks, and promote sleep. CNS depressants are addicting, and their long-term use results in tolerance, such that larger doses of the drug are needed to achieve its effects. If use of these drugs is discontinued abruptly, serious withdrawal symptoms, including seizures, can result.

Source: National Institute on Drug Abuse. (2001). *NIDA research report: Prescription drugs: Abuse and addiction* (NIH publication no. 01-4881). Bethesda, MD: U.S. Department of Health and Human Services, National Institutes of Health, National Institute on Drug Abuse.

Stimulants

Also referred to as "speed" and "uppers," stimulants such as amphetamines enhance brain activity, producing increased alertness, attention, and energy as well as elevated blood pressure and increased heart rate and respiration. Amphetamines and other stimulants can result in side effects, including insomnia, irritability, dizziness, adverse mood reactions, and loss of appetite.[a] Stimulant users sometimes attempt to counter these effects by using other drugs, such as CNS depressants or opioids. As a result, individuals who continually use stimulants are at a greater risk for developing multiple drug dependencies.[b]

Sources: [a]Mycek, M. J., Harvey, R. A., and Champe, P. C. (1997). *Lippincott's illustrated reviews: Pharmacology* (2nd ed.). Philadelphia: Lippincott-Raven. [b]Brands, B., Sproule, B., and Marshman, J. (Eds.). (1998). *Drugs and drug abuse* (3rd ed.). Toronto: Addiction Research Foundation.

Steroids

Anabolic steroids are hormones derived from the male sex hormone, testosterone. Injected, taken orally, or rubbed into the skin, they are normally used to relieve pain and rebuild muscles from physical injury.[a] They also are used to treat delayed puberty and treat some other hormonally related conditions. Misuse of steroids can retard bone growth; damage the liver, heart, and kidneys; increase blood pressure and bad cholesterol; and cause severe acne.[b] Because they are sex hormones, they can cause growth of facial hair, baldness, clitoral enlargement, menstrual changes, and a deepening of the voice in girls and women.[c] Misuse of steroids also can cause extreme mood swings, aggression, and even violence.[d] Because steroids can cause fat loss and lean muscle gain, some girls use them to achieve shapeliness and to control weight.[e] Some also use them to help reduce their breast size.[f]

Sources: [a]Irving, L. M., Wall, M., Neumark-Sztainer, D., and Story, M. (2002). Steroid use among adolescents: Findings from Project EAT. *Journal of Adolescent Health* 30 (Suppl. 4):243–52. [b]National Institute on Drug Abuse. (2004). *NIDA infofacts: Steroids (anabolic-androgenic).* www.drugabuse.gov (accessed March 5, 2004). [c]Join Together. (2000). *New Web site for information about anabolic steroid abuse.* www.jointogether.org (accessed March 5, 2004). [d]National Institute on Drug Abuse. (2004). [e]Mathias, R. (1997). Steroid prevention program scores with high school athletes. *NIDA Notes* 12(4). [f] Hormone Foundation. (2003). *Hormone abuse.* www.hormone.org (accessed September 10, 2002).

OVER-THE-COUNTER (OTC) ABUSABLE DRUGS

OTC Stimulants. These amphetaminelike drugs usually contain caffeine and/or phenylpropanolamine and are promoted as appetite suppressants or stay-awake drugs.[a] The use of these drugs is especially high among high school students who also use illicit drugs.[b] When taken in high doses, these drugs can cause an amphetaminelike high and side effects such as restlessness, insomnia, irritability, weight loss, flushed skin, and dilated pupils.[c]

Diet Pills. The use of diet pills, some of which are stimulants, is dramatically higher among girls than boys; almost one out of four senior girls has used them at some point, compared with fewer than one in ten boys.[d] Girls and women with eating disorders often abuse diet pills as well as diuretics, emetics, and laxatives,[e] which contribute to weight reduction by inducing vomiting, diarrhea, or water loss.[f]

Other OTC Drugs. Over-the-counter drugs containing nicotine and alcohol are likely candidates for misuse and abuse. For example, some teens, including some nonsmokers, misuse OTC nicotine patches, gum, and other products; of those teens who use nicotine replacement products, 18 percent are nonsmokers.[g] Cough medicines, including some cold medications, often contain alcohol—as much as 40 percent—and may be abused. In the past, a cough medicine might have contained both alcohol and codeine.[h] While codeine is no longer available in OTC medications, its predecessor, dextromethophan (DXM—often labeled DM, Tuss or Maximum Strength), can cause hallucinations and other psychedelic effects when taken in large dosages. Today, cold medications such as Robitussin, Benadryl, NyQuil, and Coricidin are the latest additions to a growing list of OTC drugs that teens abuse to get high, a practice sometimes referred to as "robotripping."[i]

Sources: [a]National Library of Medicine and National Institutes of Health. (2002). *Medline Plus medical encyclopedia: Drug abuse.* www.nlm.nih.gov/medlineplus (accessed March 5, 2004). [b]Johnston, L. D., O'Malley, P. M., and Bachman, J. G. (2001). *Monitoring the future: National survey results on drug use, 1975–2000: Volume 1: Secondary school students* (NIH publication no. 01-4924). Bethesda, MD: U.S. Department of Health and Human Services, National Institutes of Health, National Institute on Drug Abuse. [c]National Library of Medicine and National Institutes of Health. (2002). [d]Johnston, O'Malley, and Bachman. (2001). [e]The National Center on Addiction and Substance Abuse (CASA) at Columbia University. (2003). *Food for thought: Substance abuse and eating disorders.* New York: CASA. [f]Bulik, C. M. (1992). Abuse of drugs associated with eating disorders. *Journal of Substance Abuse* 4(1):69–90; Mitchell, J. E., Pyle, R. L., Specker, S., and Hanson, K. (1992). Eating disorders and chemical dependency. In Yager, J., Gwirtsman, H. E., and Edelstein, C. K., *Special problems in managing eating disorders.* Washington, DC: American Psychiatric Press. Pp. 1–14. [g]Klesges, L. M., Johnson, K. C., Somes, G., Zbikowski, S., and Robinson, L. (2003). Use of nicotine replacement therapy in adolescent smokers and nonsmokers. *Archives of Pediatric and Adolescent Medicine* 157(6):517–22. [h]National Clearinghouse for Alcohol and Drug Information. (2002). *Give 'em the facts: Prescription and over-the-counter drug abuse.* www.health.org (accessed March 24, 2002). [i]ABC News. (2002). *Robotripping: Kids overdose on cold medicine to get high.* http://abcnews.go.com (accessed December 17, 2002).

alone. One large-scale study found that over half of deaths caused by accidental overdose could be attributed to using two or more drugs in combination.[114] Both males and females who are dependent on three or more substances are more likely to have higher dependence severity, as well as to have been diagnosed with a mood disorder such as depression. Research indicates that poly-substance use is related to greater levels of novelty seeking, impulsivity, and rebelliousness.[115]

Social and Other Consequences

Considerable evidence indicates that the misuse of prescription drugs may lead to serious emotional, social, and health consequences. Seven percent of all prescription drug abusers experience emotional or mental health problems caused or worsened by their misuse of these drugs. Those who use stimulants nonmedically are the most likely to report emotional problems and problems with friends, family, or work, while tranquilizer misusers or abusers are the least likely.[116]

Marijuana

Marijuana is, by far, the most commonly used illicit drug in the United States. The main chemical component of marijuana, THC, produces sedation, mild euphoria, and mild analgesia and in high doses may intensify sensations or cause hallucinations.[a] The marijuana used today is more than twice as strong as it was in the late 1970s and early 1980s.[b] Smoking marijuana during early adolescence increases the risk of anxiety and depression in late adolescence,[c] particularly for girls and young women.[d] Long-term use of marijuana can lead to psychological addiction,[e] with withdrawal symptoms that include anxiety, irritability, and insomnia.[f] Chronic marijuana smoking also can lead to many of the same respiratory problems as tobacco smoking, including cough and phlegm, symptoms of chronic bronchitis, frequent chest colds, and several forms of cancer.[g] Prolonged use of marijuana can lead to serious lung disease.[h] Marijuana use also can impair attention and short-term memory and distort perception and judgment.[i]

Sources: [a]Pinger, R. R., Payne, W. A., Hahn, D. B., and Hahn, E. J. (1997). *Drugs: Issues for today* (3rd ed.). Boston: WCB/McGraw-Hill. [b]Office of National Drug Control Policy. (2004). *Marijuana: Factsheet.* www.whitehousedrugpolicy.gov (accessed September 22, 2004). [c]Brook, J. S., Rosen, Z., and Brook, D. W. (2001). The effect of early marijuana use on later anxiety and depressive symptoms. *NYS Psychologist* 13(1):35–40; Patton, G. C., Coffey, C., Carlin, J. B., Degenhardt, L., Lynskey, M., and Hall, W. (2002). Cannabis use and mental health in young people: Cohort study. *British Medical Journal* 325(7374):1195–98. [d]Ibid. [e]National Institute on Drug Abuse. (2002a). *NIDA infofacts: Marijuana.* www.nida.nih.gov (accessed October 26, 2001); The National Center on Addiction and Substance Abuse (CASA) at Columbia University. (2004). *Non-medical marijuana II: Right of passage or Russian roulette?* New York: CASA. [f]National Institute on Drug Abuse. (2002a). [g]National Institute on Drug Abuse. (2002b). *NIDA research report: Marijuana abuse* (NIH publication no. 02-3859). Bethesda, MD: U.S. Department of Health and Human Services, National Institutes of Health, National Institute on Drug Abuse; National Institute on Drug Abuse. (2002a); Zhang, Z.-F., Morgenstern, H., Spitz, M. R., Tashkin, D. P., Yu, G.-P., et al. (1999). Marijuana use and increased risk of squamous cell carcinoma of the head and neck. *Cancer Epidemiology, Biomarkers and Prevention* 8(12):1071–78. [h]National Institute on Drug Abuse. (2002a). [i]National Institute on Drug Abuse. (2002b).

Cocaine and Crack Cocaine

Cocaine commonly is snorted, injected, eaten, or smoked as free-base or crack cocaine. Crack cocaine is made by combining cocaine with ammonia or baking soda. When heated, it produces the crackling sound that gives it its name. While cocaine is highly addictive, crack cocaine is even more so.[a] Women become addicted more quickly to crack cocaine than men even when they are casual or occasional users.[b] Cocaine use increases heart rate, breathing rate, blood pressure, and body temperature. It can cause heart attack, heart aneurysm, or stroke.[c] Women appear to be more sensitive to the cardiovascular effects of cocaine than men.[d] Its long-term use can affect a woman's reproductive system, resulting in problems with ovulation and miscarriage.[e]

Sources: [a]National Institute on Drug Abuse. (2003). *NIDA infofacts: Crack and cocaine.* www.drugabuse.gov (accessed March 4, 2004). [b]National Institute on Drug Abuse. (1999). *NIDA research report: Cocaine abuse and addiction* (NIH publication no. 99-4342). Bethesda, MD: U.S. Department of Health and Human Services, National Institutes of Health, National Institute on Drug Abuse. [c]Siegel, A. J., Sholar, M. B., Mendelson, J. H., Lukas, S. E., Kaufman, M. J., et al. (1999). Cocaine-induced erythrocytosis and increase in von Willebrand factor: Evidence for drug-related blood doping and prothrombotic effects. *Archives of Internal Medicine* 159(16):1925–30; Vongpatanasin, W., Mansour, Y., Chavoshan, B., Arbique, D., and Victor, R. G. (1999). Cocaine stimulates the human cardiovascular system via a central mechanism of action. *Circulation* 100(5):497–502. [d]Lukas, S. E., Sholar, M., Lundahl, L. H., Lamas, X., Kouri, E., et al. (1996). Sex differences in plasma cocaine levels and subjective effects after acute cocaine administration in human volunteers. *Psychopharmacology* 125(4):346–54; National Institute on Drug Abuse. (1999). [e]Blume, S. B. (1994). Women and addictive disorders. In Miller, N. S., *Principles of addiction medicine*. Chevy Chase, MD: American Society of Addiction Medicine. Pp. 1–16; Lex, B. W. (1995). Alcohol and other psychoactive substance dependence in women and men. In Seeman, M. V., *Gender and psychopathology*. Washington, DC: American Psychiatric Press. Pp. 311–58.

Heroin

Heroin is a highly addictive drug. Injected, snorted, or smoked, it initially causes euphoria followed by periods of drowsiness and wakefulness and mental confusion. It can slow breathing to the point of respiratory failure and cause pneumonia and other pulmonary disorders. Long-term use can lead to collapsed veins, abscesses, heart infections, and liver disease. Sudden withdrawal from heroin can cause vomiting, diarrhea, insomnia, muscle and bone pain, and cold flashes, but rarely death. Withdrawal symptoms—which peak after a few days—can last up to a week. Heroin overdose can result in shallow breathing, convulsions, coma, and death.

Source: Office of National Drug Control Policy. (2003). *Heroin* [Fact sheet] (NCJ publication no. 197335). Washington, DC: Office of National Drug Control Policy.

Inhalants

The term *inhalants* comprises a wide variety of substances, normally easily obtainable, whose vapors can be inhaled to produce a mind-altering effect. Such substances include paint-thinners; gasoline; felt-tip marker fluids; aerosol sprays, such as spray paint, hair spray, and cooking spray; and gases from whipped cream canisters and butane lighters. Consequences of inhalant use can be deadly and sometimes immediate: "sudden sniffing death" occurs when prolonged sniffing, particularly of butane or other gases, results in heart failure within minutes. Death can result when inhaled chemicals force the air out of the lungs, resulting in asphyxiation. Long-term use of inhalants can result in severe and irreversible brain damage, producing symptoms similar to those of multiple sclerosis. Severe dementia and inability to coordinate movement are possible. Chronic use also results in damage to the heart, lungs, liver, and kidneys.

Source: National Institute on Drug Abuse. (2004). *Inhalant abuse: NIDA research report series.* www.drugabuse.gov (accessed September 23, 2004).

Ecstasy

Ecstasy (MDMA) acts both as a stimulant and a hallucinogen.[a] Ecstasy affects serotonin in the brain, which in turn can affect sleep, mood, appetite, sexual behavior, and memory.[b] Heavy Ecstasy users are at risk of hyperthermia, dehydration, and heart or kidney failure. Chronic, heavy use increases the risk of sleep disorders and may increase the risk of memory- and attention-related deficits.[c] Women appear to be more susceptible than men to the toxic effects of heavy Ecstasy use on the brain.[d]

Sources: [a]Office of National Drug Control Policy. (2004). *MDMA (ecstasy)* [Fact sheet] (NCJ publication no. 201387). Washington, DC: Office of National Drug Control Policy. [b]Reneman, L., Booij, J., de Bruin, K., Reitsma, J. B., de Wolff, F. A., Gunning, W. B., et al. (2001). Effects of dose, sex, and long-term abstention from use on toxic effects of MDMA (ecstasy) on brain serotonin neurons. *Lancet* 358(9296):1864–69. [c]Gouzoulis, E., Daumann, J., Tuchtenhagen, F., Pelz, S., Becker, S., et al. (2000). Impaired cognitive performance in drug free users of recreational ecstasy (MDMA). *Journal of Neurology, Neurosurgery and Psychiatry* 68(6):719–25; Morgan, M. J. (2000). Ecstasy (MDMA): A review of its possible persistent psychological effects. *Psychopharmacology* 152(3):230–48; Wareing, M., Fisk, J. E., and Murphy, P. N. (2000). Working memory deficits in current and previous users of MDMA ("ecstasy"). *British Journal of Psychology* 91(Pt. 2):181–88. [d]Reneman, Booij, de Bruin, Reitsma, de Wolff, Gunning, et al. (2001).

Methamphetamines

Methamphetamines are powerful stimulants that can be swallowed, smoked, snorted, or injected.[a] Their effects on the brain are similar to the effects of cocaine; they stimulate the release of high levels of dopamine and produce euphoria.[b] Methamphetamines—which are highly addictive—can cause wakefulness, increased physical activity, anxiety, and paranoia. They can cause heart attack, stroke, and Parkinsons-like symptoms. Overdosing can lead to hyperthermia, convulsion, and death. Because they suppress appetite, methamphetamines appeal to girls and women who want to lose weight.[c]

Sources: [a]National Institute on Drug Abuse. (2003). *NIDA infofacts: Methamphetamine.* www.nida.nih.gov (accessed March 12, 2004). [b]National Institute on Drug Abuse. (2003); Pinger, R. R., Payne, W. A., Hahn, D. B., and Hahn, E. J. (1997). *Drugs: Issues for today* (3rd ed.). Boston: WCB/McGraw-Hill. [c]The National Center on Addiction and Substance Abuse (CASA) at Columbia University. (2003). *Food for thought: Substance abuse and eating disorders.* New York: CASA.

For the most severely addicted, once hooked, a woman may find herself doing things she never imagined in order to acquire drugs. Rates of risky sex and prostitution are high among drug-abusing women, as are homelessness, unemployment, and the involvement of the foster care system. And once she stops using drugs, the effort to cope with a past history that may include physical and sexual abuse, prostitution, violence, or the loss of her home or children makes the drugs that much more appealing.

Risky Sex

The link between drugs and sex—particularly unprotected sex—is very strong, especially for teenagers. Even controlling for such factors as age, race, gender, and parents' education level (a proxy for income / socioeconomic status), teens who have used drugs are five times more likely than those who have never used drugs to have sex.[117] For example, one study found that teenage girls who used marijuana at least three times in the past month were more than twice as likely to be sexually active and 25 percent less likely to use condoms as those who had never used marijuana.[118]

Adult women drug users also are at increased risk for unprotected sex. One study found female crack users averaged 10 incidents of unprotected sex in the prior 30 days.[119] Because drug users are at increased risk of having unsafe sex and multiple sex partners, even occasional users are at high risk for contracting sexually transmitted diseases (STDs) and the AIDS virus.

Two out of three AIDS cases in American women are associated with drug abuse.[120] Even women who don't inject drugs are at high risk for AIDS if their partners do. Almost half of these AIDS cases are the result of injection-drug use, while another quarter comes from having sex with an injection-drug user. Indeed, according to the Centers for Disease Control and Prevention (CDC), 85 percent of all heterosexually transmitted AIDS cases to date have been due to sexual activity with a person who injected drugs.[121] * And because the mucous membrane of the vagina (particularly if there are cuts or sores) is vulnerable to the exchange of semen, vaginal fluid, or blood during sex, a woman appears to be more likely to get AIDS from an infected man than a man is to get AIDS from an infected woman.[122] Those women with histories of prostitution are at extremely high risk for AIDS and other STDs.[123]

*Of 62,599 adult / adolescent AIDS cases due to heterosexual contact, 25,276 were due to sex with an injection drug user, and 32,987 cases were due to sex with an HIV-infected individual where the risk was not specified. Excluding these unspecified cases, sex with an injection drug user represents 85 percent of AIDS cases due to heterosexual contact in which the risk factor through heterosexual exposure was known.

AIDS is a serious and increasing problem among women drug abusers in prison, and the rates are increasing more rapidly among women than men. Women in state prisons are twice as likely as their male counterparts to be infected with HIV (4% vs. 2%).[124] Drug users also have almost three times the risk of nonusers of contracting other STDs.[125] So, even if a female drug user escapes HIV or AIDS, she is at high risk of contracting other STDs, such as syphilis, herpes, gonorrhea, and the human papillomavirus (HPV), which can cause cervical cancer.[126]

Rape and Violence

Girls who smoke marijuana are more than twice as likely to say they have gotten into fights as those who have never smoked marijuana (44.2% vs. 18.7%). The younger a girl is when she initiates marijuana use, the likelier she is to get into fights. Whereas less than one-third (30.6%) of girls who reported first trying marijuana in their later teen years get into fights, more than half (56.3%) of those who initiated marijuana use before age 13 have been in a physical fight in the past 30 days.[127] Similar results were found for girls' use of other illicit drugs.

The majority of female drug addicts have been violently assaulted.[128] Women with drug abuse problems have, in fact, two to four times higher rates of severe partner violence than nonabusing women.[129] Not only does substance abuse increase a woman's risk of being raped or assaulted but also being the victim of such a crime increases a woman's risk of subsequent drug abuse.[130] Rape victims are significantly more likely to

DATE-RAPE DRUGS

Drug-related violence has become increasingly common on college campuses because of the recent popularity of certain club drugs, some of which are called "date-rape drugs."[a] The most common of these drugs are GHB (liquid ecstasy), Rohypnol (roofies), and ketamine (K or Special K). Because date-rape drugs are odorless, flavorless, and colorless, they easily can be slipped into a drink.[b] When combined with alcohol, these drugs can cause incapacitation or unconsciousness, and if a woman is sexually assaulted, she may be unable to recall exactly what happened to her.

Sources: [a]Wesson, D. R., Smith, D. E., Ling, W., and Seymour, R. B. (1997). Sedative-hypnotics and tricyclics. In Lowinson, J. H., Ruiz, P., Millman, R. B., and Langrod, J. G., *Substance abuse: A comprehensive textbook*. New York: Williams and Wilkins. Pp. 223–30. [b]Fitzgerald, N., and Riley, K. J. (2000). *Drug-facilitated rape: Looking for the missing pieces* (NCJ publication no. 181731). Washington, DC: U.S. Department of Justice, Office of Justice Programs, National Institute of Justice.

be drug abusers than nonrape victims. One study found that, compared to women who were never raped, rape victims were more than three times likelier to have used marijuana, six times likelier to have been cocaine users, and 10 times likelier to have used heroin and amphetamines.[131]

Prostitution

One of the most unfortunate consequences and sometimes causes of drug abuse for women is prostitution. This link between drugs and prostitution is hardly new; nineteenth-century prostitutes used opiates as a way to cope with the emotional and physical hardships of their vocations. Because these drugs can cause the disruption or cessation of menstruation, they were considered useful as a means of birth control.[132]

Estimates of the percentage of female drug users or addicts who have engaged in prostitution vary tremendously, from 18 to 72 percent.[133] Most begin using drugs prior to or at the time they become prostitutes,[134] and many take up prostitution to pay for their drugs.[135]

Drug-addicted women who exchange sex for money or drugs are more likely than other prostitutes to work on the street, and are less likely to use condoms, be able to negotiate the terms of their encounters, and to have regular clients. They are more likely to spend all the money they earn on drugs, often do not engage in prostitution when drug-free, and have more negative feelings about prostitution.[136]

Cocaine and crack users are particularly vulnerable to prostitution.[137] The shortness of the crack high creates a desperation during which the addict often is willing to do anything for the price of just one more high. The crack house setting also fosters sex-for-crack or sex-for-money exchanges.[138] Although girls represent approximately 28 percent of arrested juveniles, they account for 55 percent of all arrests for prostitution.[139]

Crime

Women who violate drug laws and commit drug-related crimes are the fastest growing segment of the prison population.[140] Before the 1960s, drug-abusing women primarily were arrested for such nonviolent crimes as prostitution, theft, and shoplifting. In the 1960s and 1970s, increasing numbers of women drug abusers were being arrested for auto theft, burglary, fraud, and embezzlement. And between 1965 and 1977, narcotic violations by women rose from just over 1 percent to over 6 percent. The total number of women in the criminal justice system increased dramatically in the 1980s and 1990s, and most of this increase was due to drug-related crimes.[141]

Women who commit crimes are more likely than male criminals to have used drugs regularly, used them daily in the month before the crime, committed the offense to raise

THE HIGH COSTS OF WOMEN IN PRISON

In Oklahoma, the arrest rate for women is 62 percent higher than the national average, and the drug-related arrest rate for women is 116 percent above the national average. However, the state spends half of the national average on drug treatment, and in fact allots only one percent of its prison budget to treatment. According to K. C. Moon, director of the Oklahoma Criminal Justice Resource Center, when the cost of placing the children of incarcerated mothers into foster care is factored in, it costs the state 31 percent more to imprison a woman than a man.

—*New York Times,* December 29, 2003

Source: Butterfield, F. (2003). Women find a new arena for equality: Prison. *New York Times,* December 29, 2003, p. A9.

money to buy drugs, and to have been under the influence of drugs at the time of the crime.[142] In 2002, approximately 67 percent of women arrestees tested positive for illicit drugs—mostly cocaine and marijuana—and 21 percent had used multiple drugs.[143]

The crack epidemic fueled an explosion in the female prison population,[144] particularly among minority women who have significantly higher rates of incarceration than white women.[145] The violent environment surrounding crack addiction pushed some women into robbery, burglary, and drug dealing.[146] By 1991, a third of female state inmates had violated drug laws, compared to a fifth of male inmates, and this does not include all women who committed their crimes while under the influence of drugs or alcohol, or who did so in order to buy drugs.[147] Although women are still less likely than men to commit violent crimes, female crack users commonly shoplift, pickpocket, sell stolen goods, and forge checks.[148]

Between 1990 and 1999, juvenile male and female drug-offense cases increased; however, the increase was much more significant for female juveniles. Specifically, drug-offense cases for females grew by 219 percent, while drug-offense cases for males grew by 161 percent.[149]

Three-quarters of female inmates are mothers of at least one child; between 4 and 15 percent are pregnant when they enter prison.[150] Those who are addicted to drugs stand to lose their children because of their drug abuse. (For more on the effects of drugs on pregnancy and children, see chapter 5.)

Without early intervention in the lives of girls and women, a new generation of children will be trapped in a cycle that includes a substance-abusing parent; prenatal exposure to tobacco, alcohol, and drugs; possible physical and sexual abuse; poverty; and psychological problems.

THE PROBLEMS THAT LEAD WOMEN TO PRISON

The problems that lead women to prison—abuse and battering, economic disadvantage, substance abuse, unsupported parenting responsibilities—have become more criminalized as contemporary society ignores the context of these women's lives. Because many of these women are poor, from minority communities and behave in ways outside middle-class sensibilities, prison has become the uniform response to problems created by inequality and gender discrimination.

—Barbara Owen, Department of Criminology, California State University, Fresno

---

Source: Owen, B. (2003). *Women in prison.* www.drugpolicy.org (accessed April 15, 2004).

Overdoses

Among women and men, prescription drugs are involved in almost one in four (23%) emergency department (ED) admissions and in an estimated 18 percent of deaths. Between 1994 and 2002, the number of opioid-related ED visits increased by 168 percent. In 2002, prescription opioids were by far the most frequently mentioned prescription drug in all drug-related deaths (17% vs. 4% for stimulants and 8% for tranquilizers). In fact, prescription opioids even surpassed cocaine and heroin as the most frequently mentioned drug involved in multiple-drug-related deaths, the most common type of drug deaths.[151]

Suicide

Psychoactive drug abuse contributes to depression, and if the problem goes untreated, the depression will worsen.[152] Although overdoses from prescription and over-the-counter drugs are responsible for most suicides and suicide attempts in adolescents,[153] illicit drugs—such as heroin, cocaine, amphetamines, and Ecstasy—are commonly used for suicide attempts as well.[154]

Drug-use disorders in adolescents are among the strongest risk factors for suicide attempts.[155] Indeed, 12 to 17 year olds who use drugs are more than twice as likely to contemplate or attempt suicide than their non-drug-using peers (25% vs. 9%).[156]

Girls who use marijuana are at increased risk for both suicidal thoughts and suicide attempts; 34.5 percent who are current marijuana users report suicidal tendencies, compared to 19.5 percent of those who never used the drug. As with alcohol, the earlier girls initiate marijuana or other illicit drugs, the greater their risk for suicidal thoughts and behaviors.[157]

Teens who use drugs other than marijuana are at even higher risk for suicide.[158] Those who abuse both drugs and alcohol are at especially high risk for intentional and unintentional drug-related deaths. Indeed, many suicide attempts and drug overdoses involve a combination of drugs, or drugs and alcohol.[159] Women and teens are especially at high risk for suicide attempts using illicit drugs.[160] Teenage girls are more than twice as likely as boys to be admitted to a hospital for acute drug intoxication—usually as a result of a suicide attempt.[161] (See chapter 6 for a discussion of drug abuse treatment.)

Advertising and the Drug Culture

Although media portrayals of smoking and alcohol use are widespread—as are advertisements for cigarettes and alcohol products—portrayals of illicit drug use are less pervasive in the entertainment media and virtually nonexistent in advertising. However, the fashion and cosmetics industries have, periodically, capitalized on the "glamour" of addiction to push its products. In addition, the commercial presence of potentially addictive prescription drugs is becoming increasingly common, particularly with the new wave of direct-to-consumer marketing of these drugs.

Advertising and Media Portrayals of Illicit Drug Use

The media played a large role in publicizing a crack cocaine "epidemic" among poor women in the 1980s.[162] In the mid-1980s, an estimated 30 to 40 percent of cocaine and crack addicts were women. Crack cocaine use was initially confined to poor, urban women and was associated with high-risk sexual activity, such as trading sex for drugs.[163] By the late 1980s media attention had focused on the possible effects of maternal crack cocaine use when pregnant, and research emerged suggesting that "crack babies" are more often born prematurely, underweight, and with poorer motor skills and behavior abnormalities including impulsiveness and moodiness.[164] More recent research, however, has found that many of these studies were faulty in design and that there actually is no unique "crack baby" syndrome.

Heroin use increased among middle and high school girls and boys between 1991 and 1996.[165] Heroin has long been associated with fashion, art, and transgression, particularly in avant-garde communities such as the Lower East Side of Manhattan in the 1970s and 1980s. But it did not receive widespread media coverage—and public outcry—until "heroin chic" emerged in popular culture in the mid-1990s as a fashion-photography trend characterized by expressionless and unhealthy-looking models. The trend was typified by a controversial 1996 ad campaign for Calvin Klein's unisex fragrance Be, which eventually was pulled due to pressure from parents and family

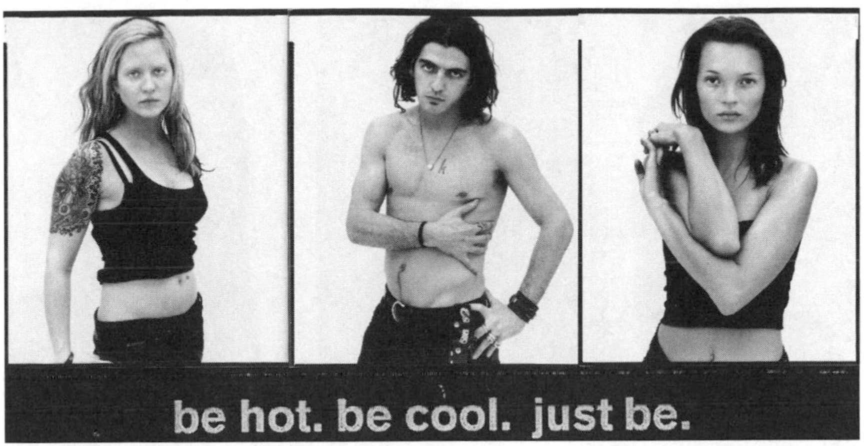

Fig. 4.1. Calvin Klein advertisement

groups. (One of the ads featured three images with the legend "be hot. be cool. just be.") The heroin-chic phenomenon coincided with a mid-1990s glut of heroin-related films (*The Basketball Diaries, Pulp Fiction, Trainspotting*)[166] and with the increased availability of a purer form of heroin that could be snorted in powder form, erasing the need for the more threatening mainline use.[167] President Clinton decried the use of strung-out looking models in a 1997 speech, saying, "the glorification of heroin is not creative, it's destructive. It's not beautiful, it is ugly. And this is not about art, it's about life and death."[168] Fashion soon cycled out of the heroin-chic trend into another, but heroin use among teen girls and boys remained stable after 1996, not declining substantially until 2000 to 2001.[169]

Fashion continues to align itself with the image and language of addiction, but this time the public is on the offensive. In 2002, Christian Dior launched an ad campaign for the perfume of its new cosmetic line, Dior Addict.[170] Along with glossy images, the campaign often coupled the word "addict" with words like "sensuality," "pleasure," and "energy," and the tagline, "Admit It." It inspired such outrage that a coalition of recovery advocacy groups created a counter "Addiction Is Not Fashionable" campaign. Under the pressure of the coalition, Christian Dior agreed to alter the way in which the perfume was marketed. Ads must now feature the full name of the product, Dior Addict, the tagline "Admit It" has been dropped, and the word "addict" alone will not be used to promote the product.[171]

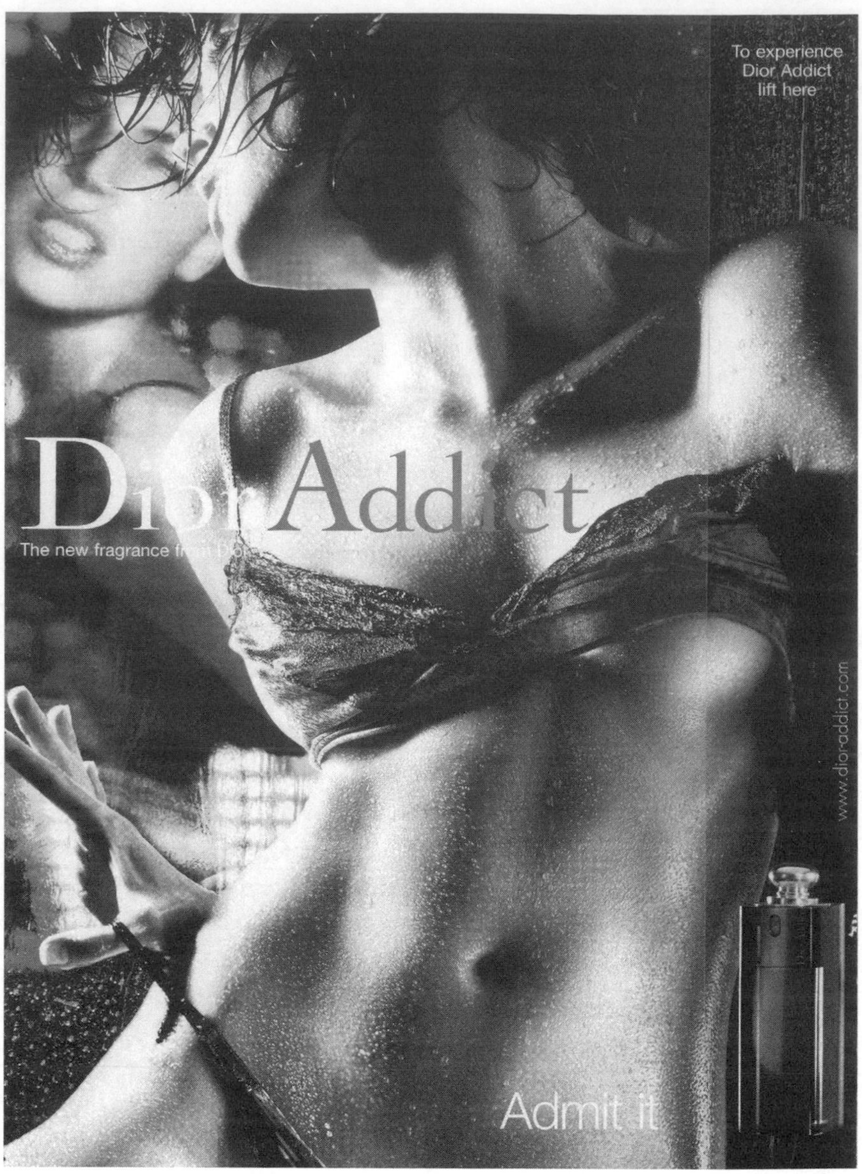

Fig. 4.2. Christian Dior advertisement

Direct Advertising

In the past, patients learned about prescription drugs primarily from their doctors and occasionally from friends or relatives, but today's consumer is far more drug-savvy, thanks to a multimedia barrage of advertisements. Pharmaceutical marketing has played an enormous role in encouraging doctors to prescribe drugs and—more recently—in encouraging patients to request them from their doctors.

The American Medical Association (AMA) fought long and hard to prevent the drugs they prescribed from being advertised directly to patients. The campaign was successful for a while, but in the 1980s the Food and Drug Administration (FDA) began lifting restrictions on the direct advertising of prescription drugs to patients.[172]

In 2000, the pharmaceutical industry spent over $2.5 billion on direct-to-consumer advertising alone, over three times the amount it spent in 1996, and this represents only 15 percent of the dollars spent on drug promotion.[173] These ads promote drugs to cure everything from social anxiety to sexual disinterest, thus further promoting the medicalization of everyday life.[174]

As patients become educated about new drugs, they are likely to demand the newest, most innovative ones available. One survey found that nearly half of respondents had talked to their doctors about a drug they had heard about through an advertisement, and in half of these cases the individuals reported that their doctor had prescribed it.[175] Some argue that these ads help educate patients and help improve doctor-patient relationships. However, others are concerned that these ads not only needlessly contribute to the already high costs of prescription drugs but also may contribute to the problem of inappropriate prescribing[176] and ultimately prescription drug misuse and abuse.

Physicians today, as in the past, continue to prescribe psychoactive drugs to women more frequently then they prescribe them to men.[177] Indeed, women are up to 48 percent more likely than men to be prescribed a narcotic, antianxiety, or other potentially abusable drug.[178] Millions of women are prescribed these drugs to treat problems related to marital status, menstruation, motherhood, and menopause. The medicalization of these normal life stages has been and continues to be widely criticized by those concerned with women's health.[179]

Widespread Availability of Abusable Prescription Drugs

Prescription drugs can easily be found in medicine cabinets in one's home or the homes of friends.[180] This is especially appealing to teenage girls because it avoids the risks of going through drug dealers and the cost of buying the drugs. Prescription drugs can be bought on the street, borrowed, stolen, or swapped—all illegal practices.[181]

Doctor shopping is a common method of obtaining prescription drugs for non-medical purposes; drug seekers go from doctor to doctor requesting prescriptions for their drugs and filling their prescriptions at different pharmacies.[182] Prescription drug abusers may falsify prescriptions or lie to physicians about a medical condition in order to obtain their drugs. Physicians and pharmacists may fail to monitor prescription forms to detect false or altered ones. Rogue Internet pharmacies are emerging as a new and largely unmonitored or regulated source of diversion for controlled drugs.[183]

Many doctors possess outdated medical knowledge and lax prescription writing habits that lead them to inappropriately prescribe potentially abusive medications. Those doctors and other health care professionals who themselves have substance abuse problems may inappropriately prescribe or dispense drugs.[184] And some unscrupulous doctors illegally sell prescriptions.[185] In addition to physicians, other health care professionals may contribute to prescription drug diversion as well by failing to provide clear information and advice on how to take a medication appropriately or to monitor prescription forms to detect false or altered ones.[186]

Major factors in the abuse of prescription drugs are that they are readily available to both teens and adults and they are generally thought to be safe because they are prescribed by doctors.[187] The more available a drug is and the less harmful it is perceived to be, the more likely it is to be used and abused.[188]

chapter 5

Pregnancy and Substance Abuse

Without addressing the stigma of addiction, biases against poor and minority women, unequal access to services and relative unavailability of services, we will make little progress toward reducing the occurrence of substance use by pregnant women.
—L. W. Roberts & L. B. Dunn, 2003

- 17 percent of pregnant women smoke, 3 percent binge drink, and 3 percent use illicit drugs.[1]
- Smoking during pregnancy is responsible for 14 percent of premature births and 10 percent of infant deaths.[2]
- Drinking during pregnancy is the single greatest preventable cause of mental retardation.[3]
- Only little more than half (54.5%) of the pregnant women who drink say that a health care provider discussed drinking during pregnancy with them.[4]
- Approximately 70 percent of women who used illicit drugs or alcohol during pregnancy failed to disclose that information during prenatal exams.[5]
- Illicit drug use during pregnancy is one of the most frequently missed diagnoses in obstetrical medicine.[6]
- Women who abuse drugs during pregnancy typically are single parents with a history of sexual or physical abuse and with little to no financial, social, or childcare support.[7]

The idea of a pregnant woman with a cigarette in her mouth, a wine glass in her hand, or a needle in her arm is deeply disturbing and even tragic. Unfortunately, this is the reality for one in four pregnant women.[8] Women who smoke, drink, or use drugs during their childbearing years face heightened risks of infertility, pregnancy complications, and adverse birth outcomes. Although this has been well documented in the scientific literature—and despite the stigma, the prevention campaigns, and the warnings on cigarette packs and alcohol bottles—some women remain in the dark about the particular effects that substance use—even of a light to moderate nature—can have on pregnancy. Other women know the risks but choose to ignore the warnings. And some women are aware of the risks but continue to smoke, drink, or use drugs during pregnancy because the associated problems they face (e.g., depression, abuse, poverty, homelessness, addiction) are so insurmountable that they are unable to stop.[9]

Approximately 17 percent of pregnant women smoke, 9 percent drink, 3 to 4 percent are heavy or binge drinkers, and 3 percent use illicit drugs.[10] Using more than one substance is very common; one study found that half of pregnant illicit drug users also smoke and drink.[11]

Smoking, drinking, or using drugs during pregnancy jeopardizes fetal development. Substance abuse during pregnancy increases the risk of miscarriages, stillbirths, premature births, low birth weight, congenital defects, and neonatal death.[12] Babies born to mothers who smoke, drink, or use drugs during pregnancy are at risk for a whole host of medical problems, some of which are life threatening. Prenatal exposure to tobacco, alcohol, or illicit drugs can create physiological changes in the brain of the developing fetus and result in mental retardation, poor cognitive skills, and conduct disorders.[13] These problems often continue into adolescence and adulthood, burdening the offspring with ailments that can be as severe as or worse than those experienced by an actual substance abuser.[14]

The estimated lifetime cost of caring for a child prenatally exposed to tobacco, alcohol, or drugs is between $750,000 to $1.4 million.* Most of the bill stems from hospital care at birth and includes the cost of complications during pregnancy and delivery, intensive care, detoxification, and neonatal care. Other costs are related to treating the physical, developmental, and emotional problems that emerge as the child gets older.[15]

That just about every woman—including those who abuse substances—wants to have a healthy baby provides the best window of opportunity to motivate and help

*This cost estimate is based on data from 35 studies; tobacco-, alcohol-, or drug-exposed babies included in this cost estimate are those born with symptoms attributable to the prenatal exposure (e.g., low birth weight, fetal alcohol syndrome).

women who are pregnant or planning to get pregnant to stop smoking, drinking, or using drugs.

Everyone's Problem

Substance abuse during pregnancy crosses all racial, economic, educational, age, and regional lines. However, studies have found that white women are more likely to smoke and drink during pregnancy, while black women and poorer women are more likely to use illicit drugs.[16] Substance abuse during pregnancy generally is higher among pregnant women who are not married, are unemployed, have less than a college education, or rely on public aid. Those who are victims of past or current physical or sexual abuse and those who live with substance users are at increased risk of using substances while pregnant.[17]

Despite that substance use during pregnancy is a problem that is relatively evenly distributed among various racial/ethnic and socioeconomic groups, poor women and minority women are likelier than white women and wealthier women to be reported to health and child welfare authorities for using substances during pregnancy.[18] They also are less likely to have access to proper prenatal care or to have health insurance coverage.[19]

Why Do Pregnant Women Abuse Substances?

A woman who abuses or is addicted to tobacco, alcohol, or drugs may find it difficult to quit despite good intentions. Locating help can be challenging, and, depending on the substance and level of use, withdrawal can be extremely difficult both physically and emotionally. Furthermore, although pregnancy may increase a woman's motivation to quit, the problems that often precipitate the use of substances—such as domestic violence, poverty, or other forms of stress—may remain or be exacerbated by pregnancy.

Accidental Exposure

In many cases the potential for harm of using substances while pregnant is unforeseen. Approximately 50 percent of all pregnancies are unplanned.[20] Among teens alone the unplanned pregnancy rate is even higher—nearly 80 percent.[21] Anywhere from 800,000 to 900,000 teenage girls between the ages of 13 and 19 become pregnant each year.[22] Even more disturbing is the fact that 55 percent of teens indicate that sex while under the influence of alcohol or drugs often is the reason for unplanned pregnancies.[23]

As many as 60 percent of pregnant women who drink do not discover their condition until after the first trimester.[24] During that time, a woman may unwittingly expose the fetus to dangerous substances. For example, children born to mothers who drink during the first trimester of pregnancy are at the greatest risk of suffering neurobehavioral deficits in perceptual, motor, memory, and attention skills.[25]

It is important to note that the intention to get pregnant may positively affect a woman's behavior. There is evidence to suggest that a woman who plans to have a child will exhibit healthier behavior (e.g., suspending smoking or drinking, taking vitamins, etc.) before becoming pregnant and in the first few months of pregnancy.[26]

Mental Health Issues

The emotional and physical demands of pregnancy make it one of the most challenging times in a woman's life. If she has come to rely on smoking, drinking, or using drugs to cope with stress and ease anxiety, quitting may be very difficult. For many women, pregnancy adds to a list of life stressors with which they already struggle. Women who have a history of mental illness are at increased risk of engaging in substance use during pregnancy.[27] One study found that women in treatment with a history of depression were more likely to increase smoking during pregnancy than those who had no such history.[28] Another study found that after learning that they were pregnant, 21 percent of depressed women (compared to 5% of nondepressed women) had at least one binge-drinking episode.[29]

Victims of Violence

Women who continue to use or abuse substances once pregnant often are victims of physical violence.[30] As many as 20 percent of all pregnant women experience abuse, which often starts or intensifies during pregnancy.[31] One study of pregnant women and new mothers entering substance abuse treatment found that 23 percent reported being physically assaulted, 16 percent reported being beaten up, 12 percent reported being assaulted with a weapon, 3 percent reported being deliberately burned, and 14 percent reported being raped.[32]

There is a strong connection between a partner's violent behavior and a pregnant woman's substance use. Being a victim of partner violence appears to increase substance abuse during pregnancy,[33] and addiction severity may be higher among substance-abusing pregnant women who are abused than among those who are not abused.[34] Among pregnant teens, those who have experienced both physical and sexual violence are more likely to smoke, drink, and/or use illicit drugs.[35]

Physical and sexual abuse are highly interrelated among pregnant women and are linked to a history of depression with suicidal thoughts.[36] One study found that pregnant women entering treatment for substance abuse who were current victims of abuse were 10 times likelier to suffer from major depression than pregnant women entering treatment who were not abused.[37] Other studies also find a higher risk of psychiatric disorders and victimization among pregnant, substance-abusing women, including post-traumatic stress disorder.[38]

Women who are abused during pregnancy are at greater risk for miscarriage and spontaneous abortion. They also tend to enter prenatal care later than other women. Negative health outcomes for the fetus associated with violence to the mother include low birth weight and premature labor.[39] Maternal substance use associated with violence during pregnancy also may harm the fetus; one study found that recent physical or psychological abuse may lead to maternal smoking and low maternal weight gain during pregnancy, which can result in low birth weight.[40] Being abused during pregnancy is related to negative views of motherhood and the baby itself.[41]

Other Factors That Increase Risk

Among pregnant women who abuse drugs, there are high rates of mental illness, homelessness, poverty, unemployment, and prostitution. Those who add alcohol to the mix appear to experience many more psychological problems.[42] A study of pregnant black women attending an urban prenatal clinic sheds some light on factors that predict continued substance use during pregnancy. Those who drank alcohol moderately to heavily during their first trimester were less educated, had lower self-esteem, were more depressed, were less happy about their pregnancy, and were likelier to use tobacco and illicit drugs than those who drank lightly or not at all in their first trimester. Those who continued to drink moderately to heavily through their third trimester were less likely to be members of a church or to attend religious activities.[43]

Homelessness is common among substance-abusing pregnant women. A survey of women in Philadelphia in the 1990s found that over 11 percent of women were homeless at some point in the three years before or the four years following the birth of a child. Rates of homelessness among women giving birth in the seven-year period varied widely by ethnicity. Twenty percent of black women were found to have been homeless during the study period compared to only 1 percent of white women.[44] Another study found that 30 to 40 percent of predominantly low-income pregnant women entering treatment for heroin, cocaine, or alcohol abuse were homeless, and 50 to 80 percent had been victims of domestic violence.[45]

Homeless pregnant substance abusers are subject to a wide variety of problems.

Compared to pregnant substance abusers with a fixed address, they have greater addiction severity, more medical problems, less social support, higher family conflict, and a greater incidence of psychiatric illness and physical and sexual abuse.[46] Both homelessness and domestic violence are related to failure to successfully complete treatment.[47]

Involvement with a substance-abusing partner is common among pregnant substance abusers. Of pregnant women entering treatment for substance abuse, 50 to 70 percent have substance-abusing partners.[48] They are more likely to have substance-abusing partners if they currently are victims of domestic violence than if they are not.[49]

Understanding the Problem

There is no one simple profile of a pregnant substance user. However, because the reproductive years—particularly the teen years and early adulthood—also constitute times of high risk for initiating and escalating the use of substances, women of this age who become pregnant are likelier than older pregnant women to smoke, binge drink, or use drugs.[50] And although women of all races, ethnicities, cultural backgrounds, and economic levels are at risk, research has uncovered certain patterns of those groups that are likelier to use particular substances during pregnancy.

Smoking

The older pregnant women are, the less likely they are to smoke. Most pregnant smokers tend to be under 25. While smoking during pregnancy has declined overall since 1990—from 19.5 percent of pregnant women in 1989[51] to approximately 17 percent in 2002[52]—the rate of smoking among pregnant teens actually has increased since 1994. Indeed, teenage girls now have the highest rate of smoking during pregnancy—almost 18 percent[53]—and older pregnant teens ages 18 to 19 have the highest rates, over 18 percent.[54] Less than 10 percent of pregnant women over the age of 30 smoke.[55]

Pregnant white women are significantly more likely to smoke (24%) than pregnant black (7%) or Hispanic (6%) women.[56] Non-high-school graduates have the highest smoking rates during pregnancy and college-educated women the lowest.[57] Women who smoke during pregnancy are more likely to drink than pregnant nonsmokers.[58]

Drinking

Unlike smoking, overall alcohol use during pregnancy is on the rise nationally. Although collecting accurate information on drinking rates among pregnant women is difficult, by the late 1990s, an estimated 20 percent of women reported drinking during pregnancy,[59] a 67 percent increase from 1991, when 12 percent of pregnant women admitted drinking.

Among adult pregnant women, drinking during pregnancy is more common among older (ages 31 to 44) than younger (ages 18 to 30) women. When teenagers are included in the mix, overall past-month alcohol use remains higher among older adult women;[60] however, binge drinking rates are higher among younger than older pregnant women. In fact, pregnant teens are more likely than women of any other age to binge drink.[61]

Pregnant women of all races are less likely to drink during pregnancy than their nonpregnant peers, and white, black, and Hispanic women report binge drinking at relatively equal rates (approximately 3%).[62]

Pregnant women entering treatment for substance abuse are less likely than nonpregnant women entering treatment to report alcohol as their primary substance of abuse (18% vs. 31%).[63]

Illicit Drug Use

As with alcohol use, it is exceedingly difficult to determine the actual number of pregnant women who use illicit drugs. Approximately 3 percent of pregnant women admit to using illicit drugs,[64] but the actual number is likely higher. One recent study found that approximately 70 percent of women who used illicit drugs or alcohol during pregnancy failed to disclose that information during prenatal exams.[65] Admitting to using illicit drugs is admitting to a crime, and pregnancy raises the stakes.

Among pregnant women aged 15 to 44 years, 3 percent reported using illicit drugs in the month prior to their interview compared with 9 percent who were not pregnant. Teens and young adults are more likely than older women to report using illicit drugs while pregnant.[66]

Black pregnant women are more likely to use illicit drugs than white pregnant women (6% and 4%, respectively), and both are likelier than Hispanic pregnant women (2%) to do so.[67] Over half of the pregnant women who use illicit drugs also drink and smoke during pregnancy.[68] Pregnant women are likelier to use marijuana or hashish (3%) or use prescription drugs nonmedically (1.5%) than they are to use cocaine (1.1%), crack (0.9%), or hallucinogens (0.2%).[69] Pregnant women entering treatment for substance abuse are more likely than nonpregnant women entering treatment to report cocaine or crack (22% vs. 17%), amphetamines or methamphetamines (21% vs. 13%), or marijuana (17% vs. 13%) as their primary substance of abuse.[70]

Sounding the Alarm

The 1950s brought "miracle drugs" to the world—antibiotics, cortisone, and the polio vaccine.[71] But during the 1960s, physicians and the general public became increasingly aware of the possible negative effects of illness and all drug use during pregnancy. Women who suffered from rubella (German measles) or who had used thalidomide to prevent nausea during their pregnancy found themselves giving birth to infants with birth defects. Soon, physicians and the public were considering that other substances could have similarly devastating effects on the fetus if taken during pregnancy.[72]

Tobacco

When the first Surgeon General's Report on Smoking and Health was released in 1964, the evidence on smoking's effects on pregnant women was just emerging. Physicians and researchers knew that pregnant women who smoked had children with lower birth weights,[73] but it wasn't until 1971, when the Surgeon General called for a large-scale campaign to educate women about the harms of cigarette smoking, that the issue became a national health problem. The evidence was mounting: more women were smoking, women found it more difficult to quit than men, the children of pregnant smokers were more likely to die before or just after birth, and the industry appeared to be ready to mount a major campaign targeted at women.[74] However, it would be another 11 years before federal recognition of the dangers would translate into warning labels on cigarette packages targeted at pregnant women.

The first general warning labels were mandated in the wake of the 1964 report on smoking. Although reluctant to ban cigarettes, the government did find that cigarette ads were "unfair or deceptive" because they failed to reveal the health risks that smoking posed.[75] Congress passed a law requiring a printed alert on all cigarette packages: "Warning: The Surgeon General has determined that cigarette smoking is dangerous to your health." (The tobacco industry had pushed hard to ensure that all warnings came from the Surgeon General and not Congress in order to reduce the industry's potential legal liability.)[76] Later legislation required cigarette companies to place the warning in all their ads.[77] Yet in 1981, despite years of public warnings by a succession of surgeons general, almost half of all women didn't know that smoking during pregnancy increased the risk of stillbirth and miscarriage.[78] The Tobacco Institute, an industry lobby group,[79] was still suggesting that there was no direct link between smoking and lung cancer or problems during pregnancy.[80]

In 1982, a number of labels that warned smokers of specific dangers, including

WARNING LABELS TARGETED AT PREGNANT WOMEN

On Cigarette Packages and Ads

"Smoking causes lung cancer, heart disease, emphysema and may complicate pregnancy."
"Smoking by pregnant women may result in fetal injury, premature birth and low birth weight."[a]

On Alcoholic Beverages

"Government warning: According to the Surgeon General, women should not drink alcoholic beverages during pregnancy because of birth defects."[b]

Sources: [a]Associated Press. (1984). Cigarette warning bill is signed by President. *New York Times,* October 15, 1984, p. A20. [b]Egan, T. (1989). A worried liquor industry readies for birth-defect suit. *New York Times,* April 21, 1989, p. A12.

emphysema, lung cancer, and premature births for pregnant women, was proposed.[81] Not only did the new labels have the support of key members of Congress but they were also endorsed by the American Lung Association, the American Cancer Society, the American Heart Association, the American Medical Society, and the American Dental Association.[82] Fearing tougher labels that directed attention to addictive properties and the connection between smoking and miscarriages, the tobacco industry gave up the fight.[83] After years of political brawling, the warnings were finally signed into law by President Reagan in October 1984.

Alcohol

In 1968, a pattern of birth defects was noted in children of mothers who drank alcohol during pregnancy,[84] and in 1973, the term *fetal alcohol syndrome* was coined to describe this pattern.[85] But it took many years before warnings appeared on alcoholic beverages. In April 1977, the director of the National Institute on Alcohol Abuse and Alcoholism (NIAAA) asked the government to warn pregnant women that drinking "more than two [alcoholic] drinks a day" could injure a fetus.[86] The birth defects caused by alcohol were noted as second only to rubella and as being greater in one year than the total number of thalidomide births. By June of that year, the National Council on Alcoholism was planning a nationwide campaign to warn women to abstain from drinking while pregnant.[87] In November, the Food and Drug Administration (FDA) asked the Treasury Department—which has jurisdiction over the Bureau of Alcohol,

Tobacco, and Firearms (BATF)—to require warning labels on alcoholic beverages.[88] * The BATF argued instead for a national education program with labeling only as a last resort.[89] Finally, in July 1981, the Surgeon General officially advised doctors that pregnant women and women who were planning to become pregnant should abstain from drinking and that doctors should alert patients to the dangers of alcohol in food and drugs.[90]

Alcohol already had been linked to Sudden Infant Death Syndrome (SIDS).[91] Studies indicated that one in 600 babies were born with severe birth defects linked to their mother's alcohol use.[92] Communities around the country responded to the increasingly incriminating body of evidence by taking the law into their own hands. New York City, for example, passed legislation that required the more than 8,000 bars, liquor stores, and restaurants with alcohol licenses in the city to post warnings that pregnant women who drink put their children at risk of birth defects. Many hailed the decision as a way to help families; others thought that the signs failed to actually inform women and showed little respect for their ability to make intelligent decisions.[93] In California, the battle over legislation to post signs went all the way to the state supreme court, where it was upheld.[94]

Finally in 1988, fifteen years after fetal alcohol syndrome was first identified, warning labels targeted at pregnant women were scheduled to appear on alcoholic beverages nationwide within a year.[95] Unlike the revised cigarette warnings, which had increased in size and were printed within a box,[96] the alcohol warnings on standard-sized bottles were written in type just as high as two stacked dimes on a contrasting background. For containers that contain eight ounces or less, the type may be as high as one dime.[97] A small 1994 study found that women were less aware of alcohol warning labels than they were of those on other products.[98]

Just as the passage of the new labels was announced in 1988, the FDA proposed new warning labels for pregnant women on aspirin bottles. Aspirin had been linked to longer labors, heavier bleeding, and abnormal clotting in mothers and their babies.[99] Within two years, the warning labels were required to be on every aspirin product on store shelves within 12 months.[100]

Illicit Drugs

The late 1960s and early 1970s also saw a wave of research demonstrating the negative effects of hallucinogens, particularly LSD, which ranged from chromosomal damage,

---

*In 1977, the FDA also called for and achieved the addition of warning labels on saccharine products after studies indicated that saccharine could be linked to bladder cancer.

to fetal and birth defects, to miscarriage. While some studies found contradictory results, the press chose to highlight the potential negative effects of LSD, an already controversial drug in the public eye. Concern about maternal heroin use became equally broad. Researchers found that infants who were born addicted to heroin suffered from a wide range of medical ailments, including tuberculosis and sexually transmitted diseases such as syphilis. That such infants were primarily born to poor, black women made the plight of the addicted infant instantaneous fodder for television and print media,[101] reaching its height in the 1980s with concern for "crack babies."

Consequences

The actual physical effects of substance use or abuse on a developing fetus can be devastating. No substance is benign, and some of the most widely used substances (i.e., cigarettes and alcohol) can have the most destructive effects.

Smoking

If a smoker becomes pregnant, she and her fetus face a whole host of potential problems, ranging from miscarriages to birth defects.[102] Smoking increases the flow of carbon monoxide to the fetus and decreases placental blood flow, putting the baby at risk for growth retardation, low birth weight, premature delivery, spontaneous abortion, and other complications of pregnancy and delivery.[103] If a smoker does carry her baby to term, she increases the baby's risk of stillbirth, neonatal death, or SIDS.[104] As many as 14 percent of premature deliveries and 10 percent of all infant deaths are associated with tobacco use during pregnancy.[105] In fact, the Centers for Disease Control and Prevention (CDC) predicts that the elimination of maternal smoking would result in a 10 percent reduction in all infant deaths, a 12 percent reduction in deaths from perinatal conditions, and a significant reduction in the risk for adverse reproductive outcomes, including difficulties in becoming pregnant, infertility, premature rupture of membranes, preterm delivery, and low birth weight.[106]

Smoking during pregnancy also increases the likelihood of a baby being born with congenital defects such as cleft lip or cleft palate.[107] Babies born to mothers who smoke both during and after pregnancy have a 44 percent increased risk of chronic ear infections.[108] One study found that a woman who smokes during a first pregnancy also has an increased risk of early-onset breast cancer.[109]

HEALTH CONSEQUENCES FOR SMOKING MOTHERS AND THEIR CHILDREN

Mother

- Cancer
- Ectopic pregnancy
- Miscarriage

Baby

- Stillbirth
- Low birth weight
- Sudden infant death syndrome (SIDS)
- Cleft palate and cleft lip
- Chronic ear infections
- Tonsillitis
- Asthma
- Bronchitis
- Pneumonia
- Fire-related death and injury
- Behavior disorders during childhood and adolescence
- Obesity and diabetes in adulthood

Sources: Office of the Surgeon General. (2001). *Women and smoking: A report of the Surgeon General* (GPO item no. 0483-L-06). Washington, DC: U.S. Government Printing Office; Pollack, H., Lantz, P. M., and Frohna, J. G. (2000). Maternal smoking and adverse birth outcomes among singletons and twins. *American Journal of Public Health* 90(3):395–400; Richter, L., and Richter, D. M. (2001). Exposure to parental tobacco and alcohol use: Effects on children's health and development. *American Journal of Orthopsychiatry* 71(2):182–203.

A Healthy Future Up in Smoke

Many of the problems that result from smoking during pregnancy may not show up for years. Prenatal exposure to maternal smoking, for example, can lead to decreased lung function, putting a child at risk for lung disease in adulthood.[110] Children born to mothers who smoke (at least one cigarette per day) also are at increased risk of becoming obese and developing diabetes later in life.[111] Women who smoke during pregnancy pass on cigarette-related carcinogens to their fetuses, making their children more susceptible to the development of cancer later in life.[112]

Children prenatally exposed to tobacco also appear to suffer from a variety of intellectual, behavioral, and psychological problems, including lower IQ and poor verbal, reading, and math skills.[113] Toddlers of smoking mothers tend to exhibit more negative behavior—such as risk taking and rebelliousness—than other toddlers.[114] Smoking during the last trimester of pregnancy has even been linked to children's future criminal behavior, arrest rates, and psychiatric hospitalization.[115] As they grow older, children of smoking mothers are at increased risk for smoking and alcohol use in adolescence, behavioral disorders, and drug abuse.[116] The risk of smoking and drug abuse for girls whose mothers smoked regularly during pregnancy is even greater than for boys.[117]

Clearly, the link between prenatal exposure to smoking and these later negative health and behavioral outcomes is a complex one. For example, how much a woman smokes while pregnant can be related to the value she places on the pregnancy and the consequent lifestyle variables that can influence the health of the baby, including nutrition, caffeine use, drug use, exposure to stress, and quality of prenatal care. More generally, women who smoke during pregnancy might differ from non-substance-using women in many ways, any of which might contribute to the ostensible relationships found between prenatal tobacco use and adverse childhood outcomes. That said, there is a strong association between prenatal tobacco use and negative physical and mental health consequences for children at various stages of development.

BREASTFEEDING AND SMOKING. Nicotine and cotinine (the urinary metabolite of nicotine) have been found in the breast milk of smoking mothers and have been shown to decrease milk production and interfere with a baby's weight gain. Breastfed babies of smoking mothers also face the additional risk of being exposed to secondhand smoke.[118]

SECONDHAND SMOKE. Regardless of whether or not they breastfeed, when mothers resume smoking they expose their babies to secondhand smoke. These babies are, in effect, going from smoke-filled wombs to smoke-filled rooms. Secondhand or environmental tobacco smoke (ETS) is especially harmful to babies and children.[119] ETS appears to cause and exacerbate childhood asthma. Smoking in the home also greatly increases the risk of such respiratory diseases as bronchitis and pneumonia in young children.[120] Indeed, secondhand smoke increases the risk of developing serious respiratory disease during the first two years of a child's life.[121] There is some evidence that secondhand smoke can hinder a child's ability to learn[122] and even cause cavities.[123]

Unfortunately, over a third (37.4%) of children (27 million) live in a household where a parent or other adult uses tobacco.[124] Children from lower-income homes and children living in the South are more likely to be exposed to ETS than other children. Black and Hispanic parents are less likely to allow smoking in their homes than are other parents.[125]

DRINKING DURING PREGNANCY

The bottom line is that women should not drink during pregnancy. We cannot say that there is a safe level of drinking during pregnancy.
—Jennifer Willford, Ph.D., University of Pittsburgh School of Medicine

Source: Gordon, S. (2004). *Studies warn of dangers of drinking in pregnancy: Confirm detrimental but not always obvious effects on babies.* www.healthscoutnews.com (accessed March 29, 2004).

Drinking

Drinking during pregnancy can result in a range of serious consequences—from miscarriage and fetal death to fetal alcohol syndrome. The risk of miscarriage during the second trimester, for example, has been found to be twice as high among those who have up to two drinks a day compared to those who do not drink at all. And heavy drinking is even more strongly associated with late miscarriage and neonatal death.[126]

HOW MUCH IS TOO MUCH? While heavy alcohol use clearly is dangerous for the developing fetus,[127] there is increasing evidence that even light (less than three alcoholic drinks per week) to moderate drinking (at least three drinks per week but less than one drink per day) also can cause serious problems.[128] Heavy drinking (five or more drinks a week) women have three times the risk of having both first trimester miscarriages and stillbirths compared to those who drink less than once a week.[129] Children prenatally exposed to light to moderate drinking are at increased risk of having memory and learning problems.[130]

Because a safe level of drinking during pregnancy has not been established, the Surgeon General, the U.S. Department of Agriculture, the U.S. Department of Health and Human Services, the American College of Obstetricians and Gynecologists, and the American Academy of Pediatrics all recommend that women abstain from alcohol during pregnancy and when trying to get pregnant.[131]

BOTTLE BABIES. The negative effects of alcohol on fetuses have been known for thousands of years. In the Bible, Samson's mother was warned against drinking during her pregnancy.[132] And Aristotle noted that, "Foolish drunken or harebrain women for the most part bring forth children like unto themselves."[133]

Infants born to mothers who drink alcohol during pregnancy—even light to moderate amounts—are significantly smaller in weight, height, and head circumference than babies born to nondrinking mothers.[134] Tragically, over 40,000 children are born

PRENATAL EXPOSURE TO ALCOHOL: LONG-TERM PROBLEMS

Hyperactivity and attention deficits
Childhood depressive symptoms
Memory and information-processing difficulties
Poor problem-solving skills
Deficits in abstract thinking and flexibility
Significant weakness in arithmetic skills
Lower IQ scores
Problems with linguistic, perceptual, and motor development

Source: Richter, L., and Richter, D. M. (2001). Exposure to parental tobacco and alcohol use: Effects on children's health and development. *American Journal of Orthopsychiatry* 71(2):182–203.

each year who experience negative health effects associated with prenatal exposure to alcohol.[135] And some of the negative effects of prenatal exposure to alcohol might not show up for years. These include antisocial and delinquent behavioral problems during adolescence and young adulthood, including poor impulse control, poor social adaptation, inappropriate sexual behavior, trouble with the law, problems with employment, and alcohol or drug problems.[136]

Other childhood problems associated with prenatal exposure to alcohol include hyperactivity and attention deficits, childhood depressive symptoms, memory and information processing difficulties, poor problem-solving skills, impaired planning and response inhibition, deficits in abstract thinking and flexibility, significant weakness in arithmetic skills, lower IQ scores, problems with linguistic, perceptual, and motor development, and varying degrees of mental retardation.[137] However, for many children, the consequences of alcohol use during pregnancy often are dramatically apparent at birth.

FETAL ALCOHOL SYNDROME (FAS). The most visible and serious result of drinking during pregnancy is fetal alcohol syndrome (FAS). FAS is characterized by growth deficiency, facial malformations, mental retardation, and central nervous system dysfunction.[138] Children with FAS have problems with learning, memory, attention, problem solving, speech, and hearing. Other problems associated with FAS include skeletal malformations, visual and auditory deficits, altered immunological function, and behavioral problems.[139]

Up to 8,000 babies born in the U.S. each year have FAS[140]—or approximately 6 percent of all babies born to women who drink alcohol regularly during pregnancy.[141] Many experts believe that FAS is underreported because many of the symptoms are not obvious at birth, many children with FAS are not seen in medical settings where a

CHARACTERISTICS OF BABIES WITH FAS

Small eyes
Small, flat cheeks
Short, upturned nose
Growth retardation
Cleft palate
Central nervous system dysfunction

Source: March of Dimes. (2002). *Drinking alcohol during pregnancy.* www.marchofdimes.com (accessed September 30, 2002).

proper diagnosis can be made, and some physicians are reluctant to label children as having FAS or label their mothers as being alcoholics.[142]

Since FAS was first identified, evidence has grown that its consequences endure throughout life. Although the physical signs of FAS may become less distinctive with age, developmental problems associated with intelligence, memory, and attention persist. Indeed, FAS is the leading cause of preventable mental retardation in the Western world.[143] Children who are diagnosed with FAS have an average IQ of 68.[144]

The estimated annual cost of caring for individuals with FAS, including medical treatment, foster care, residential care related to mental retardation, special education services, incarceration, and lost productivity—is almost $4 billion. Preventing only one case of FAS could save approximately $2 million over that person's lifetime.[145]

If a woman has one child with FAS, she has up to a 70 percent chance of having another.[146] Whether or not a child of a mother who drank during pregnancy will develop problems depends to a great extent on the amount of alcohol the mother consumed and the period and length of time during pregnancy when the fetus was exposed to alcohol. Other factors play a role in determining which babies are affected; even when

OUTDATED DATA

Only 17 percent of the obstetrical textbooks published over the past forty years recommend that women abstain from alcohol during pregnancy; the majority of the textbooks either present conflicting data, do not make a recommendation about drinking, or do not address the issue.

Source: Loop, K. Q., and Nettleman, M. D. (2002). Obstetrical textbooks: Recommendations about drinking during pregnancy. *American Journal of Preventive Medicine* 23(2):136–38.

FETAL ALCOHOL EFFECTS

Some babies display some but not all of the characteristics of FAS. These babies are often referred to as having fetal alcohol effects (FAE). This term also has been used recently to describe children who have all the signs of FAS, but who have milder symptoms.[a] Ten times more children are born with FAE than FAS.[b]

Sources: [a]Centers for Disease Control and Prevention. (2002). *Fetal alcohol syndrome: Frequently asked questions.* www.cdc.gov (accessed September 30, 2002). [b]March of Dimes. (2002). *Drinking alcohol during pregnancy.* www.marchofdimes.com (accessed September 30, 2002).

controlling for the amount of alcohol a woman drinks, the chances of having a FAS baby are significantly increased in alcohol-abusing women who live in poverty, have low levels of education, and get late or no prenatal care.[147]

Children born with Fetal Alcohol Effects (FAE), a milder version of FAS, may have fewer physical signs of alcohol exposure but face the same developmental challenges as those born with FAS.[148]

The full range of possible outcomes due to maternal alcohol use during pregnancy, from birth defects to full-blown FAS, is referred to as fetal alcohol spectrum disorder (FASD).[149] Many factors can contribute to the severity of effects experienced by a child prenatally exposed to alcohol, such as how much alcohol he or she is exposed to, the pattern of the mother's drinking, the stage of pregnancy during which the drinking occurred, the use of other drugs, and the mother's nutrition and prenatal care.[150] The duration of alcohol exposure during pregnancy determines the extent of impairment in children's attention, language, and memory skills up to early adolescence.[151]

Animal research suggests that there may be a genetic component that determines the extent of damage caused by prenatal alcohol exposure. Women who are more sensitive to alcohol's effects may be more likely to have a child with more severe motor deficits if they drink during pregnancy, particularly during the third trimester.[152] Despite research that suggests that fetal alcohol disorders occur along a continuum, with the most severe effects associated with the heaviest prenatal exposure, even light to moderate exposure to alcohol before birth can result in long-term effects on children in terms of physical size, behavior, intellect, physical defects, and future alcohol problems.[153]

A MATTER OF TIME. Prenatal exposure to alcohol appears to affect a fetus differently at each stage of fetal development. Heavy alcohol use in the first trimester is associated with abnormal facial features such as those seen in FAS children.[154] Consuming an average of two drinks or more per day during the first trimester of pregnancy is associated with severe neurobehavioral deficits in children's perceptual, motor, memory, and attention outcomes.[155] However, growth retardation and central nervous system problems can occur from prenatal exposure to alcohol at any point during pregnancy.[156] Alcohol exposure is associated in the second trimester with spontaneous abortion and in the third with poor growth.[157] The fetus's brain is at greatest risk of being damaged from alcohol exposure during the last trimester of pregnancy. During this period, the brain undergoes rapid development, and alcohol exposure is most likely to lead to nerve cell death. Just one episode of excessive drinking (defined in this study as drinking for several hours in a single drinking episode) during the final trimester could be enough to damage the brain of a fetus.[158] Other research shows that as few as two cocktails consumed by the mother during this period can cause nerve cells in the fetus's brain to die.[159]

FROM BOTTLE TO BREAST. The potential problems associated with alcohol use do not end with pregnancy. While pregnant women are warned against drinking alcohol, some nursing mothers still may be advised by medical professionals to drink beer or other alcohol, and many women do. This advice often is based on the assumption that alcohol will facilitate an increase in milk production and help relax the new mother and her mammary glands—thus facilitating nursing. An old wives' tale promotes beer-enhanced milk to calm a fussy baby, help the baby sleep better, and enhance the nutritional value of breast milk.[160]

These assumptions are not supported by fact and may be dangerous. Studies show that alcohol increases prolactin secretion, a necessary hormone for breast-milk production;[161] however, it decreases the oxytocin level, which relates to reduced milk production and ejection.[162] In fact, studies on lactating women seem to indicate that alcohol slightly suppresses milk production and that there is a decrease in a baby's intake of breast milk during the three to four hours after its mother has had a drink. As far as helping the babies sleep better, alcohol in breast milk seems to have the reverse effect and disrupts a baby's sleep-wake cycle after nursing.[163]

The long-term effects of small quantities of alcohol on babies are still unknown. When nursing mothers drink even small amounts of alcohol, the alcohol gets into the breast milk and may affect the babies.[164] Whether or not these small amounts can be harmful to babies is the subject of much debate. One study conducted in the 1980s found that babies of nursing mothers who drink at least once a day may be at increased risk of delayed motor development.[165] Two decades later, however, the same researcher could not replicate the findings.[166]

Some nursing women pump their breasts and discard the milk after they've had a drink believing that the subsequent milk they produce will be alcohol free. However, as

NURSING CONFUSION

When her son was a few days old, health writer Elizabeth Agnvall asked her pediatrician if it was alright to have a glass of wine at night. According to Agnvall, her pediatrician replied, "What!? This baby is a couple of days old and you're asking me if you can have a drink? Absolutely not." When asked about when the baby was older, she said, "Maybe in a few months, when he's sleeping through the night, you can have an occasional glass of wine late at night after your last nursing." According to Agnvall, "This advice confused me, since numerous books and articles in parenting magazines said that an occasional alcoholic drink . . . was acceptable. In fact, my obstetrician/gynecologist had told me she sometimes recommended that women have a glass of wine while nursing to help them relax."

—Elizabeth Agnvall, writer, *Washington Post*

Source: Agnvall, E. (2003). The breast milk cocktail. *Washington Post*, March 18, 2003, p. HE01.

long as there is a measurable amount of alcohol in a woman's blood, newly produced breast milk will contain some alcohol.[167] Because of the extraordinary body of evidence about the harmful effects of alcohol, the American Academy of Pediatrics (AAP) recommends that nursing mothers avoid alcohol altogether while nursing.[168]

Indeed, there is reason to be cautious. In addition to the known severe effects of alcohol on fetal development, recent research has found that alcohol can cause permanent brain damage during adolescence, when the brain is undergoing tremendous change—albeit less than can be found in infants.[169] It is reasonable, therefore, to assume that babies are even more vulnerable to alcohol exposure.

Illicit Drug Use

Pregnant women use a variety of illicit drugs, including marijuana, cocaine, and hallucinogens, as well as abuse prescription drugs. The negative consequences of these drugs on a developing fetus depend largely on the particular drug of abuse, the quantity consumed, and the mode of consumption (e.g., swallowed, injected, snorted).

MARIJUANA. Many of the effects of prenatal exposure to marijuana are similar to those of prenatal exposure to tobacco. Increased carbon monoxide levels and reduced oxygen flow place the fetus at risk for future neurological and cognitive deficits, such as diminished verbal and memory skills.[170] Marijuana use during pregnancy can cause low birth weight and neurobehavioral abnormalities and has been linked to irritability and tremors among newborns[171] and jitteriness in children. Older children whose mothers were heavy users of marijuana during pregnancy have an increased risk of hyperactivity, impulsivity, and delinquency.[172]

COCAINE. Because cocaine use decreases oxygen and nutrition flow across the placenta to the fetus, prenatal exposure to cocaine increases the risk of a number of adverse outcomes including spontaneous abortion, stillbirths, premature delivery, low birth weight, and growth retardation.[173] Babies who were prenatally exposed to cocaine often are born with smaller heads than other babies, possibly indicating smaller brains.[174] Once born, the babies can suffer from intracranial hemorrhages, seizures, and respiratory distress.[175] Cocaine-exposed infants also may experience symptoms of irritability, hyperactivity, problems with sleep and feeding,[176] and attention and short-term memory problems.[177] Ironically, because some women believe that cocaine initiates labor and eases the pain, they may use cocaine intentionally to relieve the discomfort of pregnancy and to induce labor, exacerbating the above risks.[178]

As with the research on prenatal exposure to tobacco or alcohol, it often is difficult to disentangle the unique effects of prenatal exposure to a drug like cocaine from the risks posed by a drug-abusing mother. For example, mothers who use cocaine while pregnant typically also have poor prenatal care, poor nutrition, and often are poly-drug users, making it difficult to isolate the unique adverse effects of the exposure to the drug itself. Because of this ambiguity, other previously assumed effects of prenatal exposure to cocaine (i.e., effects on postnatal growth, mental and motor development, and language skills) might actually be a function of the child's environment and prenatal exposure to tobacco, alcohol, or other drugs.[179]

One notable example of the detrimental effects of over-attributing childhood problems to prenatal exposure to a drug is the widespread concern regarding the group of children who came to be known as "crack babies" as a result of the "crack epidemic" of the 1980s.[180] Years later, research suggests that there is no syndrome or pattern of problems associated with prenatal cocaine or crack exposure, and certainly no conclusive

"CRACK BABY"

Those two words almost cost me an education. It's crazy how powerful two words can be.
—College student previously known as a "crack baby"

Source: Shipp, E. R. (2004). Living down the label of "crack baby" [Editorial]. *New York Daily News,* March 28, 2004, p. 48.

evidence that a set of symptoms is due solely to prenatal exposure rather than to other environmental influences. Despite this, the myths surrounding "crack babies" have resulted in a large group of highly stigmatized children who, with appropriate attention and care, are able to grow up without significant physical or mental deficits.

OPIATES / NARCOTICS. Prenatal exposure to opiates, such as heroin and methadone, can cause a newborn to experience severe withdrawal symptoms. Opiates have been linked to premature delivery, miscarriages, and increased risk of SIDS.[181]

Infant withdrawal symptoms—which can last for several months—include respiratory problems, restlessness, disturbed sleep, difficulty with feeding, vomiting, diarrhea, fever, and excessive crying.[182] Newborns experiencing withdrawal are "difficult" babies; their cries are high-pitched and frequent, they are more likely to be irritable, and they often are sick.[183] They even have been described as less cuddly than other babies. For mothers already struggling with drug addiction and the problems that often accompany it, such as depression, anxiety, or limited resources, a "difficult" infant might be too much to handle.[184]

As with cocaine research, many of the studies that have been conducted on the effects of opiates on developing fetuses did not account for factors such as maternal polysubstance use, lack of prenatal care, and poor nutrition, all of which can complicate the study of the effect of maternal drug use on infant outcomes. Other complications include medical disorders common in pregnant opiate addicts, such as hepatitis, tuberculosis, bacterial infections, HIV, and STDs.[185] Indisputable, however, is that prenatal

"HELPING" HER BABY THROUGH WITHDRAWAL

Her baby cried and seemed out of sorts. Nothing would settle her down. So, Jacqueline Rosetta Edwards did the only thing she knew to do: she fed heroin to her four-month-old daughter. Edwards told the police that she had been hooked on heroin and cocaine for a dozen years and assumed her daughter was addicted as well. Instead of seeking medical help, she decided that small amounts of heroin would help the baby through withdrawal. "She said she gave it to the child to try to ease the withdrawal and calm it down because it would cry a lot and carry on," said the police department's Lt. Albert Scott. Age 28, she appeared in court to answer charges of drug distribution and felony neglect and abuse.[a] Edwards received a ten-year prison sentence and three years probation. She will be required to serve at least 85 percent of the term.[b]

Sources: [a]Baker, P. (1995). Virginia mother allegedly gave heroin to her baby. *Washington Post,* May 10, 1995, p. D3. [b]Heroin fed to baby. (1995). *Washington Post,* August 29, 1995, p. C4.

METH-USING MOTHER ARRESTED FOR MURDER

A six-week-old baby girl died from methamphetamine poisoning after being breastfed by her mother, a methamphetamine abuser. The mother claimed she tried to rid the breast milk of the methamphetamines she snorted or smoked by pumping her breasts several times before feeding her daughter. Obviously, it didn't work. After a two-year investigation, the mother was arrested for felony child abuse two years after the baby's death. She faces 10 to 24 years in prison if convicted.

Source: Biggs, P. (2002). *Mom charged in baby's meth death: Drug in breast milk killed 6-week-old in '00.* www.azcentral.com/arizonarepublic (accessed December 23, 2002).

opiate exposure can elicit a clear withdrawal syndrome in the newborn, affecting central nervous, autonomic, and gastrointestinal systems.[186]

STIMULANTS. Prenatal use of stimulant drugs can increase the risk of miscarriages, stillbirths, premature births, and congenital birth defects.[187] They also can cause intrauterine growth retardation and decreased head circumference. Growth and neurobehavioral problems can occur later in childhood among those whose mothers used stimulants in combination with tobacco, alcohol, or other drugs.[188]

HIV/AIDS

Pregnant drug-abusing women, especially those who inject their drugs, put themselves and their babies at risk for HIV/AIDS. Worldwide, up to 30 percent of HIV-positive women transmit the infection to their children through pregnancy or breastfeeding.[189] In the United States, because of the implementation of a standard of HIV testing and drug therapy for HIV-positive mothers, transmission of the infection from mother to child decreased from 16 to 25 percent in the early 1990s to less than 2 percent in the year 2000.[190] Although most if not all cases of prenatal transmission of HIV infection could be prevented via testing and medication, 280 to 370 infants are born infected with the AIDS virus in the United States each year.[191] Most of these are born to mothers, often illicit drug users, without access to prenatal care.[192] Hispanic women and children are by far overrepresented among cases of maternal and infant HIV infection.[193]

A Window of Opportunity

Although there is no better window of opportunity than pregnancy during which to motivate a woman to stop smoking, drinking, or using drugs, there remain many obstacles. A substance-abusing pregnant woman faces a double stigma; she is damaging not only her own body but also that of her fetus.[194] A study of drug-using new mothers found that even their fellow drug users criticized or ostracized them and dealers sometimes refused to sell them drugs.[195] The stigma attached to substance abuse during pregnancy may lead some women to deny their substance abuse or its harmful effects or to avoid seeking help.[196]

When women who are addicted to tobacco, alcohol, or drugs discover that they are pregnant, they are faced with serious choices ranging from quitting, to continuing as before, to terminating the pregnancy. Some women may try to cut back or switch to a different substance that they believe to be safer for the developing fetus. Substance-abusing women often are ambivalent about having a baby in the first place because of concerns that they may not be financially, physically, or emotionally capable of caring for a child. Many substance-abusing women have other children at home, and the burden of one more child may be too much.

Pregnant women who seek treatment for alcohol or drug addiction face additional problems, such as financial, social, and legal barriers. Custody concerns, for example, are a major deterrent, especially for women who stand to lose other children at home. For these reasons, pregnant substance abusers are less likely than other pregnant women to seek prenatal care.[197]

Quitting Smoking

Only about one in four pregnant women manages to quit smoking,[198] but women who smoke are more likely to quit while pregnant than at any other time in their lives.[199] Some women succeed in quitting on their own when they discover that they are pregnant. These "spontaneous quitters" tend to be better-educated women who are light smokers and have few friends who smoke.[200]

Pregnant women who continue to smoke once they discover that they are pregnant are likelier than spontaneous quitters to be heavier smokers, less affluent, less educated, and unemployed. They also are more likely to lack stability and support and to have more emotional, financial, and familial problems.[201] A partner's smoking status has been found to be one of the major determinants of whether a woman will quit smoking successfully and continue to abstain in the postpartum period.[202] Women not interested in quitting tend not to know or believe that smoking can harm a fetus.[203]

Table 5.1 Signs of Substance Use Disorders in Pregnant Women

Medical	*Obstetric*	*Behavioral/Personal*
Anemia	Abruptio placentae	Child abuse/neglect
Arrhythmias	Congenital anomalies	Chronic unemployment
Bacterial endocarditis	Fetal distress	Difficulty concentrating
Cerebrovascular accident	Fetal alcohol syndrom	Domestic violence
Hepatitis B and C	Poor prenatal care	Family history of substance abuse
HIV seropositivity	Preterm labor and delivery	Frequent visits to emergency department
Myocardial ischemia or infarction	Preterm membrane rupture	Inappropriate/bizarre behavior
Pancreatitis	Reduced fetal growth	Incarceration
Poor dental hygiene	Spontaneous abortion	Noncompliance with appointments
Poor nutritional status	Stillbirth	Prostitution
Septicemia	SIDS	Psychiatric history
Sexually transmitted diseases		Restless, agitated, demanding
Tuberculosis		Slurred speech, staggering gait
		Substance-abusing partner

Source: Bolnick, J. M., and Rayburn, W. F. (2003). Substance use disorders in women: Special considerations during pregnancy. *Obstetrics and Gynecology Clinics of North America* 30(3):545–558. Reprinted with permission from European Society of Elsevier.

The benefits of quitting smoking during pregnancy can be dramatic and measurable. For example, babies born to women who stop smoking during the first trimester are likely to have similar birth weights and body measurements to babies born to nonsmoking mothers. Low birth weight, which is the single best predictor of infant mortality,[204] could be reduced by 17 to 26 percent by eliminating smoking during pregnancy.[205] Quitting smoking even late in pregnancy can have significant benefits because the most negative effects of smoking on birth weight occur during the third trimester.[206]

There are measurable results for society as well; for each dollar spent on smoking cessation for pregnant women, more than six dollars is saved in neonatal intensive care costs and the cost of long-term care associated with low birth weight babies.[207]

Unfortunately, too often physicians do not seize upon the opportunity to counsel smoking pregnant women about the need to quit and about smoking cessation options. One national survey of nearly 800 physicians who treated pregnant patients found that while the pregnant patient's smoking status was identified in 81 percent of visits, smoking-related counseling was provided in only 23 percent of visits.[208]

Quitting Drinking and Drugs

Stopping drinking or using drugs at any point during pregnancy helps prevent or minimize many of the adverse consequences of prenatal exposure to these substances.[209] Women who occasionally drink or use illicit drugs may be able to stop on their own without the need for professional intervention. However, when a pregnant woman who is addicted to alcohol or drugs quits abruptly, there can be serious ramifications for her and her baby. Because severe withdrawal symptoms such as delirium tremors and convulsions can occur, alcohol- and drug-dependent pregnant women need detoxification and treatment that involves careful medical supervision.

Unfortunately, only between 5 and 10 percent of pregnant substance abusers receive treatment. In addition to the fear of losing their children, barriers include employment concerns; lack of insurance, stable housing, transportation, and childcare; long waiting lists; and absence of pressure to enroll in treatment. A recent study of pregnant substance abusers found that those who enrolled in a day treatment program tended to have more severe crack-related and other drug problems, a prior history of drug treatment, and more psychological problems than nonenrollees. Enrollees also tended to have more children than nonenrollees. Black women who had been physically or sexually abused during pregnancy were more likely to enroll in treatment than other women. Women with more serious legal problems—such as pending court dates or being on parole or probation—also were more likely to enroll than those without such legal pressure.[210]

There is no doubt that treatment works for many pregnant substance abusers. A national study of 50 residential programs for pregnant and parenting women found that 60 percent of the women were *completely* alcohol- and drug-free during the six months following treatment. Although an additional 13 percent of women relapsed at some point after discharge, they were completely substance free during the 30 days preceding the interview at the sixth-month mark. Women who had been in the treatment programs also demonstrated improvement in personal relationships and economic well-being, as well as reduced drug-related and other criminal behavior. Parenting status also improved significantly after treatment; the women were more likely to keep custody of their children, less likely to have children in foster care after treatment, and less likely to have children removed from their care by local child protective services than before treatment. But the most significant and heartening benefits are to the babies themselves; a recent study found that for pregnant women in residential treatment for alcohol or drug abuse, the risk of infant mortality was reduced by 67 percent, premature births by 70 percent, and low birth weight by 84 percent. Babies of pregnant black women who received treatment had the greatest risk reduction.[211] (See chapter 6 for additional discussion of treating pregnant substance abusers.)

Relapse

Approximately one-third of pregnant women who manage to quit smoking relapse *before* their babies are born.[212] Relapse rates are estimated to be as high as 80 percent in the first year after delivery.[213] Risk factors affecting postpartum relapse include lack of confidence at midpregnancy regarding one's ability to continue to refrain from smoking and concern about weight gain.[214] Weight gain is one of the major factors for relapse for both pregnant[215] and nonpregnant[216] young women who quit smoking. Other factors linked to relapse include having a partner who smokes and having friends who smoke. One study found that most pregnant women who quit had resumed smoking within 30 days of giving birth, and most of these women tended to start smoking again in the presence of other smokers.[217] Another study found that bottle-feeding, as opposed to breast-feeding, was the most important predictor of postpartum relapse.[218] Unfortunately, very little research exists on alcohol or drug use relapse among pregnant women.

Legal and Ethical Issues

The legal and ethical aspects of substance abuse and pregnancy involve emotionally charged yet unresolved issues. At stake is a woman's right to autonomy, confidentiality, and the right to consent to and refuse treatment versus the larger public health goal of having women give birth to healthy babies. Pregnant women who fear punitive actions for abusing substances may avoid acknowledging their problem, seeking prenatal care, or seeking substance abuse treatment, particularly if they have other children who are in custody of child protective services or living in foster care. However, the promise of being reunited with their children can serve as an incentive for pregnant substance-abusing women to seek treatment.[219]

Criminalization and Treatment

Some states have attempted to criminalize prenatal substance abuse or make it grounds for terminating maternal rights.[220] Thirteen states require that health care professionals report prenatal substance abuse and/or screen pregnant women for such abuse. Thirteen states allow for the termination of parental rights if a pregnant woman is a

FAIR TRADE?

Children Requiring a Caring Kommunity (CRACK) is a controversial program that offers drug-addicted women and men $200 if they agree to be sterilized or placed on long-term birth control. Founded in 1997, the New York–based organization now has chapters in several other cities. So far, more than 1,000 women and 24 men have taken them up on their offer. Critics say the program targets and exploits poor women and women of color and accuse the program of selective breeding and racism.

Sources: Join Together. (2003). *Addicted individuals in N.Y. offered cash for sterilization.* www.jointogether.org (accessed March 4, 2004); Kigvamasud'Vashti, T. (2002). *Fact sheet on positive prevention / CRACK (Children Requiring a Caring Kommunity).* www.cwpe.org (accessed March 4, 2004); Project Prevention-Children Requiring a Caring Community. (2004). *Project Prevention-Children Requiring a Caring Community: Statistics.* http://cashforbirthcontrol.com (accessed March 4, 2004).

substance abuser, and three states authorize civil commitment of these women.[221] Twenty-four states mandate alcohol or drug treatment for pregnant substance abusers.[222] To date, no state has passed a law that specifically criminalizes using drugs during pregnancy; however, pregnant substance abusers have been charged with such crimes as "fetal abuse," child abuse and neglect, delivering drugs to a minor, corruption of a minor, and even assault with a deadly weapon and manslaughter.[223] The good news is that seven states have given pregnant women priority access to treatment, and 19 states have created or fund treatment programs for pregnant substance abusers.[224]

Approximately 250 women in 30 different states have been prosecuted for substance abuse during pregnancy,[225] but all convictions, except one in South Carolina, have been overturned. The supreme court of South Carolina maintained that a viable fetus was a person deserving of legal protection and therefore prenatal substance abuse constituted criminal child abuse.[226] In the early 1990s in South Carolina, women who tested positive for illicit drug use were reported to the police and the local prosecutor. A woman could avoid arrest and prosecution only if she complied with mandatory prenatal care and substance abuse treatment. Unfortunately, the mandated treatment was not comprehensive and did not provide transportation or childcare, the lack of which is a common barrier to effective treatment.[227] Furthermore, South Carolina ranks among the lowest of all states in spending on substance abuse prevention.[228] The U.S. Supreme Court, in *Ferguson v. Charleston,* found that the policy was coercive in that it used law enforcement to force patients into treatment and was particularly problematic because the patients did not provide informed consent to be tested or to provide test results to law enforcement.[229]

Other states, such as Minnesota, have required physicians to report suspected drug use by pregnant women and authorized involuntary civil commitment to prevent pregnant women from continuing to use substances of abuse. South Dakota and Wisconsin's child abuse and neglect statutes have been amended to include fetuses, and Virginia requires social services to intervene in cases of pregnant women known to be abusing alcohol or illicit drugs.[230]

Punitive laws can have the unintended consequence of making it difficult for pregnant substance abusers voluntarily to seek treatment.[231] These women often do not have a relationship with a physician that they trust and are reluctant to seek help if they fear arrest or losing their children, or if they are ashamed of their substance abuse. The majority of substance-abusing pregnant women who need treatment are single parents of multiple children who receive little to no financial, social, or childcare support from the fathers of their children. They often suffer from multiple addictions and have other physical and mental health problems.[232] About two-thirds have experienced sexual or physical assault.[233] Furthermore, reporting and prosecution of pregnant substance abusers appear to disproportionately affect minority and poor women.[234]

Many medical professional organizations have opposed coercive or punitive policies imposed on pregnant substance-abusing women, including the American Public Health Association, the American Medical Association, the American College of Obstetricians and Gynecologists, and the American Society of Addiction Medicine.[235] Alternative recommended approaches to helping pregnant substance-abusing women quit and remain drug-free involve expanding access to clinical treatment facilities and redesigning programs to be more comprehensive and to attend to the social and economic difficulties that many substance-abusing pregnant women face.

However, because of financial constraints and public support for more punitive approaches, others have argued that a public health model is needed to address this problem—one that focuses on preventing women from abusing substances or engaging in other unhealthy behaviors while pregnant and one that focuses on the larger community. A preventative, public health approach would attempt to reduce community violence, enhance safety and health education, and provide for women's basic financial and social needs—such as adequate access to healthcare and childcare—which can reduce stress and the subsequent risk for substance abuse.

pter 6chapter 6chapter 6chapter 6chapter 6

Getting Over the Influence

Today we know that when a woman abuses alcohol or drugs, the risk to her health is much greater than it is for a man. Yet there is not enough prevention, intervention, and treatment targeting women. It is still much harder for a woman to get help. That needs to change.
—Betty Ford, former First Lady, 1995

- Almost one in three substance abusers in treatment is a woman.[1]
- Women who quit smoking greatly reduce their risk of dying prematurely.[2]
- In 2003, 5.7 million women who needed treatment for an alcohol problem and 2.4 million women who needed treatment for an illicit drug problem did not receive it.[3]
- Women are more likely than men to be in treatment for abusing heroin and cocaine and less likely than men to be in treatment for alcohol or marijuana abuse.[4]

In 2003, six million women (ages 12 and older) were alcohol abusers or alcohol dependent, yet only 763,000 received treatment, leaving a treatment gap of over 5.2 million women. That same year, 2.6 million women were abusing or dependent on illicit drugs, yet only 651,000 received treatment, leaving a treatment gap of nearly two million women. Ninety-two percent of women do not receive needed treatment for alcohol and drug problems.[5] This is due in part to the lack of available treatment options that meet the needs of women; only 38 percent of treatment facilities have special women-only programs, while even fewer (19%) offer programs for pregnant or postpartum women.[6]

Substance abuse treatment for women received little attention prior to the 1970s.[7] Historically, substance abuse was seen as a male problem,[8] and, as a result, treatment programs were and continue to be designed primarily for men and by men. Over the past 30 years, however, research on the causes, consequences, and treatment of substance abuse in women has increased significantly. We now know that drugs affect women differently than men, and because women's life roles, responsibilities, and opportunities differ, their treatment needs differ as well. We also are beginning to understand the special role biology and social influences play in girls' and women's substance use. We know that women are more likely to seek substance abuse treatment in mental health facilities rather than specific substance abuse treatment programs, probably because of the high rates of co-occurrence of substance abuse and mental health problems in women.[9] Yet, research that specifically addresses the treatment needs of substance-abusing girls and women and the effectiveness of the programs that treat them remains in short supply.[10]

Developing the most appropriate treatments for women is not the only issue. Access to treatment also is a tremendous problem. Women often face many obstacles when it comes to identifying, accessing, and completing a treatment program. Concerns about children—especially when custody and childcare issues are in play—lack of social support from partners, other family members, or friends; lack of health insurance or financial resources necessary to cover the cost of treatment; and lack of transportation to and from treatment facilities all factor into the success of a woman's attempt at recovery.

Who Gets Through the Door?

Girls

Girls and boys abuse or are dependent on substances at similar rates (about 9%), but only 1.1 percent of girls and 1.7 percent of boys received treatment for alcohol or drug problems in 2003. In that year, 357,000 teens (139,000 girls) ages 12 to 17 received treatment for alcohol or illicit drug abuse.[11] About 1 in 4 teens was admitted for marijuana abuse and 1 in 10 for abuse of drugs other than marijuana. Over half the teens in treatment are being treated for both marijuana and alcohol abuse, and about 1 in 10 for alcohol abuse alone.[12]

The number of teens in treatment has increased 20 percent since 1994, largely as a result of referrals from the criminal justice system.[13] Many of these referrals reflect increased marijuana dependence.[14] While boys are more likely than girls to enter treatment through the criminal justice system,[15] girls are likelier to enter treatment through self-referral or referral by parents. However, increasing numbers of girls are being referred to treatment through the juvenile justice system as well.[16]

Among teens in drug treatment, nearly twice as many girls as boys have a history of sexual or physical abuse (57% vs. 31%), with 36 percent of girls (vs. 16% of boys) reporting abuse in the year prior to treatment.[17] Nearly twice as many girls in drug treatment who have a history of sexual abuse began using alcohol before the age of 11 compared to those with no history of abuse (39.5% vs. 22.3%).[18]

Adult Women

Of the approximately 1.5 million people in publicly funded substance abuse treatment, almost one-third are women.[19] Women are more likely than men to be in treatment for the use of drugs such as cocaine and heroin; men are more likely to be admitted to treatment for alcohol and marijuana abuse. Cocaine is reported as the primary substance of abuse by 22 percent of women (vs. 14% of men) entering treatment. Women also are more likely than men to report heroin and other opiates (19% vs. 16%) as well as stimulants (7% vs. 4%) as the primary substance for which they are seeking treatment (Table 6.1).[20]

Women in treatment are more likely than their male counterparts to have sought treatment in the past, to have mental health problems, to be victims of physical or sexual abuse,[21] to have attempted suicide, and to have other health problems besides addiction. Their economic perch is perilous as well. They are less likely than men in treatment to be high school graduates.[22] Upon entering treatment, almost half of women (45% vs. 34% of men) are not in the labor force.[23]

The racial differences that exist in tobacco, alcohol, and drug abuse also extend to

Table 6.1 Women and Men in Treatment for Substance Abuse

Primary Substance of Abuse	*Women*	*Men*
Alcohol	40%	53%
Cocaine	22	14
Heroin	19	16
Marijuana	7	10
Stimulants	7	4

Source: Data from Substance Abuse and Mental Health Services Administration, Office of Applied Studies. (2001). *The DASIS report: Women in substance abuse treatment.* Rockville, MD: Substance Abuse and Mental Health Services Administration. P. 2.

Table 6.2 Primary Substances of Abuse among Women Admitted to Treatment, by Race

Race	*Alcohol*	*Marijuana*	*Stimulants*	*Opiates*	*Cocaine*
White	24%	12%	11%	19%	11%
Black	9	12	1	19	36
Mexican	14	14	22	25	11
Puerto Rican	7	10	1	49	14
American Indian/ Alaska Native	29	13	11	10	7
Asian/Pacific Islander	13	18	30	12	10

Source: Data from Substance Abuse and Mental Health Services Administration, Office of Applied Studies. (2003). *Treatment episode data set (TEDS), 1992–2001: National admissions to substance abuse treatment services.* DASIS series S-20. DHHS publication no. SMA 03-3778. Rockville, MD: Substance Abuse and Mental Health Services Administration. Pp. 115–18.

treatment. In 2002, white women accounted for 19 percent of all treatment admissions, followed by black women (7%). A woman's primary substance of abuse varies greatly by her race and, among Hispanic women, her or her family's country of origin (Table 6.2).[24]

Once admitted, women tend to spend less time in treatment than men.[25] Although women are more likely than men to have many of the risk factors for relapse, such as low self-esteem, depression, and anxiety,[26] clinical studies show that women's abstinence rates after treatment are equally good if not better than that of men (except in smoking cessation).[27]

Pregnant Women

Approximately 4 percent of pregnant substance abusers enter treatment. Cocaine/crack is the primary substance of abuse for 22 percent of admissions among pregnant women entering treatment (vs. 17% of admissions among other women). After cocaine, amphetamine/methamphetamine (21%), alcohol (18%), marijuana (17%), heroin (15%), and other opiates (2%), respectively, are the primary substances of abuse among pregnant women entering treatment.[28]

Pregnant substance-abusing women are more likely than other substance-abusing women to be admitted to residential and outpatient treatment and less likely to be admitted to detoxification treatment.[29] A recent study uncovered certain characteristics of pregnant women who enroll in day treatment programs. The study found that these women tended to have more severe drug problems, a prior history of drug treatment, and more psychological problems than those who declined treatment. Enrollees also had more children than nonenrollees and were likelier than nonenrollees to have more serious legal problems—such as pending court dates or being on parole or probation.[30]

Older Women

While older women are particularly susceptible to the effects of substance abuse, less than 1 percent of the approximately two million older women (defined here as women over age 59) who might benefit from treatment for alcohol abuse receive it.[31] Women represented only 19 percent of the 50,700 adults over the age of 55 admitted to publicly funded substance abuse treatment in 1999.[32]

Older women in treatment tend to have been older than their male counterparts when they began their drug or alcohol abuse. More than one in four older women report that their first abuse episode occurred after the age of 30. Older men, on the other hand, report that their first abuse episode occurred around the age of 17. As baby boomers age, the number of older adults needing and receiving treatment is expected to increase.[33]

How We Got Here: The History of Substance Abuse Treatment for Women

In the late 1700s, Dr. Benjamin Rush, the "father of American psychiatry," was the first American doctor to propose that "intemperate individuals" be medically treated.[34] However, it wasn't until late in the nineteenth century that some doctors started viewing addiction as a disease rather than primarily as a moral failing. At this time, substance abuse treatment methods mostly involved helping an addict withdraw from a drug either slowly—often with the use of alcohol or narcotics—or abruptly, as some doctors preferred.[35] Because such treatments were difficult to administer at home—especially since drugs were readily available in most households—treatment facilities sprang up across the nation. The American Association for the Study and Cure of Inebriety (AACI) was a professional association of such facilities, and one of its founding principles was to proclaim addiction as a disease. Most did not accept women because some addiction experts believed that women addicted to alcohol or drugs were too difficult to treat; by the time they presented for treatment, their addiction was far more severe because of the social pressure on women to hide their drinking.[36]

The First Treatment Centers for Women

The Martha Washington Societies were the first addiction treatment centers specifically designed for women. Founded in the early 1840s, these programs were organized

SURGICAL MEASURES

During the nineteenth century, the surgical removal of a woman's uterus and ovaries was sometimes recommended as a cure of last resort for alcoholism.[a] In fact, the practice of sterilizing alcoholic women continued until the 1950s.[b]

Sources: [a]Sandmaier, M. (1992). *The invisible alcoholics: Women and alcohol* (2nd ed.). Blue Ridge Summit, PA: TAB Books. [b]Straussner, S. L. A., and Brown, S. (Eds.). (2002). *The handbook of addiction treatment for women*. San Francisco: Jossey-Bass.

by women for women with drinking and drug problems. Women's temperance groups also started treating women in what were called *industrial homes*.[37] Most residential treatment programs—also referred to as *inebriate asylums* or *farms*—did not start treating women with drinking problems until the later part of the nineteenth century.[38] Some residential treatment facilities added women's sections to existing programs, while others built facilities exclusively for women. Programs that included women had separate quarters for males and females, with separate entrances to help protect their privacy. Some of these facilities not only segregated the women but also condemned any fraternization between the sexes; women were seen as a threat to men. One doctor, for example, believed keeping women from men was necessary because women could easily hide bottles of liquor and other banned substances in their dresses and smuggle them to the male patients.[39]

Sanitariums and Asylums

By 1910 there were about 100 private sanitariums in the United States that offered specialized treatment for addicts—but only for those who could afford their often-hefty fees. Many of the "treatment experts" opening sanitariums, including Harvey Kellogg (later of cereal fame)—were savvy businessmen, while others, such as Dr. Leslie E. Keeley, were enterprising physicians. Keeley was the first to open a national chain of addiction treatment centers that specialized in nicotine, alcohol, and narcotic addiction. Between 1892 and 1893, almost 15,000 addicts—both women and men—were treated at the famous if controversial Keeley Institutes.[40] Keeley lectured across the country and distributed pamphlets and a newsletter, the *Banner of Gold*. Pictures of the "Keeley Baby"—a baby born to an addicted mother—helped promote the program. Keeley's treatment for addicts involved bichloride of gold, a substance purportedly

ADDICTION GOLD STANDARD

While chemical evaluation of Keeley's "Bichloride of Gold" found considerable inconsistencies in the preparations, most analyses found such ingredients as alcohol, ginger, ammonia, willow bark, and hops. Some assays uncovered traces of coca, atropine, and strychnine, and some even found traces of gold.

Source: Morgan, H. W. (1981). *Drugs in America: A social history, 1800–1980.* Syracuse, NY: Syracuse University Press.

containing gold that would cure alcohol and drug addiction. The use of bichloride of gold became highly controversial and was opposed by the American Medical Association (AMA) because Keeley refused to disclose the contents. After the death of Dr. Keeley in 1900, the popularity and existence of his institutes waned.[41]

Alcoholics Anonymous

Nineteenth- and early-twentieth-century women with drinking and drug problems faced many of the same obstacles to getting treatment that women today face. In addition to the shortage of treatment programs for women, the stigma of addiction kept many from seeking the help they needed. Women suffering the effects of alcohol addiction also were viewed differently than men; the causes of their drinking problems were often thought to be the result of "women's problems," domestic violence, or too much independence rather than "willful intemperance." The view that women "drunks" were different from and a threat to men persisted well into the twentieth century and resulted in their initial exclusion from Alcoholics Anonymous (AA) meetings. In the early years of AA (1930s–1940s), most members were uncomfortable being around women with drinking problems, and many members doubted that women could even *be* alcoholics. When women finally were able to attend meetings, they sat on the other side of the room from the men whose wives were often threatened by the increasing numbers of single and divorced women in attendance.

By the mid 1940s, AA had acknowledged that women who abused alcohol had special problems—such as social isolation—and special needs. In the 1940s, separate women's groups emerged that provided an opportunity to discuss without embarrassment "women's issues" such as menstruation, menopause, and men. Unfortunately, separate women's groups did not end the controversy nor reduce the stigma; women

WHY WOMEN SHOULD NOT BE ALLOWED IN AA

In a 1946 AA newsletter, a male member noted the following reasons why women should not be allowed in AA meetings:

1. The percentage of women who stay in AA is low.
2. Many women form attachments too intense—bordering on the emotional.
3. So many women want to run things.
4. Too many women don't like women.
5. Women talk too much.
6. Women are a questionable help working with men and vice versa.
7. Sooner or later, a woman-on-the-make sallies into a group, on the prowl for phone numbers and dates.
8. A lot of women are attention-demanders.
9. Few women can think in the abstract.
10. Women's feelings get hurt too often.
11. Far too many women cannot get along with the non-alcoholic wives of AA members.

Source: A.A. Grapevine (1946, October). 3(5):1,6. Quoted in White, W. L. (1998). *Slaying the dragon: The history of addiction treatment and recovery in America.* Bloomington, IL: Chestnut Health Systems / Lighthouse Institute.

attending these groups often were accused of being lesbians or were viewed as wild. The negative image of and attitudes toward women with drinking problems deterred many from seeking the help they needed.

Women ultimately were welcomed into AA. Today, an estimated one out of three members is a woman. Since its inception, women have been major forces in shaping the organization into what it is today: "the largest and most enduring mutual-aid society of recovered alcoholics in human history."[42]

Criminalization of Addiction

Women became the driving force behind the temperance movement in the nineteenth century. One of the most visible organizations, the Women's Christian Temperance Union (WCTU), was formed in 1873 and proclaimed that the use of alcohol resulted in a great many evils, including the physical, emotional, and financial abuse of women by men. Through the distribution of pamphlets and infusing their message into school curricula, the WCTU successfully reached out to the masses—by 1890, the WCTU had over 7,000 branches with more than 150,000 members. The use of alcohol was further socially stigmatized in 1893 when the Anti-Saloon League (ASL) emerged and lent support to the message of the WCTU.[43] Ultimately, the temperance movement was successful—prohibition outlawed the manufacture, sale, and distribution of alcohol in 1919. But prohibition did not make it illegal to consume alcohol, and it did not put an end to either private or public drinking. Yet, for alcoholics, the proliferation of anti-alcohol messages resulted in immense social stigma that prevented many from seeking and obtaining treatment.

Following prohibition and World War I, there was great concern that there would be a huge increase in the number of addicts in the United States. After the passage of the Harrison Act in 1914—which made it a crime for doctors to prescribe narcotic medications to maintain an addict's habit—the federal government and others were concerned that female addicts might turn to prostitution or petty crime in order to get money for their drugs. To address these concerns, 44 ambulatory drug clinics were established in major cities across the nation. By legally selling drugs to patients at low or no cost, these clinics offered female patients an alternative to criminal acts by providing them with the opportunity to withdraw gradually rather than go "cold turkey."[44] Drug clinics began to proliferate, with women comprising one-quarter to one-third of the patient population. However, an estimated one to four million addicts—about a quarter of whom were women—were left untreated and had to fend for themselves.[45]

From June to December 1919, the New York City program treated over 1,500 women, 23 percent of the registered addict population. Three-quarters of the women were white and over half were under 30 years old. The clinic also had 800 pregnant addicts in 1920, the year it was forced to close by the Treasury Department. While drug maintenance programs proved quite successful in preventing crime and cutting down on "black market" sales of drugs, attitudes toward addicts and addiction became increasingly repressive.[46]

In 1920, the narcotics unit of the Treasury Department launched a campaign to close these programs because there were reports that some addicts received more drugs than they needed and sold the rest on the streets. That, coupled with the fact that many clinics were understaffed or poorly run—and the concern about rising crime—turned the public and most physicians, including the AMA, against maintenance and other ambulatory drug programs. Most programs were closed by 1921 and were replaced by inpatient programs. When these programs proved unsuccessful, it was recommended that addicts be placed under custodial care in institutions, sometimes for life.[47]

Those addicts who wanted treatment and could afford it went to private sanitariums; those who could not often wound up in state mental hospitals or prisons. Some patients underwent rapid detoxification, while other more fortunate addicts were able to withdraw gradually. Once again, an assortment of serums and potions—and various

SOUTHERN COMFORT

Narcotic maintenance programs continued to exist into the 1960s, especially in the South. A survey of Kentucky addicts published in 1969 found that 87 percent of the state's female addicts had received narcotics from physicians at some point during their addiction and more than half were placed permanently on narcotic maintenance.

Source: Brecher, E. M., and Editors of *Consumer Reports Magazine.* (1972). *Consumers Union report on licit and illicit drugs.* www.druglibrary.org (accessed December 28, 2001).

other treatments such as hypnosis and hydrotherapy—were used to help ease withdrawal and cure those addicted to drugs. The vast majority of addicts, though, received no treatment. Rather, they resorted to stealing, prostitution, and other crimes to get the money they needed to buy the drugs they could get only through the drug underworld.[48]

As the criminalization of addiction became firmly established, addicts increasingly were incarcerated, and federal prisons began to overflow with them. To handle the problem, two federal "farms" were established in Texas and Kentucky in the 1930s. These "farms"—which treated voluntarily admitted addicts as well as convicted addicts—actually were modified prisons with strict security measures and barred windows. In addition to detoxification, they offered individual and group therapy and job training. The largest—in Lexington, Kentucky—did not begin admitting women until 1941.[49] These two facilities treated almost 15,000 women (18% of their admissions) between 1941 and 1965. At first, the majority of women in the facilities resembled the female addicts of the previous century; they primarily were middle-aged, white, rural, Protestants who were iatrogenically (medically) addicted to morphine.[50] By the mid-1950s, over 25 percent of admissions at the Lexington farm were women; and nurses addicted to prescription opioid painkillers made up a large part of the female patient population.[51]

But the face of the female addict gradually changed over the next quarter century; women in federal treatment facilities became more likely to be black, addicted to heroin, and either convicted of narcotic-related crimes or engaging in prostitution.[52] Rather than having initially used morphine for medical reasons, by the 1960s most of the female addicts began to use heroin for "kicks" or curiosity. Although at that time, most of the women at Lexington were voluntarily admitted, about one-quarter reported having sold drugs and about one-half admitted that they had been prostitutes. Unfortunately, addiction treatment in the federal farms proved as unsuccessful as all the previous cures. In 1967, these two facilities were turned into addiction research centers. The former head of the women's division at Lexington, psychiatrist Dr. Marie Nyswander, later became the codeveloper of methadone maintenance therapy.[53]

In 1970, while the proportion of female heroin addicts increased from 18 to 30 percent, women continued to find themselves underrepresented in drug treatment programs. As drug abuse became more of a public problem, the number of federally funded methadone programs grew from just 16 in 1969 to 926 in 1973. While women made up 10,000 of the 42,000 methadone patients, their needs for multiple services still were not being met. By 1974, a federal public law mandated special consideration of women's needs in prevention and treatment programs. As a result of the research conducted after the passage of that law, a number of treatment programs for drug-addicted women were created and implemented beginning in the 1980s.[54]

Despite continuing perceptions of people with substance use disorders as criminals or as morally weak, there have been tremendous advances in the substance abuse field regarding the science of addiction. Many substance abuse researchers have come to recognize addiction as a brain disease. Imaging studies and measures of the chemical and other physiological changes that take place in an individual's brain as she progresses from substance use to abuse to addiction underscore the physiological aspects of addiction and the consequent need to approach it as a health condition and treat it accordingly. Although the increase in knowledge about substance abuse and addiction has advanced significantly our understanding of these problems and how to treat them, long-standing biases against individuals with substance use disorders have sustained the low priority of treating addiction and the resulting tremendous gap in substance abuse treatment.

Closing the Treatment Gap

The first step in closing the treatment gap is to educate the American public to recognize substance abuse as a public health problem that can respond to treatment. Although millions of Americans suffer from chronic, relapsing health conditions, including diabetes, hypertension, asthma, and addiction, addiction relapse alone is viewed as an indication that treatment does not work. To change this erroneous perception and to begin to give individuals suffering from addiction a chance to recover, the country must take three important steps consistent with a comprehensive public health approach: train healthcare providers to identify, diagnose, and treat addiction or refer for treatment; build a solid infrastructure for treating addiction, including a range of evidence-based programs tailored to client needs and provided in a manner consistent with standards of education, training, practice, and accountability; and assure parity for health care provider reimbursement for time spent addressing addiction.

The Role of Health Care Professionals

Physicians and other health care professionals have an important role to play in diagnosing and referring girls and women with substance abuse problems to treatment. Women typically see their doctors more frequently than men do. Gynecologists may see girls and women multiple times a year for birth control, STD screening, pregnancy, and other conditions, so they have a unique opportunity to discuss substance abuse with their patients and refer them to treatment if a problem is detected.

Yet, physicians are *less* likely to consider and diagnose abuse and addiction in women than in men.[55] The reasons for this are complex. Because of the stigma of abuse, a woman may try and hide her problem or seek help for the medical or psychiatric symptoms associated with her substance abuse—such as digestive difficulties, insomnia, or depression—rather than for the problem itself. These symptoms can mask the signs of alcohol and drug abuse from a doctor who might prescribe drugs to treat the symptoms rather than refer a patient for drug or alcohol treatment.[56]

Teenage girls rely heavily on their doctors and other health care professionals for information about their health.[57] Unfortunately, primary care providers often fail to counsel adolescents about substance use and abuse. One study found that while 72 percent of doctors asked patients 11 to 21 years old whether they smoked, less than 2 percent of office visits involved counseling and information about smoking.[58] Another large survey found that fewer than 30 percent of girls said their doctors discussed smoking, drinking, or drug use with them.[59] A study of California primary care physicians found that over 90 percent of physicians screened their younger and older adolescent patients for high blood pressure more frequently than they screened for smoking and drug use.[60]

CASA's *Missed Opportunity: National Survey of Primary Care Physicians and Patients on Substance Abuse* found that when presented with the classic symptoms of illicit drug use in teenagers, 41 percent of pediatricians failed to mention drug abuse as a potential diagnosis, even when offered five opportunities to suggest a potential diagnosis. When presented with these symptoms in a fictional female patient, pediatricians were more likely to diagnose depression (63%) than drug use (51%). However, when presented with these symptoms in a fictional male patient, pediatricians were more likely to diagnose drug use (64%) than depression (52%). Even worse, the survey found that 94 percent of primary care physicians (excluding pediatricians) failed to include drug abuse among the five diagnoses they offered when presented with early symptoms of alcohol abuse in an adult patient. Female physicians were seven times likelier to identify substance abuse in a male patient (27%) than in a female patient (4%), while male physicians mentioned substance abuse about equally for the hypothetical male (7%) and female (5%) patients.[61]

The physician's role is especially critical for older women because these women may be unaware of their increasing vulnerability to the effects of alcohol and drugs, and the potentially lethal interaction of the two. Some older women may be isolated from family and friends who otherwise might detect the early signs of substance abuse and intervene. Some physicians feel substance abuse treatment for older women is not effective. A survey of physicians conducted for CASA's study on substance abuse among older women shows that less than 1 percent of primary care physicians even considered a substance abuse diagnosis when presented with the typical early symptoms of alcohol and prescription drug abuse in an older woman. Only three out of five (62%) physicians believe that substance abuse treatment is somewhat or very effective for older women. This lack of confidence in treatment discourages some physicians from addressing the problem at all.[62]

Screening

One of the barriers to physician screening for substance abuse in their young female patients is a lack of a widely accepted and practical screening tool. Certain youth substance abuse screening tools are inappropriate for primary care settings because they take too long to administer or they focus solely on alcohol use.[63] Others, although appropriate for adults, have been found to be ineffective for youth.[64]

AN EXAMPLE OF A BRIEF SCREENING TOOL: THE CRAFFT

- Have you ever ridden in a Car driven by someone (including yourself) who was "high" or had been using alcohol or drugs?
- Do you ever use alcohol or drugs to Relax, feel better about yourself, or fit in?
- Do you ever use alcohol or drugs when you are by yourself, Alone?
- Do you ever Forget things you did while using alcohol or drugs?
- Do your Family or friends ever tell you that you should cut down on your drinking or drug use?
- Have you ever gotten into Trouble while you were using alcohol or drugs?

Source: Knight, J. R., Sherritt, L., Shrier, L. A., Harris, S. K., and Chang, G. (2002). Validity of the CRAFFT substance abuse screening test among adolescent clinic patients. *Archives of Pediatrics and Adolescent Medicine* 156(6):614.

Another problem is a lack of adequate assessment tools for women; existing tools tend to focus on alcohol- and drug-related issues that are more common among men—such as legal and job troubles—rather than those more relevant to many women—such as family conflict, violence, sexual abuse, and reproductive problems. Even doctors who screen women for drug or alcohol problems may not uncover a substance abuse problem. For example, screening instruments measuring the quantity and frequency of drinking tend not to be gender specific, and screening often does not take into account women's different metabolism of alcohol. Physicians also may fail to adjust for women's declining tolerance for alcohol with age. In one CASA survey, physicians cite lack of time, patients' feelings of denial, physicians' lack of knowledge, and patients' and physicians' discomfort discussing the problem as the biggest barriers to effective screening for substance abuse in their daily practice.[65]

Coming To Terms

Coming to terms with drug or alcohol abuse isn't easy. Some in need of treatment may feel that their drug or alcohol use is under control. Others may believe that they just don't fit the definition of an alcoholic or an addict. They may hold down jobs and have families and feel they cope rather well.

Denial doesn't end with the substance abuser. Family members and friends also may ignore the signs of drug or alcohol abuse.[66] Unfortunately, when this happens, it makes admitting having a problem and seeking help all the more difficult.

Even those who admit that they have a problem and are highly motivated and determined to get help might have significant barriers to overcome. Women entering treatment are more likely than men to be living with a drug-using partner and to be responsible for the care of children.[67] If a partner is a substance abuser, he or she may not support treatment. Family and friends also might oppose or fail to support treat-

DENIAL

You know you have a problem long before you seek a solution to it. You think you can master it yourself, you think you can stave it off with either abstinence or strong will or, quite frankly, pacts with God . . . I was incredibly secretive, very proud, very much in denial . . . I didn't really understand what it was going to take to beat my addiction . . . I kept thinking I could strong arm it, abstain for a period of time.
—Jamie Lee Curtis, actor and recovering substance abuser

Source: Curtis, J. L., personal communication, April 9, 2003.

CHOOSING TREATMENT

There was an opening for [the treatment program]. But the only hardest part was I had to choose one kid. So [child welfare] came and got my 10-month-old, and my two-year-old came here. It's not fair . . . because he's only a baby, he didn't deserve all this. I had to do it by myself . . . just what I thought would be best.
—Felicia, age 20, patient, residential treatment program for pregnant and parenting women

Source: Jessup, M. A., Humphreys, J. C., Brindis, C. D., and Lee, K. A. (2003). Extrinsic barriers to substance abuse treatment among pregnant drug dependent women. *Journal of Drug Issues* 33(2):294.

ment. For women with small children, lack of childcare is a serious obstacle to seeking treatment.[68] The treatment process can be emotionally grueling and may require a woman to be away from her family for many hours a day or for many weeks. If she works, time away from her job may adversely affect her income. For some women, fear of losing their children to the child custody system upon admission that they have a problem makes them apprehensive about entering treatment.[69]

In fact, it is unfortunate that many of the same risk factors that drive women to begin abusing substances also keep them from beginning or successfully completing treatment. For instance, partner abuse, homelessness, and depression have been found to predict how successful residential treatment programs are for female substance abusers.[70] And, while many women with substance abuse problems have experienced physical or sexual abuse, among women in substance abuse treatment a history of sexual abuse actually is associated with fewer incidences of substance abuse treatment (but more incidences of general mental health treatment).[71] Such women may not be getting the specialized addiction treatment they need despite having this key risk for substance abuse.

Barriers to treatment can be especially high for substance-abusing pregnant women and mothers. Like other substance-abusing women, pregnant women who experience poverty, homelessness, or incarceration might place substance abuse rehabilitation low on their list of priorities. Many pregnant women fear prosecution for endangering fetal health by engaging in substance abuse and, therefore, may avoid medical professionals and other authorities capable of providing prenatal care or treatment referrals. They also fear losing custody of their baby and older children if they admit to having a problem and accept treatment. Such concerns can be quite valid; substance-abusing pregnant women report limits on the number of children that programs will allow them to bring into residential treatment programs, forcing others to be cared for by family, friends, or the foster-care system.[72]

BARRIERS TO TREATMENT FOR WOMEN

External Barriers

- Inadequate training of health professionals
- Opposition by family or friends
- Inadequate financial resources and insurance
- Comprehensive services not in a single location
- Lack of child care facilities
- Male-oriented treatment services

Personal or Internal Barriers

- Denial of the problem
- Guilt and shame
- Fear of stigmatization
- Fear of leaving or losing children
- Fear of losing job

Source: Beckman, L. J. (1994). Treatment needs of women with alcohol problems. *Alcohol Health and Research World* 18(3):206–11.

Lack of infrastructure is a formidable problem to achieving effective treatment, and each year the addiction problems of millions go untreated. Unlike health services for other relapsing conditions, we know very little about the current infrastructure of the nation's treatment system. What we do know is troubling. In addition to the general lack of treatment resources for women and men alike, there are no national standards of education, training, practice, or accountability for the full range of treatment providers. Many service delivery units—the basic elements that make up the treatment system—appear to have extraordinarily short life expectancies, disappearing before a client has an opportunity for effective treatment. Service delivery units appear to be plagued by chronically high rates of staff turnover at leadership and direct services levels.[73] These problems with the treatment system itself may contribute to the difficulty women face in achieving recovery.

Then there is the issue of cost. Some women can't afford or are denied treatment because they don't have health insurance coverage. Even if a woman has insurance, there is no guarantee that the insurer will cover the treatment costs. CASA's survey of physicians found that of those who have tried to refer older adult patients to substance abuse counseling or treatment, one-fifth said that a managed care organization or insurance company refused to cover the costs of the referral.[74] Indeed, among treatment facilities that offer special programs or special services for women, self-payment is the

BARRIERS TO TREATMENT FOR PREGNANT SUBSTANCE ABUSERS

- Denial of problem
- Guilt or shame about the problem
- Fear of losing custody of children
- Fear of prosecution and incarceration
- Lack of transportation
- Lack of child care
- Long waiting list
- Lack of obstetric and pediatric services

Sources: Ashley, O. S., Marsden, M. E., and Brady, T. M. (2003). Effectiveness of substance abuse treatment programming for women: A review. *American Journal of Drug and Alcohol Abuse* 29(1):19–53; Coletti, S. D. (1998). Service providers and treatment access issues. In Wetherington, C. L., and Roman, A. B., *Drug addiction and the health of women* (NIH publication no. 98-4290) (237–43). Rockville, MD: U.S. Department of Health and Human Services, National Institutes of Health, National Institute on Drug Abuse; Gordon, S. M. (2002). *Women and addiction: Gender issues in abuse and treatment.* www.caron.org (accessed March 19, 2004).

most widely accepted form of payment. Only a small proportion of these facilities accept state-financed health insurance, federal military insurance, or Medicare.[75] While many of the barriers to treatment are manifestations of complex personal and social issues, something as simple as a lack of adequate transportation can end a woman's hopes of entering treatment.

Smoking: The Number-One Preventable Killer

Of all forms of substance abuse, smoking is by far the most prevalent, with nearly 28 million women in the United States reporting that they are current smokers.[76] It also is the number-one preventable cause of death. The number of relatively low-cost options available to women who want to stop smoking is much greater than the number of resources available to those who seek treatment for an alcohol or other drug problem. Smoking cessation options are quite variable and fairly accessible, ranging from self-help methods to brief therapies to over-the-counter and prescription medications. The real hurdles are motivating smokers to seek out these options, stick to cessation programs, and maintain their abstinence from tobacco once they have quit successfully.

The majority of smokers in the United States want to quit smoking;[77] however, the desire to quit tends to be somewhat stronger among women than among men. Eighty

DECIDING NOT TO SMOKE

I did the patch. I smoked on the patch. I did hypnosis. I tried everything until that morning it felt like an elephant was sitting on my chest. And so I said, here's the deal. You're alive so you can make decisions. You can decide to smoke and continue to feel this way, or you could not.
—S. Epatha Merkerson, actor and former smoker

Source: Merkerson, S. E., personal communication, November 21, 2003.

percent of women say they want to quit smoking compared to 72 percent of men.[78] Teenage girls who smoke also may have a slightly stronger desire to stop smoking cigarettes than their male peers. Among current smokers, 59 percent of girls in middle school (vs. 52% of boys) and 63 percent of girls in high school (vs. 59% of boys) report wanting to stop smoking cigarettes. Middle school (66%) and high school (63%) girls are significantly likelier than boys of those ages (55%) to have attempted to quit smoking in the past year.[79]

Unfortunately, many female smokers who attempt to quit fail. One study found that 45 percent of twelfth-grade girls who smoked daily had tried to quit but were unsuccessful.[80] Adult women, like girls, tend to be less successful at quitting than men.[81] And even those women who do successfully quit may resume smoking again.[82] Relapse is likeliest to occur in women facing stressful life events.[83]

For women and men, the main barrier to smoking cessation is physical addiction to the nicotine in tobacco products.[84] Females and males share many similarities in the factors promoting their smoking behavior,[85] their motivations for wanting to stop, their readiness to stop, and their general awareness of smoking's harmful effects.[86] Nevertheless, certain factors beyond physical addiction are especially important in promoting smoking or hindering smoking cessation in women. For example, smoking is reinforcing to women because of the physical effects of nicotine and because of the subjective sense of comfort and relaxation derived from the act itself; these subjective experiences are not as reinforcing for men.[87] Because women are responsive to these non-nicotine-related reinforcing effects of smoking, quitting appears to be more difficult for them.

It's Never Too Soon—or Too Late—to Quit Smoking

Women who quit smoking considerably reduce their risk of dying prematurely as well as gain more immediate health benefits. The sooner one quits, the better. Women who quit smoking at younger ages experience relatively greater benefits than those who quit later. A person who quits smoking before age 35 can almost completely eliminate the risk of mortality associated with smoking.[88] Indeed, women who quit at 35 are expected to live almost seven years longer than women who continue smoking. But even quitting much later in life has considerable benefits; women who quit smoking at 65 increase their life expectancy by almost four years compared to those who continue to smoke.[89]

Within a year of quitting smoking, a woman reduces her smoking-related risk of heart disease by 50 percent. Within five years, her smoking-related risk of heart disease can disappear altogether.[90]

Although an older woman who quits smoking cannot completely undo the damage done by years of smoking, she can make great strides in restoring her health, avoiding paralyzing disabilities, protecting her ability to live independently, and enhancing the quality of her life. Not only do mortality rates decline, the risk of developing lung- and other smoking-related cancers and heart attacks also are reduced.[91]

Weighing the Pros and Cons of Quitting

Most women want to quit smoking because they are concerned about their health. However, fear of weight gain often outweighs their desire for a healthy future and is a major reason why many women fail to quit. While women who quit smoking do tend to gain more weight than those who continue, the health risks of smoking far outweigh the risks of the weight gain.[92]

Women are more afraid than men of gaining weight during smoking cessation.[93] Research confirms that this fear is somewhat justified, as women do tend to gain more weight after cessation, either as a percentage of their pre-quit bodyweight or in actual pounds.[94] Moreover, young women are far more likely than young men to report that

FIVE STEPS TO SUCCESSFUL QUITTING

1. Get ready to quit by setting a quit date.
2. Get support from family, friends, health care providers, and support groups.
3. Learn new skills and behaviors to distract you from smoking.
4. Get medication and follow directions carefully.
5. Be prepared for difficult situations or relapse.

Source: Adapted from U.S. Department of Health and Human Services. (2000). *You can quit smoking: Consumer guide.* www.cdc.gov/tobacco (accessed February 24, 2004).

ADDITIONAL BENEFITS OF QUITTING SMOKING

- Quitting reduces the risk of developing cataracts.[a]
- Quitting reduces the risk of macular degeneration, the leading cause of blindness among seniors.[b]
- Quitting reduces the risk of dying after undergoing angioplasty to open blocked arteries.[c]
- Quitting six to eight weeks before undergoing surgery reduces the risk of post-operative complications.[d]

Sources: [a]Weintraub, J. M., Willett, W. C., Rosner, B., Colditz, G. A., Seddon, J. M., and Hankinson, S. E. (2002). Smoking cessation and risk of cataract extraction among US women and men. *American Journal of Epidemiology* 155(1):72–79. [b]American Academy of Ophthalmology. (2004). *There's hope for people with age-related macular degeneration.* www.aao.org (accessed February 27, 2004). [c]American Heart Association. (2004). *Persistent smokers skip full benefit of angioplasty.* www.americanheart.org (accessed February 27, 2004). [d]Moller, A. M., Villebro, N., Pedersen, T., and Tonnesen, H. (2002). Effect of preoperative smoking intervention on postoperative complications: A randomised clinical trial. *Lancet* 359(9301):114–17.

smoking is a dieting strategy and that weight gain is a cause of smoking relapse.[95] Indeed, 80 percent of women smokers relapse following treatment.[96]

Unfortunately, efforts to address adult women's weight concerns in smoking cessation programs have met with mixed success.[97] Better strategies are needed to address the concerns of weight gain and other barriers to successful smoking cessation for many women. The combination of cognitive-behavioral therapy (CBT) and smoking cessation medication may prove especially effective.[98]

Social Support

Social support from one's family or friends improves the chances of success in quitting for women and men.[99] Social support may be particularly beneficial to girls and women who are trying to quit.[100] Girls are more likely than boys to respond well to smoking cessation programs that include support from family members or the peer group.[101] Support from a spouse or partner has been shown to be an important factor in quitting attempts and success. In general, however, husbands tend to provide less effective support for their wives who are trying to quit than wives give their husbands.[102] In recent years, support services are increasingly being offered through telephone hotlines and Web sites.

Smoking Cessation among Pregnant Women

Pregnancy is a key window of opportunity during which to encourage women to quit smoking. Most pregnant women are concerned about having a healthy pregnancy and avoiding causing harm to their fetuses. However, many pregnant women who decide to quit during pregnancy perceive their abstinence as temporary and resume smoking after delivery. Within one year of delivery, 70 percent of pregnant women who quit smoking relapse, with most resuming smoking within six months of delivery.[103]

Typical care for pregnant smokers includes a doctor's recommendation to stop smoking along with a referral to certain self-help materials or smoking-cessation programs. If these interventions are unsuccessful, additional or alternative treatments are considered. For pregnant smokers who are unable to quit with the help of clinical or self-help interventions, pharmacotherapy may be used. Where pharmacotherapy is involved, the treatment provider and pregnant woman must determine that the risks and unknown effects of a given pharmacotherapy on the woman and her fetus are less than the risks of continued smoking.[104] While studies have demonstrated that nicotine itself presents risks to the fetus,[105] Bupropion SR (Zyban)—a first-line of defense in smoking cessation pharmacotherapy—has been shown to cause seizures in one out of every 1,000 patients.[106] The effectiveness of Bupropion SR and other pharmacotherapies in treating tobacco dependence in pregnant women and the risks of use to both mother and the fetus are unknown and require further research.

Effective Treatment

An effective smoking cessation program would address the predictors of smoking initiation as well as known barriers to quitting that are unique to girls and young women. Currently there exists very little research examining effective smoking cessation programs specifically for girls and young women. There also is little research that examines their preference for or success with various smoking cessation treatments.

Nevertheless, research suggests that smokers treated with a combination of nicotine replacement therapy (NRT), pharmacotherapy, cognitive-behavioral therapy, and the provision of social support stand the best chance of successfully quitting.[107] More research is needed, however, to determine whether there are gender differences in effective smoking cessation strategies.

SMOKING CESSATION METHODS

"Cold Turkey"

One common approach to quitting smoking is simply to stop using cigarettes altogether. Up to 88 percent of women quit in this way.[a] While quitting "cold turkey" seems to work well for some, evidence is mounting that the most effective way to quit is by using a combination of professional interventions.[b]

Sources: [a]American Cancer Society. (2001). *Preparing to quit.* www.cancer.org (accessed February 25, 2002). [b]Office of the Surgeon General. (2001). *Women and smoking: A report of the Surgeon General* (GPO Item No. 0483-L-06). Washington, DC: U.S. Government Printing Office; U.S. Department of Health and Human Services. (2000). *You can quit smoking: Consumer guide.* www.cdc.gov/tobacco (accessed February 24, 2004).

Self-Help

Self-help methods are the most common means by which smokers try to quit. These methods range from quitting without any aids to fairly intense self-administered cessation strategies. Self-help methods usually involve written materials on coping strategies and the importance of preparing for a quit date. The methods can be used alone or in combination with other forms of smoking-cessation aids or interventions. The written materials pose an advantage in that they can be tailored to specific target audiences, including adolescent girls and pregnant women, and they can be disseminated easily. Materials can be strategically placed in locations where girls and women tend to congregate, such as schools, houses of worship, beauty salons, grocery stores, mass transit, shopping centers, community centers, or doctors' offices.

Sources: Lando, H. A., and Gritz, E. R. (1996). Smoking cessation techniques. *Journal of the American Medical Women's Association* 51(1–2):31–34, 47; Office of the Surgeon General. (2001). *Women and smoking: A report of the Surgeon General* (GPO item no. 0483-L-06). Washington, DC: U.S. Government Printing Office.

Brief Clinical Interventions

Minimal clinical interventions are designed to be integrated easily into routine care by doctors and other health care practitioners during office visits.[a] The U.S. Public Health Service has recommended a brief intervention of "five A's" for physicians and other health care practitioners to incorporate into their practices. The "five A's" (Ask about tobacco use; Advise to quit; Assess willingness to make a quit attempt; Assist in quit attempt; and Arrange for follow-up) are consistent with guidelines established by the National Cancer Institute as well as the American Medical Association. They require three minutes or less of a practitioner's time to implement. Brief interventions have been shown to improve significantly the smoking cessation success rates of both women and men.[b]

Sources: [a]Fiore, M. C., Bailey, W. C., Cohen, S. J., Dorfman, S. F., Goldstein, M. G., et al. (2000). *Treating tobacco use and dependence: Clinical practice guideline* (GPO item no. 0491-B-17). Washington, DC: U.S. Government Printing Office; Kendrick, J. S., and Merritt, R. K. (1996). Women and smoking: An update for the 1990s. *American Journal of Obstetrics and Gynecology* 175(3, Pt. 1):528–35. [b]Fiore, Bailey, Cohen, Dorfman, Goldstein, et al. (2000).

Intensive Clinical Interventions

Intensive clinical interventions involve multiple-session group, individual, or telephone counseling. These interventions tend to appeal to women more than men. Women also appear to be more interested than men in smoking cessation groups that offer mutual support through a buddy system as well as in participating in treatment meetings over a longer period of time.

Source: Office of the Surgeon General. (2001). *Women and smoking: A report of the Surgeon General* (GPO item no. 0483-L-06). Washington, DC: U.S. Government Printing Office.

Pharmacological Treatments

Both prescription and over-the-counter drugs can help women quit smoking. These drugs can be taken orally, nasally, or through skin patches. Some FDA approved pharmacological treatments are available only by prescription (sustained-release Bupropion, nicotine inhaler, nicotine nasal spray, some nicotine patches), while others (i.e., nicotine gum and some nicotine patches) are available over the counter.

Source: U.S. Department of Health and Human Services. (2000). *You can quit smoking: Consumer guide.* www.cdc.gov/tobacco (accessed February 24, 2004).

Community-Based Interventions

Community-based interventions focus on engaging entire communities in intervention activities to reduce smoking. They may use a variety of strategies to engage the community, including media campaigns, educational programs, face-to-face interventions, telephone-quit lines, and environmental modification. These interventions have shown mixed rates of success and few differences in quit rates between women and men.

Sources: Office of the Surgeon General. (2001). *Women and smoking: A report of the Surgeon General* (GPO item no. 0483-L-06). Washington, DC: U.S. Government Printing Office; Secker-Walker, R. H., Flynn, B. S., Solomon, L. J., Skelly, J. M., Dorwaldt, A. L., and Ashikaga, T. (2000). Helping women quit smoking: Results of a community intervention program. *American Journal of Public Health* 90(6):940–46.

Alcohol and Drug Treatment

Therapeutic approaches for assisting people to quit smoking are more accessible than many of those available for assisting people who are addicted to alcohol or drugs. This may be due, in part, to the numerous barriers women face in receiving effective alcohol and drug treatment—which typically require more extensive, time-consuming, and costly interventions than most available smoking cessation programs. Studies specifically examining the effectiveness of various therapies for treating women are scarce.

Strategies for treating alcohol or drug abuse can involve self-help approaches or programs run by professionals. Treatment can be long-term or brief, inpatient or outpatient, and can involve individual therapy, group therapy, pharmacotherapy, or a combination of several approaches.[108]

ALCOHOL AND DRUG ABUSE BEHAVIORAL TREATMENT AND RECOVERY APPROACHES

Self-Help / Twelve-Step Programs

Twelve-step recovery programs allow substance abusers to share their experiences and concerns with other individuals attempting to recover from addiction. Recovery from substance abuse via twelve-step programs is likeliest to occur among women who combine such self-help approaches with other forms of treatment, such as psychotherapy or pharmacotherapy. Alcoholics Anonymous (AA), and its drug-related offshoots such as Narcotics Anonymous, is the best known of these programs.

Source: O'Connor, L. E., Esherick, M., and Vieten, C. (2002). Drug- and alcohol-abusing women. In Straussner, S. L. A., and Brown, S., *The handbook of addiction treatment for women* (75–98). San Francisco: Jossey-Bass.

Brief Clinical Interventions

Brief clinical interventions are suited primarily for people who have alcohol or drug problems but not dependency. Primary care physicians or other health care professionals usually deliver brief interventions that typically involve five or fewer office visits in which the patient is given information about the negative effects of excess drinking or of drug use. Patients also are given practical advice and strategies for cutting down on substance use as well as referrals to community agencies and other resources. Brief interventions have been used effectively in other settings besides practitioners' offices, such as trauma centers, emergency rooms, and on college campuses.

Source: National Institute on Alcohol Abuse and Alcoholism. (2000). New advances in alcoholism treatment. *Alcohol Alert* 49.

Behavioral and Psychosocial Therapies

Behavioral therapies attempt to reduce substance abuse by changing behavior. Commonly used strategies include cognitive-behavioral therapy and motivation-enhancement therapy.[a]

- *Cognitive-Behavioral Therapy* (CBT). Cognitive-behavioral therapists help patients change their drinking or drug use behaviors by learning how to identify situations that put them at high risk, rehearsing strategies to be used in those specific situations, and learning to recognize and cope with cravings for alcohol or drugs.[b]
- *Motivation-Enhancement Therapy* (MET). MET works to motivate the client to change her behavior by using her own resources.[c] The therapist first makes an assessment to determine the type and severity of the patient's substance use problem and then provides feedback that is designed to motivate change in substance use behavior. Over several sessions, the therapist and patient work closely together to maintain or increase the patient's motivation to change. MET has been shown to be very effective in overcoming resistance to entering treatment.[d]

Sources: [a]National Institute on Alcohol Abuse and Alcoholism. (2001). *Alcoholism: Getting the facts* (NIH publication no. 96-4153). Rockville, MD: U.S. Department of Health and Human Services, National Institutes of Health, National Institute on Alcohol Abuse and Alcoholism. [b]Fuller, R. K., and Hiller-Sturmhofel, S. (1999). Alcoholism treatment in the United States. *Alcohol Research and Health* 23(2):69–77; Winters, K. C. (1999). Treating adolescents with substance use disorders: An overview of practice issues and treatment outcome. *Substance Abuse* 20(4):203–25. [c]Fuller and Hiller-Sturmhofel (1999). [d]National Institute on Alcohol Abuse and Alcoholism. (2000). New advances in alcoholism treatment. *Alcohol Alert* 49.

Therapeutic Communities

Therapeutic communities (TCs) are residential substance abuse treatment programs that foster personal and social responsibility in patients via peer influence and group therapy. Self-help and "mutual self-help"—in which individual patients assume partial responsibility for the recovery of their peers—are important aspects of the TC treatment process.[a] Patients who successfully complete treatment in a TC show reductions in drug and alcohol use, criminal behavior, unemployment, and symptoms of depression.[b]

Sources: [a]De Leon, G. (2000). *The Therapeutic Community: Theory, model and method.* New York: Springer. [b]National Institute on Drug Abuse. (2002). *Therapeutic community* (NIH publication no. 02-4877). Rockville, MD: U.S. Department of Health and Human Services, National Institutes of Health, National Institute on Drug Abuse.

PHARMACOLOGICAL TREATMENTS FOR ALCOHOL AND DRUG ABUSE

A variety of drug therapies to treat addiction have been available over the years, with new ones continually emerging. While there are many pharmacological treatments for opioid abuse, drug therapies targeted at addiction to prescription stimulants and depressants lag far behind. Examples of the primary alcohol treatment and opioid treatments available include:

- *Antabuse.* Antabuse (Disulfiram) is a drug that produces an extremely unpleasant reaction in patients who consume even small amounts of alcohol while under treatment. If a person takes Antabuse and drinks alcohol, she becomes violently ill and experiences the symptoms of a severe hangover. When used alone, without proper supportive therapy, Antabuse is unlikely to have lasting effects on chronic alcohol abuse.
- *Naltrexone.* Naltrexone is a narcotic antagonist that blocks opioid receptors in the brain, preventing a woman from getting high or feeling euphoric when using opioids. Although it was originally used to treat dependence on illicit opioid drugs, it was recently approved by the FDA as a treatment for alcoholism. It blocks alcohol's ability to stimulate the body's natural opiates,[a] removing the craving for alcohol. It must be taken regularly and is effective only when used in combination with behavioral therapies.[b]
- *Methadone.* Since the 1970s, methadone maintenance has been widely used to treat heroin addiction.[c] Methadone works by occupying the same opioid receptors in the brain as heroin; however, its use does not result in the same uncontrolled, compulsive, and disruptive behavior. Although patients become physically dependent on the drug, the dependence is not associated with the adverse psychological and physical effects of illicit opioids, allowing the patient to change her behaviors and function more adaptively.[d]
- *LAAM.* Levo-alpha-acetyl-methadol (LAAM), like methadone, is provided through certified clinics to treat opioid dependence.[e] LAAM lasts longer than methadone and is administered less frequently. Because of its slower onset and sustained action properties, LAAM poses a lower risk for abuse than methadone.[f]
- *Buprenorphine.* Buprenorphine is used to reduce the symptoms associated with opioid dependence.[g] It is unique in that trained physicians may administer the drug in an outpatient office setting rather than the usual clinic setting. The medication regimen that patients must follow is less burdensome than with other treatments, making taking the drug more convenient, potentially enhancing patient compliance.[h]

There also are alternative strategies such as faith-based programs, acupuncture, and hypnosis. The most common forms of treatment for substance abuse and addiction are behavioral and psychosocial therapy and pharmacotherapy. Unfortunately, there exists little gender-based research that assesses the relative benefits of these various approaches for women versus men. Some programs do offer gender-specific interventions (separat-

Sources: [a]Volpicelli, J. R. (2000). *Medical treatments for alcohol dependence.* www.uphs.upenn.edu (accessed March 23, 2004). [b]National Institute on Alcohol Abuse and Alcoholism. (2001). *Alcoholism: Getting the facts* (NIH publication no. 96-4153). Rockville, MD: U.S. Department of Health and Human Services, National Institutes of Health, National Institute on Alcohol Abuse and Alcoholism. [c]Brecher, E. M., and Editors of *Consumer Reports Magazine.* (1972). *Consumers Union report on licit and illicit drugs.* www.druglibrary.org (accessed December 28, 2001). [d]Office of National Drug Control Policy. (2000). *Methadone* [Fact sheet] (NCJ publication no. 175678). Washington, DC: Office of National Drug Control Policy. [e]Substance Abuse and Mental Health Services Administration. (2002). *NIDA research and SAMHSA physician training combine to put care for opiate dependence in hands of family doctor* [Press release]. Rockville, MD: U.S. Department of Health and Human Services. [f]Office of National Drug Control Policy. (1996). *Treatment protocol effectiveness study.* www.ncjrs.org (accessed October 31, 2003). [g]U.S. Food and Drug Administration, Center for Drug Evaluation and Research. (2002). *Subutex and suboxone: Questions and answers.* www.fda.gov (accessed October 15, 2002). [h]Substance Abuse and Mental Health Services Administration. (2002).

ing men from women), but these are not necessarily gender-sensitive; that is, most do not take into account the unique psychosocial and physiological needs of women.

Although new pharmacological interventions are being developed (primarily to treat addiction to alcohol and opioid dependence), more research clearly is needed to determine what works best for women in treatment for substance use disorders. The current predominant approach for treating those suffering from alcohol or drug addiction is psychosocial in the form of cognitive and/or behavioral therapies.

Designing and Implementing Programs That Work

Once a woman gathers the courage to admit that she has a problem and enters treatment, and once the obstacles to actually receiving such treatment are removed, she—or those referring her—must choose an appropriate program. Ideally, she will have a choice of programs that are sensitive to the needs of women in general as well as her personal needs.

The success of women-oriented programs in treating substance abuse may be due in part to their ability to reduce the barriers around entering and remaining in treatment.[109] For example, women-only programs may attract girls and women with a history of sexual and physical abuse, and women who may fear being ridiculed or humiliated in co-ed groups, such as gay women or prostitutes.[110] To be successful, treatment programs should address women's physical, mental, and social needs.[111] This includes offering services for women in a supportive, nonjudgmental manner.

Programs that are gender-specific, age appropriate, and ethnically, culturally, and linguistically sensitive are likelier to be successful, as are those that offer comprehensive inpatient and outpatient treatment and comprehensive medical services that address reproductive health, sexuality, relationships, and victimization.[112] The likelihood of successful treatment increases with the availability of varied counseling services (including individual, group, and family therapy), vocational and educational training, and childcare for those who need it.

Beyond mental and physical aid are real structural issues. Residential programs that allow women to live with their infants and young children are likelier to keep patients in treatment longer. Drug-free, safe housing and, for some women, financial support and transportation services (e.g., cab vouchers, bus tokens) make it more likely that a woman will complete treatment. However, these services are not readily available in all or even most treatment programs. A 1998 survey, for example, found that only 36 percent of programs offered transportation to their facilities.[113]

Because addressing the physical, mental, social, and structural needs of women in treatment is associated with decreased substance use, improved mental and physical health, reduced risk of HIV, and higher rates of employment,[114] there is a growing emphasis on developing programs that do so.[115] Unfortunately, while the costs for effec-

ADDITIONAL COMPONENTS NEEDED FOR EFFECTIVE TREATMENT FOR WOMEN

- Food, clothing, and shelter
- Transportation
- Job counseling and training
- Legal assistance
- Literacy training and educational opportunities
- Assertiveness training
- Couples counseling
- Family-planning services
- Parenting training
- Medical care
- Childcare
- Social services
- Social support
- Family therapy
- Psychological assessment and mental health care

Source: Adapted from National Institute on Drug Abuse. (2001). *NIDA infofacts: Treatment methods for women.* www.drugabuse.gov (accessed January 22, 2002).

tive treatment are high, public and private financial resources are low. Insurance coverage for treatment often is inconsistent and insufficient. Until policy makers prioritize this important health benefit, much of what we know about effective treatment may not be available to women in need.

Treating Young and Old

Treating girls and older women for substance abuse presents special challenges. During adolescence, girls go through enormous physical, hormonal, and emotional changes that can increase stress while challenging their coping abilities. And because girls are more likely than boys to have experienced physical and sexual abuse,[116] traditional male-dominated programs—especially those that use confrontational approaches—may be less appropriate for survivors of such abuse.[117]

Many of the life stresses that lead to substance abuse in girls and young women are intricately connected with other problems, such as co-occurring psychiatric disorders, emotional difficulties, dysfunctional family relations, and parental abuse of alcohol or drugs. Each of these issues, when pertinent to the patient, must somehow be addressed in the treatment setting.[118] Early intervention is key.[119]

IMPORTANT FEATURES OF TREATMENT SERVICES FOR GIRLS

- Early screening
- Food, shelter, and clothing
- Transportation
- Literacy training and educational opportunities
- Physical and sexual abuse assessment and counseling
- Family counseling
- Legal assistance
- Social services
- Prenatal care
- Family-planning services
- Parenting training
- Childcare
- Mentoring
- Psychological assessment and mental health care

Source: The National Center on Addiction and Substance Abuse (CASA) at Columbia University. (2003). *The formative years: Pathways to substance abuse among girls and young women ages 8–22.* New York: CASA.

IMPORTANT FEATURES OF TREATMENT SERVICES FOR OLDER WOMEN

- Age-specific group treatment offered in a supportive and nonconfrontational environment that builds the person's self-esteem
- A focus on coping with depression, loneliness, and loss
- A focus on rebuilding social support networks
- A content and pace of treatment appropriate for the individual
- Staff who are interested and experienced in working with older adults
- Case management, providing access to services, including medical services, for elderly persons

Source: Blow, F. C. (1998). *Substance abuse among older adults: Treatment Improvement Protocol (TIP) Series 26* (DHHS publication no. SMA 98-3179). Rockville, MD: U.S. Department of Health and Human Services, Public Health Service, Substance Abuse and Mental Health Services Administration, Center for Substance Abuse Treatment.

Older women have treatment needs that programs tailored for younger women usually do not address, yet fewer than one in five substance abuse programs in the United States offers services specifically designed for older adults, let alone older women.[120] Many older women who receive treatment for substance abuse may be receiving improper care. For example, older women may be in greater denial of the problem and experience guilt because of it.[121] As with younger women, confrontational approaches may hinder rather than aid recovery by making an older woman more reluctant to remain in treatment.[122] In addition, in a co-ed group setting, older women are likely to defer to men, and personal issues that women find difficult to discuss in front of men might fail to be addressed.[123]

Treating Pregnant Women

Access to appropriate services and adequate prenatal care are key components of any course of substance abuse treatment for pregnant women, as is effective communication between obstetricians and addiction treatment professionals. Providing comprehensive services in a nonjudgmental, supportive environment encourages women to receive the treatment they need in order to have a healthy pregnancy.

Regardless of the substance being used, withdrawal symptoms can be a threat to the health of a mother and her fetus. It is best for pregnant women to gradually withdraw from their substance of abuse under medical supervision—preferably in consul-

KEY COMPONENTS OF SUCCESSFUL SUBSTANCE ABUSE TREATMENT PROGRAMS FOR PREGNANT WOMEN

- Comprehensive medical services
- Gender-specific services that also are ethnically and culturally sensitive
- Services offered in a nonjudgmental, nonpunitive, nurturing manner
- Services that avoid confrontational treatment approaches
- Vocational and educational services
- Drug-free, safe housing
- Financial support services
- Pediatric follow-up and early intervention services
- Case-management services
- Transportation services
- Childcare services
- Counseling services

Source: Mitchell, J. L. (1995). *Pregnant, substance-using women: Treatment Improvement Protocol (TIP) Series 2* (DHHS publication no. SMA 95-3056). Rockville, MD: U.S. Department of Health and Human Services, Public Health Service, Substance Abuse and Mental Health Services Administration, Center for Substance Abuse Treatment.

tation with an obstetrician—in an inpatient setting. Such precautions allow for the withdrawal status of the mother and fetus to be monitored carefully.[124]

Some physicians recommend that pregnant women avoid pharmacotherapies for alcohol or drug treatment because it is possible that their use will result in birth defects. Thus, as with the use of any substance during pregnancy, the benefits and risks of use must be assessed and clearly understood by the mother before treatment begins. For example, while Antabuse is an effective aversion pharmacotherapy for nonpregnant individuals, it has been associated with so many birth defects that women who conceive while using it are advised to seek counseling before deciding to continue their pregnancies.[125]

Methadone is the recommended pharmacotherapy for pregnant women who are addicted to opioids such as heroin. Many women cannot quit cold turkey; withdrawal might cause fetal death or early delivery. Although there is some debate about the safety of prenatal methadone exposure,[126] it is generally agreed that the effects are preferable to continued opioid use or detoxification. Because the dose is controlled and constant, fetuses are not subject to the erratic opioid exposure and withdrawal that might come from a pregnant woman's uncontrolled heroin use. A maintenance dose of methadone might quell dangerous behavior such as prostitution or injection needle use, which put the mother and fetus at risk for infections such as HIV. Moreover, a pregnant woman being maintained on methadone has frequent contact with medical personnel, increasing the likelihood that she will receive adequate prenatal care.[127]

There is little evidence regarding the safety and effectiveness of using drugs to medically withdraw pregnant women who use cocaine. Some treatment facilities will use antidepressants for the first five days of an expectant mother's stay in order to treat the depression that results from cocaine withdrawal, with the goal of reducing the high dropout rate that occurs during this period of time. Mothers who need such drugs for a longer period of time generally suffer from more serious forms of depression requiring psychiatric evaluation. Bromocriptine, a drug used in the treatment of menstrual abnormalities, has been shown to offer relief from cocaine cravings. However, its use during pregnancy is not recommended because its degree of efficacy and short- and long-term effects on the fetus are unknown.[128]

To encourage pregnant women to receive treatment for a substance abuse problem and to retain them once they are enrolled, a variety of personal, social, and health services should be available for pregnant and postpartum women.[129] Ideally, in addition to substance abuse treatment, other services would include childbirth preparation and education, infant care and feeding classes, breastfeeding support, parenting classes, fathers' groups, nutrition classes, and crisis intervention. Unfortunately, as is true in treating women more generally, such specialized services for pregnant women are costly and largely unavailable.

Finding the Will and the Resources to Make a Difference

This country spends an inordinate amount of money carrying the burden of untreated addiction. In state government alone, 13 percent of budget expenditures go to dealing with the consequences of untreated addiction; yet only about one-half of one percent of state spending is on treatment.[130] A widely held belief is that alcohol and drug abuse treatment does not work. This belief is fostered by the fact that, for many people, substance abuse is a chronic, recurring disease that typically is not responsive to the short-term, haphazard interventions generally available. Unless a substance abuser is independently wealthy and surrounded by a caring and consistent social support system, obtaining effective and lasting care is improbable. In contrast, individuals suffering from other chronic, recurring diseases—such as hypertension, diabetes, or asthma—are able to obtain consistent and effective care without incurring the sense of hopelessness and waste that is engendered by substance abusers.

Despite public sentiment, decades of research have shown that treatment can work and can be cost-effective, yielding a significant return on investment in the form of avoided costs in the prison, mental health, medical, child welfare, and public assistance systems and net economic benefits generated by productive, law-abiding citizens.[131] Yet, for treatment to be effective, it must be readily available, tailored to fit the needs of the individual patient, and part of a comprehensive program that addresses associated medical, psychological, social, and economic needs. Only through well-designed and well-implemented comprehensive and consistent treatment can we hope to stem the burdensome societal consequences of substance abuse.

Currently, access to treatment is severely limited for the majority of those who need it. Effective, evidence-based treatment programs cannot be found in many parts of the country, and, for those who can physically access these programs, paying for them is difficult. Few health insurance programs cover substance abuse treatment, and most of those that do provide only limited coverage for short-term help. For example, the U.S. Public Health Service has recommended that private and public health insurers cover smoking cessation programs—many of which are known to be clinically effective and cost-effective. Nevertheless, only seven states' Medicaid programs (Florida, Indiana, Kansas, Maine, Minnesota, Oregon, and West Virginia) cover comprehensive cessation treatment, and no state requires private insurers to cover such treatment.[132]

To close the treatment gap, we have to not only address the different barriers to treatment and the treatment needs of girls and women but also assure that providers are well trained, services are available and accessible, and treatment costs are covered by health insurers or public benefits. If not, the hopeless cycle of addiction and relapse does not stand a chance of being interrupted.

Of course, the best way to avoid the need for treatment and its associated costs is to effectively prevent the onset of substance abuse. We know what works in prevention, and we know that prevention, like treatment, provides substantial returns on the investment. Only through effective prevention that is implemented early and consistently from childhood through adulthood, targeting the unique vulnerabilities of women and capitalizing on key opportunities for intervention, can we hope to reduce the problem of substance abuse and the corresponding need for accessible and affordable treatment services.

chapter 7chapter 7chapter 7chapter 7chapter 7

Prevention and Policy Opportunities across the Life Span

A person who reaches age 21 without smoking, abusing alcohol or using drugs is virtually certain never to do so.
—Joseph A. Califano, Jr.

- Girls who talk with their parents about substance abuse are less likely to smoke, drink, or use drugs than other girls.[1]
- Girls who are engaged in school are less likely to initiate drinking than girls who are not.[2]
- Girls often cite antidrug advertising as sources of information on drugs and reasons not to take them.[3]
- Brief physician counseling sessions about the dangers of substance abuse can reduce alcohol use in women by up to 31 percent.[4]

Although millions of girls and women are at risk throughout their lives, appropriate, research-based, and effective prevention efforts tailored specifically to the unique needs of girls and women are in desperately short supply. The broad-based prevention programs that rely on a general curriculum aimed at the largest group possible and the programs specifically targeted at those at high risk for substance use take a unisex approach. Such prevention programs—largely developed without regard to gender, and often with males in mind—fail to influence the behavior of millions of females.

As girls grow up and women age, there are many opportunities to intervene before they engage in substance use. The best window of opportunity for prevention is during childhood, before a girl begins to experiment with tobacco, alcohol, or drugs; before unhealthy attitudes, beliefs, and behaviors have set in; and before she is inundated with pro-substance-use messages from peers and the media. Parents are the greatest prevention resource available, perhaps even more so for girls than for boys. When they are engaged and involved in their children's lives and model behavior that sends a strong message about the inappropriateness of substance use for their children, the power of other influences wanes.

Once prevention efforts are implemented in grade school, additional intervention is needed. Research clearly shows that one-shot or limited interventions are not successful if they are not followed up by regular, consistent, and age-appropriate interventions throughout a child's schooling—from grade school, through middle school, high school, college, and beyond. The school is the ideal place for much of this prevention activity to take place, since nearly all children regularly attend school and are essentially a "captive audience."

For children who do not attend school regularly, young women who have dropped out of school at an early age, and adult women who have completed their education, effective prevention efforts can be provided by a parent, health professional, community leader, or member of the clergy. Even appropriate and effective messages on television or in movies and magazines can educate and motivate girls and women to avoid starting to smoke, drink, or use drugs, or to stop that use if it has already begun.

A Life-span Perspective

Effective prevention efforts should be tailored to the specific risks women face at different life stages as well as to factors universal to women of all ages, such as low self-esteem or violence. As the principal influences on and circumstances surrounding women's substance use evolve and change with age, so too should interventions to prevent that use or keep it from becoming dangerous and unhealthy. Just as it is never too late to quit smoking, drinking, or using drugs, it is never too late to intervene to keep a girl or woman from taking that first step down the destructive path of substance abuse.

Girls

A child who reaches age 21 without smoking, abusing alcohol, or using drugs is far less likely to become dependent than peers who use and abuse substances as teens. Therefore, prevention efforts must focus on how to get girls through their teen and young adult years without smoking, abusing alcohol, or using drugs.

Opportunities for prevention are more abundant for girls living at home with their families than for any other age group. Parents are the first line of defense against substance use. Parents, teachers, physicians, clergy, and other concerned adults are likely to be more effective if they know what to look for. As described in previous chapters, girls are more likely than boys to be depressed, have eating disorders, and be sexually or physically abused, all of which increase the chances of substance abuse. Girls are likelier than boys to use alcohol and drugs to improve their mood, enhance sex, and reduce inhibitions.

College Women

Substance abuse, particularly in the form of binge drinking, has become increasingly common among college women. While college students are no more likely than people their age who are not in college to use substances of abuse,[5] the transition from high school to college brings with it the greatest increase in smoking and marijuana use among young women.[6] College women, like all women, are more likely to face the combined specter of substance abuse and depression. The possibility of being a victim of rape, particularly date rape, becomes much likelier when college women drink or use drugs. Students, parents, school administrators, professors, and counselors must be awake to the chilling implications of female students' high levels of smoking, alcohol abuse, illicit drug use, and prescription drug misuse. When planning and implementing prevention initiatives, they must take into account the unique motivations that young women have for using these substances and the unique complications and consequences for women of using these substances.

Due to its widespread nature, alcohol use and abuse in particular has received attention from parents, schools, and the government. To truly make strides in preventing underage drinking and alcohol abuse among college students, school administrators, students, community leaders, alcohol producers and retailers, law enforcement professionals, and policy makers will have to recognize the problem's scope and severity and make prevention a priority by dedicating sufficient attention and resources to it. On a larger scale, the culture of alcohol that predominates on many college campuses must be overturned in order to reduce the problem instead of just cleaning up its consequences.

Other Young Adults

Although substance use and other risky behaviors often peak in the twenties* and generally occur at higher rates among young adults who are not in college than among college students,[7] there has been little research on prevention initiatives for young adults who do not go to college at all, as well as for those who already have graduated. Researchers may overlook these high-risk individuals because they are not as readily available for studies as are college students, and because the years between adolescence and the early twenties traditionally have not been regarded as a separate life stage in developmental theory.[8]

However, the years between high school and the assumption of traditional adult roles carry particular risks and concerns in terms of substance use and abuse for women, regardless of educational status. Many women are relatively unencumbered during these years, often living outside their parents' home but not yet settled in new families of their own. For instance, in 1970, the median age for marriage was approximately 21 for women, while the 2002 census reveals that only 26 percent of women aged 20 to 24 have been married. That number rises to approximately 60 percent for women ages 25 to 29 and jumps to 77 percent for women ages 30 to 34.[9] Therefore, a substantial proportion of women in their twenties are now living independently from the demands and responsibilities of their own parents as well as from marriage and parenthood. This becomes significant when considering that among young adults, marriage and parenting are associated with reduced substance use.[10] Today, financial means and a lack of familial responsibility among women in their twenties may contribute to their high levels of substance use.

Adult Women

Unlike for girls and young women, for adult women the devastating consequences of substance abuse are no longer far in the future. During the years between schooling and retirement, women become custodians of their own health more than ever. The best way to prevent dangerous substance use is to make available to adult women all the information they need to make informed choices.

Each woman should know the immediate effects of smoking on appearance, lung function, and cardiovascular disease; how women metabolize alcohol differently than

---

*For example, according to the latest National Survey on Drug Use and Health, tobacco use, alcohol use, binge drinking, and illicit drug use all are more prevalent among women aged 18 to 25 than among those aged 12 to 17 or those 26 and older.

men; how women suffer substance-related illnesses more rapidly than men; how alcohol and certain drugs suppress sexual response and cause or aggravate sexual dysfunction; how substance use is an inefficient and often counterproductive means of easing tension or stress; and how alcohol or drug use can make a woman more susceptible to unwanted sexual advances, rape, and violence.

Although women at risk for substance abuse in their adult years may not be as easy to reach as teens in school, opportunities for targeted prevention do exist and can be found by examining risk factors that mark women's substance abuse and addiction. Factors such as a family history of alcohol or drug abuse; abuse and violence during childhood, adolescence, or adulthood; depression; and substance abuse by a partner serve as warnings for women.[11] Getting the word out shouldn't be difficult. Women at risk can be found in physicians', dentists', and psychologists' offices, mental health clinics, support groups for children of alcohol abusers, domestic violence shelters, family planning clinics, jails, childcare centers, supermarkets, aerobics classes, and churches. All of these sites and situations offer opportunities for prevention.

Older Women

Substance abuse prevention among older women must take into account the challenges of identifying the problem. Often mistaken for other conditions or hidden by women themselves, substance abuse in older women can be difficult to detect.

As is true for younger women, the best way to prevent substance abuse and addiction in older women is to provide them with all of the information necessary for them to be the custodians of their own health. For instance, older women who smoke should know the benefits of quitting at or after age 60, and the likely consequences if they do not. Unfortunately, women who are still smokers later in life significantly underestimate their risk of dying prematurely as a result of their nicotine addiction.[12] Older women also should be apprised of the dangers of late-onset alcoholism and psychoactive drug use. They may believe that alcoholism is a danger that they left behind with their youth, or that they have never been and will never be susceptible to drug abuse. However, the challenges of the last decades of life can combine with other risk factors to lead older women to drinking, prescription drug abuse, and addiction. The good news is that there are benefits to overcoming abuse and addiction at any stage of life; however, if older women aren't made aware of these benefits, the quality of their lives could be diminished by the effects of nicotine, alcohol, or drug dependence.

Who Should Intervene and How?

Parents and other family members, friends, teachers, colleagues, health care providers, community leaders, and clergy members are key influencing agents in a girl or woman's decision to begin or continue to use substances, or to seek help in stopping. The media and policy makers also have important roles in helping to prevent substance abuse among women.

Parents and Families

Families—especially parents—hold the most important keys to children's decisions about substance use.[13] It may seem to parents that their daughters are inundated from all sides with pressures to smoke, drink, and use drugs and that the relative influence of parents is severely restricted; yet, this is hardly the case. Teens consistently report that parents are the most important consideration in their decision whether or not to smoke, drink, or use drugs.[14] Almost half of teens who never used marijuana credit their parents with their decision.[15] When asked what risks they associate with drug use, teens consistently rank "disappointing their parents" as a major risk. Unfortunately, one out of three parents mistakenly believe that talking to their children about drugs will not have much influence over their drug use.[16]

Parents who smoke, abuse alcohol, or use drugs themselves, or those for whom alcohol or drug abuse runs in the family, must recognize that their daughters are at higher than average risk for substance use. Other warning signs of increased risk reside in girls' own personalities and proclivities. Parents should be alert for signs of substance use if their daughters are depressed, anxious, eating too little or too much, or exhibiting signs of low self-esteem. Parents also should know that early puberty and other life stresses, such as moving often or transitioning from middle to high school, could hike the risk of substance use.[17]

Girls' behavior and performance in school also can provide clues to concerned parents. Girls who are rebellious or have conduct problems are likelier to use substances, as are girls who fare poorly academically. Moreover, parents should make sure they know who their daughters' friends are and try to ascertain whether their peers use cigarettes, alcohol, or drugs, as peer substance use is one of the leading risk factors for substance use in an individual child.[18]

Parents also should be aware of the cultural messages their daughters receive about substance use through television, movies, and advertising. While there is a fine line between monitoring and policing their children's actions, parents should be aware of the enormous impact these messages can have on their daughters' attitudes and be-

A CHECKLIST FOR PARENTS

- Set rules and expectations and enforce consequences.
- Don't accept drinking or drug use as rites of passage.
- Send clear messages about substance use.
- Discuss the negative consequences of substance use.
- Give your daughter perspective on media messages.
- Don't show your daughter that it takes a cigarette or drink to relax.
- Know your daughter's friends and where they go.
- Monitor use of TV and Internet.
- Eat dinner together.

Source: Adapted from The National Center on Addiction and Substance Abuse (CASA) at Columbia University. (2002). *Teen tipplers: America's underage drinking epidemic.* New York: CASA.

haviors and make sure to counteract pro-substance-use messages with accurate and healthful messages of their own.

Parents have a wide variety of tools at their disposal to protect their daughters against substance use and the pressures and concerns that might influence their daughters in that direction. Parents who create loving and healthy home environments, who expect their daughters to stay substance-free, who communicate honestly and openly, who set a good example, who are willing to use reasonable discipline when necessary, who know where their daughters are going and with whom, and who practice a family ritual as deceptively simple as just eating dinner together most nights are armoring their daughters against pressures to use substances and providing them with the tools they need to remain healthy.

Parents and families can take the following specific steps to help prevent girls from engaging in substance abuse.

SET HIGH EXPECTATIONS AND MAKE THEM KNOWN. Many parents are pessimistic about the likelihood that their children will refrain from drug use. Forty-one percent of parents report that future drug use by their teen is likely, but only 11 percent of teens believe they are likely to use drugs in the future. Perhaps unsurprisingly, teens whose parents think future drug use is "very likely" are more than three times likelier to smoke, drink, and use drugs than teens whose parents say future drug use is "not likely at all."[19]

COMMUNICATE OPENLY, CONSISTENTLY, AND HONESTLY. How parents communicate with their children and what they communicate by their words and actions can play a significant role in determining whether or not children use tobacco, alcohol, or drugs.[20] Positive parent-child relationships, including open and honest communication, warmth, and support, protect against substance use and abuse. Teenage girls tend to communicate more regularly and more openly with their parents—especially their mothers—than do boys.[21] Those girls who feel they can communicate openly and honestly with their parents are less likely than other girls to smoke, drink, or use drugs,[22] as are those who discuss with their parents the specific dangers of tobacco, alcohol, and drugs.[23]

SHOW DISAPPROVAL AND EXERCISE DISCIPLINE. Strong parental disapproval of substance use helps protect children from smoking, drinking, and using drugs.[24] For example, more than five times as many teens (46.6%) who say their parents would neither approve nor disapprove of their smoking one or more packs of cigarettes a day are current smokers compared to teens who say their parents would strongly disapprove (8.5%).[25] More than one-third of the girls and young women interviewed for CASA's *Formative Years* survey said that their parents "didn't really care or mind" when they found out that their daughters were smoking, drinking, or using drugs. This is in stark contrast to the beliefs of girls whose substance use had not yet been found out by their parents; less than five percent of girls predicted that their parents wouldn't care or mind if they found out their daughters were engaging in substance use (Figure 7.1).[26] Girls who perceive their parents as either highly disapproving of substance use—or who believed there would be disciplinary consequences if they engaged in substance use—get high less frequently and experiment with fewer drugs than other girls.[27]

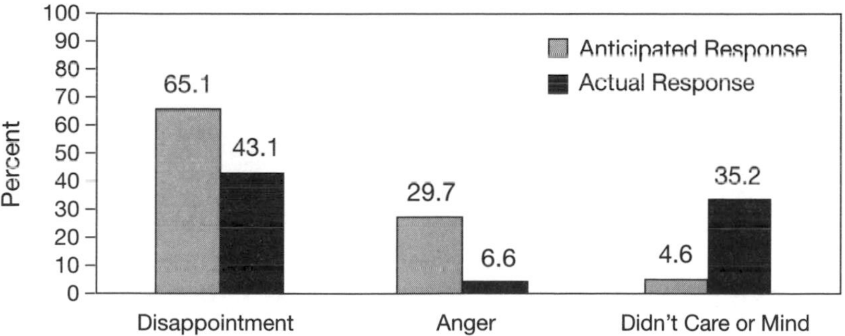

Fig. 7.1. Actual versus anticipated responses from parents on learning of daughters' substance use. *Source:* The National Center on Addiction and Substance Abuse (CASA) at Columbia University. (2003). *The formative years: Pathways to substance abuse among girls and young women ages 8–22*. New York: CASA. P. 56.

MONITOR BEHAVIOR. Parents are likelier with daughters than with sons to make sure that they know where their daughters are and with whom, to make family rules clear, to discuss instances of misbehavior, to praise achievements, and to refrain from disparaging them. Parents generally are less likely to allow their daughters to get away with misbehaving.[28] Girls whose parents monitor their activities and become involved in their everyday lives are at decreased risk of smoking, drinking, and using drugs. Highly involved parents tend to check homework, set curfews, and monitor friendships; the more often parents set clear rules for teens and enforce them, the less likely teens are to use drugs.[29]

SET A GOOD EXAMPLE. Children whose parents set good examples by avoiding substance use and conveying consistent messages against it are at substantially reduced risk of smoking, drinking, or using drugs. On the other hand, parents who smoke, abuse alcohol, or use drugs are more likely to have daughters and sons who do the same.[30] However, even those parents who smoke, drink, or use drugs should not throw up their hands helplessly. When substance-using parents convey strong anti-substance-abuse messages to children, they too can have an impact.[31]

BE AWARE OF THE RISKS. Parents who are knowledgeable about the risk factors for substance use in their children will be better equipped to offer firm yet reasonable guidance and to monitor carefully their children's behavior. Although some of the risks—such as depression or delinquent behaviors—are relatively obvious, others are less intuitive. For example, CASA's recent survey on teens and their parents found that teens who have more than $50 a week in spending money—in allowance or wages—are more likely to smoke, drink, and use marijuana than teens with less disposable income. This relationship is stronger in teen girls than teen boys.[32] High levels of stress and boredom also are implicated in increased risk for substance use among teens.[33]

PRACTICING WHAT YOU PREACH

If you don't want them to drink . . . but the message is, "this is what mommy does every single night," . . . when they go out into the world it's not going to be so foreign for them to say, "my mom drinks every night, I can drink every night." It really has to do with practicing what you preach.
—Jamie Lee Curtis, actor and recovering substance abuser

Source: Curtis, J. L., personal communication, April 9, 2003.

EAT DINNER TOGETHER. The family dinner contributes to and reinforces family bonds. CASA's research consistently demonstrates that teens who eat dinner with their families frequently (five to seven nights per week) are at half the risk of substance use as teens who have family dinners infrequently (two nights per week or less).[34] A study of urban minority sixth graders found that frequently eating dinner with the family was associated more strongly with less delinquency among girls than among boys, highlighting the importance of family dinners for protecting girls from substance use and other risky behaviors.[35]

For adolescent girls, eating dinner with family also can be beneficial in combating eating disorders, which are strongly associated with teenage substance use.[36] Parents have the opportunity to model healthy eating attitudes and behaviors and to monitor their daughters' eating behaviors during family meals. They also have a forum in which to help their daughters learn to value their attributes and develop a sense of comfort with their appearance, as well as to combat unhealthy societal messages.

FAMILIES OF COLLEGE WOMEN. Some parents may be under the mistaken impression that their opinions do not influence their children's behavior once they have begun the relatively autonomous lifestyle that college offers. Although there is limited research available, an emerging interest in this area has begun to reveal important examples of how parents can positively influence their college-age children.

For example, when parents talk to prospective college students about the dangers of binge drinking, how to deal with peers who drink, and how to recognize signs of a drinking problem, their children are less likely to drink, get drunk, and hold positive attitudes toward alcohol during their freshman year.[37] A recent CASA survey of college students found that, contrary to what most parents believe, 70 percent of students said that their parents' concerns or expectations either somewhat (30%) or very much (40%) influence whether or how much they smoke, drink, or use drugs. Those students who said they were more influenced by their parents' concerns or expectations smoked, drank, binge drank, and used marijuana significantly less than those who were influenced less by their parents.[38] Simple mother-teen conversations about how alcohol gets in the way of making true friends and how drinking makes problems worse instead of better decrease the chances that a college student will develop positive beliefs about alcohol, such as the belief that it enhances social behavior. Because having such positive beliefs is, in turn, associated with negative drinking consequences such as experiencing blackouts or regretting a sexual situation, such conversations can have a very real and quantifiable impact on the college student's quality of life.[39] Parents should make sure to talk to their daughters about how to handle drinking and other substance abuse in college *before* they leave home—as well as during the college years—

because the greatest increase in substance abuse among girls and young women occurs during the transition from high school to college.[40]

FAMILIES OF ADULT WOMEN. Older adults with alcohol or drug problems are less likely than younger adults to be socially disruptive, so their substance abuse is easier to overlook.[41] Family members may not recognize that aberrant behavioral symptoms stem from a substance abuse problem, and, even if they do, it can be deeply painful to admit that one's mother, grandmother, wife, or sister is an alcohol or drug abuser. Family members can help prevent substance use from turning into abuse and dependence by being alert to signs of trouble and by assisting older adults in getting treatment for substance abuse or for depression or other problems that might put them at high risk for substance abuse.

Schools and Colleges

For prevention efforts to be effective in the short and long terms, schools have to consider the prevention of substance use and abuse to be an integral part of the academic agenda rather than a small, isolated effort that takes place sporadically in single classroom sessions or school assemblies. Substance use prevention need not supplant traditional classroom learning. Rather, prevention efforts can be incorporated, at least in part, into regular academic activities. Although schools are overburdened and overwhelmed with competing priorities for the time, attention, and resources of students and teachers, schools do have the opportunity and responsibility to reinforce anti-substance-use messages that begin in the home or to provide such messages to those who do not receive them at home. Prevention is a school's business even if only because early prevention is key to ensuring academic success and to avoiding other consequences of student substance abuse, including conduct problems and school dropout.

ELEMENTARY, MIDDLE, AND HIGH SCHOOLS. Features of the school environment—school structure and policies, academic goals, curricula, teacher qualifications and attitudes, administrative support, level of parental and community involvement, availability of extracurricular activities, and the general characteristics of the student population—influence substance use among students. However, to provide girls with the most effective prevention efforts possible, teachers, administrators, and staff must know the signs and symptoms of substance use and be on the lookout for related problems.

Most current school-based prevention programs are narrowly defined, targeting only peer pressure, inaccurate beliefs, or low self-esteem. These programs fail to take into account the tremendous influence of parents, schools, communities, health care providers, the media, religious institutions, and government policies on girls and young women. Comprehensive programming that touches on all the key influencing agents in a child's life, while more difficult to implement, will be far more effective. Furthermore, most current programs are not culturally sensitive, delivering the same messages to girls of very different racial, ethnic, and cultural backgrounds. Prevention efforts should be sensitive to differences that affect substance abuse risk among black, white, Asian, and Hispanic girls, and recent immigrant girls or daughters of immigrants.

Few existing prevention programs are designed specifically for girls.[42] Even for those schools that do not implement gender-specific programming, certain factors unique to girls should be considered in their prevention efforts. School staff should be aware of the academic and social pressures many female students experience in order to provide them with effective means of stress management that do not involve self-medication. CASA has learned from numerous focus groups conducted with female elementary, middle, and high school students as well as with college students that girls and young women feel enormous pressure to succeed in school, and many describe substance use as a means of relieving some of the stress associated with this pressure. In fact, research shows that girls are more likely than boys to respond to stress with substance use, particularly smoking.[43]

Paying special attention to the needs of girls at risk—including those with learning disabilities, eating disorders, conduct problems, depression or anxiety, histories of physical or sexual abuse, poor academic performance, poor coping skills, or early sexual behavior, and those with a family history of substance use or other mental health problems—is the key to identifying and intervening early in the development of problem behavior. Because of their extensive contact with young people, schools are in a unique position to provide early identification, assessment, referral, and follow-up to those in need of support services. Zero-tolerance policies, which can mean suspension or expulsion for possession of tobacco, alcohol, and drugs, may inadvertently exacerbate the problem. The severe consequences may discourage teachers, parents, and other students from reporting a problem. Expulsion may simply transfer it from one place to another; if a private school cannot handle the problem, a child may be moved to a public school.[44] On the other hand, a connection to school helps girls avoid substance abuse and other delinquent behavior. School failure is more closely linked with delinquency for girls than for boys.[45] Life transitions—such as puberty, particularly early puberty, frequent moves from one home or neighborhood to another, or parental divorce—also are signs and times of increased risk of substance use in girls.

Schools should try to help students transition successfully between elementary and middle school and middle and high school. The move from elementary to middle school marks the greatest increase in girls' belief that smoking and drinking are ways to be rebellious and disobey adults, and the transition from middle school to high school marks the greatest increase in girls' belief that drinking alcohol is "cool."[46] Schools that help students move through these transitions by planning substance-free social activities, involving parents, and providing support and counseling if needed can help prevent student substance use.

A school environment that encourages students to set high yet attainable academic goals will encourage students to avoid substance use that interferes with the attainment of these goals. Encouraging students to become involved in extracurricular activities not only provides the opportunity for youth to broaden their interests and enrich their lives but also helps reduce key risk factors for substance use—boredom, delinquency, and low self-esteem.

Clear and consistent expectations for student behavior, particularly with regard to substance use, are critical for decreasing the likelihood that students will bring drugs to school, use drugs in school, or urge their friends to use drugs. Schools that provide clear and consistent expectations for student behavior, high levels of student attachment to schools, and clear messages about the unacceptability of tobacco, alcohol, and drug use are likely to witness improvements in students' academic performance and reductions in the numbers of students (and perhaps teachers and other staff members) engaged in substance use.

COLLEGES AND UNIVERSITIES. Too often, substance use prevention efforts end years before a girl goes to college—a time when she is likeliest to smoke, drink, and use drugs. Specific prevention messages obtained in grade school or high school may be outdated or no longer relevant to a college woman, leaving her open to the new pressures and circumstances she might face at a particularly vulnerable time in her life.

Although many students attending college no longer are minors, colleges and universities should not abdicate all responsibility for helping to protect their health and well-being. Mechanisms should be in place to identify and reach out to students who are abusing alcohol or drugs or are at high risk for doing so. College policies regarding substance use on and off campus should be made known to all students, faculty, staff, and administrators, and those policies should be enforced consistently and effectively.

Certain student characteristics that are linked to higher risk for substance abuse should be known to college administrators and addressed accordingly. College women at higher risk for alcohol use, for example, tend to be younger; freshmen are particularly likely to drink. Sorority members also are more likely than nonmembers to drink, binge drink, and use marijuana.[47] Screening should be done for students whose drinking could result in negative consequences, as well as for students who may already be on the road to alcohol abuse and addiction. Schools should be prepared to connect those students with appropriate treatment professionals.

Recent research has recommended a three-pronged approach to prevent abuse of alcohol, the substance that has received the most attention on college campuses due to the widespread nature of its abuse and its deadly consequences. To be effective, colleges should target individuals in the general student population and in the at-risk population, and shape campus policies and campus-community relations to create a supportive prevention environment.[48]

However, efforts to target individual students or even the larger student body will be relatively ineffective unless schools work to change the larger environment in which students learn and live. A general "culture of drinking" pervades campus society, tempting students to engage in unhealthy drinking behavior on and off campus. The formation of campus-community coalitions is one of the most promising vehicles for promoting environmental change. Schools should collaborate with their surrounding community to limit the availability and accessibility of alcohol.

Possible strategies include limiting the density of alcohol retail outlets in the surrounding community; restricting the hours of sale; prohibiting low-price alcohol promotions, such as "ladies' nights"; banning all alcohol advertising on campus from alcohol manufacturers or local alcohol retail establishments; offering alcohol-free social events; and ensuring consistent enforcement of campus and community alcohol policies and laws.

Too often, schools use haphazard approaches to preventing or controlling student substance use, many of which have not been tested for effectiveness.[49] To avoid this, schools should implement a reliable and valid system for monitoring, reviewing, and improving upon the effectiveness of their strategies and programs. Strategies and programs should be continually evaluated using rigorous research techniques. Schools allocate tremendous resources to researching and evaluating multiple aspects of their student bodies, funding streams, systems, and programs; substance use prevention should receive the same level of attention.

Physicians and Health Care Workers

Physicians, dentists, nurses, and other health professionals can have an enormous influence on a woman's quality of life by helping to identify, prevent, monitor, and provide treatment for substance use and related problems throughout the life span.

THE ROLE OF THE PHYSICIAN IN PREVENTING SUBSTANCE ABUSE IN WOMEN OF ALL AGES. Unfortunately, many primary care physicians fail to screen their patients carefully for substance abuse and, even more alarming, are likely to misdiagnose it. This is a true missed opportunity because research shows that even brief interventions can be effective in helping patients quit smoking or reduce their alcohol and drug use. Brief interventions may be particularly effective for women: one controlled study evaluated the impact of two 10- to 15-minute sessions in which physicians provided counseling and advice to encourage patients to reduce their alcohol use. Twelve months after the intervention, women reported reducing alcohol use by 31 percent and men reported cutting back by 14 percent.[50] Even dentists often can detect signs of a substance use or eating disorder during a routine checkup.

Medical schools, licensing boards, public and private insurers, and physicians must work together to make substance abuse training and screening a priority. In order to bring the level of physician care up to standard in terms of preventing substance abuse in women, greater institutional support must be provided in medical schools and in insurance companies, both public and private.[51] Without adequate training, funding, and available treatment resources, physicians will continue to miss the opportunity to prevent substance use and abuse in women.

INTERVENTION FOR GIRLS AND YOUNG WOMEN. Doctors have a built-in forum for providing education and screening that could effectively prevent substance use in teen girls. Health professionals should obtain family histories of substance abuse with all new patients and be alert to the increased risk of substance use in girls whose parents have smoked or abused alcohol or drugs. Health professionals are in a unique position to identify not only substance use risk but also behaviors and experiences associated with increased risk, including depression, anxiety, weight concerns, and risky sexual behavior, as well as one of the most pernicious risk factors for substance abuse in girls: sexual or physical abuse.[52]

Unfortunately, physician screening for adolescent substance use is uncommon. Fewer than one-third of pediatricians report asking about alcohol and drug use for over 80 percent of their patients 12 years old and over.[53] Studies show that even when physicians do screen for substance use, they are unlikely to provide guidance to their young patients.[54] One of the barriers to physician screening for adolescent substance abuse is the lack of a widely accepted screening tool.[55] However, even without the perfect screening instrument, concerned physicians can simply take a few minutes at each session to talk with their teenage patients about substance use and related risks and behaviors.

COLLEGE HEALTH CARE AND COUNSELING CENTERS. Campus health and counseling centers have a role to play in preventing substance use and abuse, particularly among young women. College women who have been raped report significantly higher levels of cigarette smoking, heavy drinking, and marijuana use,[56] and research consistently shows that substance abuse and depression are more likely to co-occur among women than men.[57] College campus health and counseling centers that encounter women who have been raped or who are struggling with depression should make sure to screen them for substance abuse risks and problems and to intervene if necessary.

The majority of students referred to substance abuse counseling for misbehavior are male (78%), but the majority of students referred after a substance-abuse-related medical emergency are female (57%). This disparity suggests that current intervention systems, at least at some colleges, are more suited to identifying at-risk students via disruptive substance-related behaviors such as vandalism or assault, which are more likely to occur among males. Female substance abusers exhibiting less overt risk behaviors and consequences may not be referred to counseling until alcohol poisoning or overdose has compromised their health.[58] It is possible that if college health and counseling centers more frequently screen at-risk females for alcohol and other substance abuse, they will begin to catch problems before they spiral out of control.

PREVENTING SUBSTANCE ABUSE DURING PREGNANCY. Pregnancy is a golden opportunity for physicians to interrupt risky substance use behavior before it causes too much damage to either the pregnant woman or her fetus. The best time to prevent smoking, drinking, and drug use is before conception, and as mentioned in chapter 5, many health organizations suggest that women abstain from cigarettes, alcohol, and drugs during their childbearing years. During the first trimester, when many women do not even realize they are pregnant, the fetus is particularly susceptible to the effects of tobacco, alcohol, and drugs. The association of alcohol and illicit drug use with amenorrhea (ceasing menstruation) may make it difficult for some women to use missed periods to determine if they are pregnant.

Prevention of fetal alcohol syndrome (FAS) requires educating all women of child bearing age about the dangers of alcohol use during pregnancy, as well as identifying and treating alcohol-abusing women before they become pregnant. One way that doctors and other health professionals can identify a woman at risk for having a child with FAS is to evaluate her older children. The chance that an alcohol-abusing woman will have a child with FAS is about 6 percent; however, if her first child was born with FAS, the odds jump to 70 percent for the next child.[59]

When efforts to deter tobacco, alcohol, or drug use before conception fail, discouraging continued substance use or abuse among pregnant women and, if necessary, referring them to treatment can reduce the risk of further damage to the fetus. A woman who stops smoking, drinking, or using drugs during pregnancy can improve the overall health of the fetus and increase the birth weight. Fortunately, CASA's survey *Missed Opportunity* found that physicians are more vigilant about screening for substance use in their pregnant patients: more than 87 percent say they discuss tobacco use with almost all of their pregnant patients, and more than 78 percent discuss alcohol use and drug use, including illegal, over-the-counter, and prescription drugs.[60]

OLDER WOMEN. Physicians, as trusted professionals, are in the perfect position to educate older female patients about the benefits of smoking cessation, safe use of alcohol and prescription drugs, and the consequences of abuse; to encourage them to reduce excessive use of these substances; and to prescribe pharmaceuticals with prudence.

Unfortunately, while most physicians screen patients on their first visits for smoking and alcohol, prescription drug, and over-the-counter drug use, their attention to such sensitive issues usually begins and ends there. Among women 65 and over who had a checkup within the last year, only 17 percent said their physician had asked about drinking.[61] Despite heavy use of prescription drugs by older adults, some physicians devote less attention to drug counseling for them than for younger adults. Even well-educated older adults lack adequate information about the safe use of their prescription drugs.[62]

Doctors' extraordinary influence places on them the responsibility to spot signs of substance abuse in older female patients and encourage them to seek appropriate treatment. Research shows that brief physician counseling to encourage older women to reduce risky drinking, address a drinking problem, or quit smoking increases the chances she will do so. Unfortunately, many physicians fail to meet their responsibility.

Physicians may not correctly identify substance use problems in older women for a variety of reasons. Knowledge plays a part. When asked to define what constitutes problem drinking, physicians do not differentiate between older and younger women, or between men and women. The average number of drinks per day that physicians say would constitute problem drinking are virtually equal for women age 60 and over, women age 40 to 60, and men age 40 to 60. Attitudes and opinions influence physician behavior as well;[63] and even more so than younger women, the older female patient may do her best to conceal or deny a problem with alcohol or drugs, complicating the physician's ability to identify and treat it.

So what should physicians be doing to identify trouble in older patients? One clue might be an unexpected response or no response to a prescribed medicine. If a physician is prescribing tranquilizers, sedatives, or antidepressants for anxiety, insomnia, or depression without treating the underlying alcohol problem that is causing the symp-

QUESTIONS PHYSICIANS CAN ASK THEIR OLDER FEMALE PATIENTS TO SCREEN FOR PRESCRIPTION DRUG ABUSE

- Do you see more than one health care provider regularly? Why?
- Have you switched doctors recently? Why?
- What prescription drugs are you taking? Are you having any problems with them?
- Where do you get your prescriptions filled? Do you go to more than one pharmacy?
- Do you use any nonprescription medications? If so, which, why, how much, how often, and how long?

Source: The National Center on Addiction and Substance Abuse (CASA) at Columbia University. (1998). *Under the rug: Substance abuse and the mature woman.* New York: CASA.

toms, the therapy is unlikely to succeed, and the prescription in combination with alcohol may endanger the patient.

Older women rely most heavily on primary care physicians for treatment of depression; few ever see a mental health specialist.[64] The risk of inappropriate prescribing for depression is greatest among primary care doctors; they are most likely to prescribe psychoactive medications without documenting the mental disorder that is prompting the prescription.[65] The lack of mental health counseling may compromise the treatment of women's depression. In turn, allowing the depression to persist hikes the risk of substance abuse and addiction for these women. If the patient seems confused about her prescriptions, sees more than one doctor, uses more than one pharmacy, or seems reluctant to discuss her drug use, closer assessment is warranted.

Pharmacists can assist in prevention by monitoring an older woman's prescriptions and notifying her and her physicians of duplication or unsafe combinations of medications.[66] However, physicians, pharmacists, and other health care workers often fail to provide clear information and advice on how to take a medication appropriately.[67] According to a national survey of primary care physicians and patients, 47 percent of physicians reported finding it difficult to discuss prescription drug abuse with their patients.[68] This is partly because health care professionals often are not well educated about the dangers and signs of prescription drug misuse, abuse, and addiction.[69] That more than one out of six Medicare beneficiaries receives an inappropriate prescription is unacceptable.[70]

To avoid dangerous reactions to mixing alcohol and a drug, or two or more drugs, health professionals should monitor older female patients' drinking habits and medications before writing prescriptions. Such an assessment may be required at each visit because an older adult's prescription drug regimen tends to change frequently.[71] Because older women who take several medications at once may have difficulty remembering what they take and when, some doctors suggest trying the "brown bag" approach in which they ask the patient or her caregiver to fill a brown paper bag with everything in her medicine cabinet.[72] The doctor then can use this inventory to discern what the patient is taking and how often. A woman's pharmacist also can help inform her of the safe use of a drug and the risks of using it in combination with alcohol.[73]

Unfortunately there are no custom-made screening tools to detect alcohol or prescription drug problems in older women. Physicians can choose from two diagnostic tools that have been proven to be reasonably effective in detecting alcohol problems among older adults of both sexes: the CAGE questionnaire and the MAST-G (Michigan Alcohol Screening Test—Geriatric Version). Because an effective screening tool for prescription drug abuse among older adults does not exist, physicians must use their diagnostic intuition and communication skills to detect signs of trouble with prescriptions.

Advertising and the Entertainment Media

Girls and women increasingly have become advertising targets for tobacco products and alcoholic beverages. Manufacturers have linked cigarettes with thinness and rebellion and alcohol with independence and sexual freedom. In movies and television, positive or consequence-free depictions of cigarette, alcohol, and even illicit drug use may demonstrate to girls and women that substance use is fun, or at least not harmful.

Advertisers and the entertainment media should refrain from linking smoking and drinking with unrealistically thin images of women, or with sex appeal, as well as refrain from presenting glamorous images of women smoking and drinking. If female characters do smoke or drink, the negative consequences of such conduct should be depicted.

Advertisers should not promote or advertise alcohol on college campuses, where significant portions of students are underage. Alcohol industry sponsorship of campus events and alcohol promotions and advertising on campus send students the message that alcohol use is acceptable and not inconsistent with academic and athletic goals. If advertisers will not do so voluntarily, schools should ban all alcohol advertising and promotions on campus.[74]

Because smoking is legal for the majority of college students, a troubling new development is the direct promotion of cigarettes and smokeless tobacco by tobacco companies to students. These promotions include handing out free lighters or packs of cigarettes and sponsoring social events at fraternities, bars, clubs, or campus venues.[75] Although there is a limit to what colleges can do to prevent tobacco promotions in neighborhood bars or clubs, tobacco companies should be prohibited from marketing directly to students at college-sponsored events, college bars, or fraternity/sorority parties.

Substance abuse prevention campaigns, which convey their messages through television, radio, or print ads, are making an effort to counteract pro-smoking and drinking media messages targeting women, particularly adolescents. These campaigns can help counter the ads that play up the sex appeal and attractiveness of smoking women. Some of the media prevention campaigns use attractive, non-substance-using famous women. Female athlete Venus Williams, popular singer Jessica Simpson, and actor Brooke Shields convey anti-substance-use messages and try to serve as positive role models for girls and young women. Other television, radio, and print campaigns use fear tactics; they try to discourage substance abuse by pointing out the damage that tobacco, alcohol, and drugs do to women's bodies. The Office of National Drug Control Policy and the Partnership for a Drug-Free America have a National Youth Anti-Drug Media Campaign that includes various radio, television, and print advertisements targeted to young people, teachers, and parents. For example, one print ad features Simpson stating that she "doesn't smoke weed." The smaller print states, "Respect, goals and motivation are not things I want to lose over drugs."[76] A Partnership for a Drug-Free America ad shows a lively young woman pictured against a backdrop of her own death certificate showing that she died from Ecstasy. The fine print says, "Ecstasy is not a recreational drug. It's a lethal drug. It killed Danielle."[77]

The *Truth* antismoking media campaign was launched by the American Legacy Foundation in 2000 with funding from the Public Education Fund, which was established by the tobacco industry in the wake of the Master Settlement Agreement (MSA) between tobacco companies and the states. The campaign provides youth with facts about nicotine addiction and the tobacco industry's marketing practices.[78] Young girls frequently cite antidrug advertising campaigns as well as certain family television programs as sources of information about drugs and reasons not to take them.[79]

Many of these prevention efforts were and still are developed with the help of teens. One such program, *At Face Value*—which is sponsored by the Task Force for Tobacco-Free Women and Girls in New York State—vividly demonstrates the impact smoking can have on a woman's appearance. The underlying message of the program, that staying tobacco-free can help a woman be wrinkle-free, was the result of a statewide school essay contest. Through computer imaging, a young girl's face is shown next to her face in 30 years; the pictures show what she will look like if she never smokes compared with if she becomes a heavy smoker. Preliminary results have been promising.[80]

Some campaigns emphasize the toll substance abuse can take on a girl's family and social life. Although many of these media prevention campaigns clearly are memorable and emotional, their long-term impact remains unclear.[81] More research is needed about the efficacy of prevention media campaigns on young people in general and on girls and young women in particular.

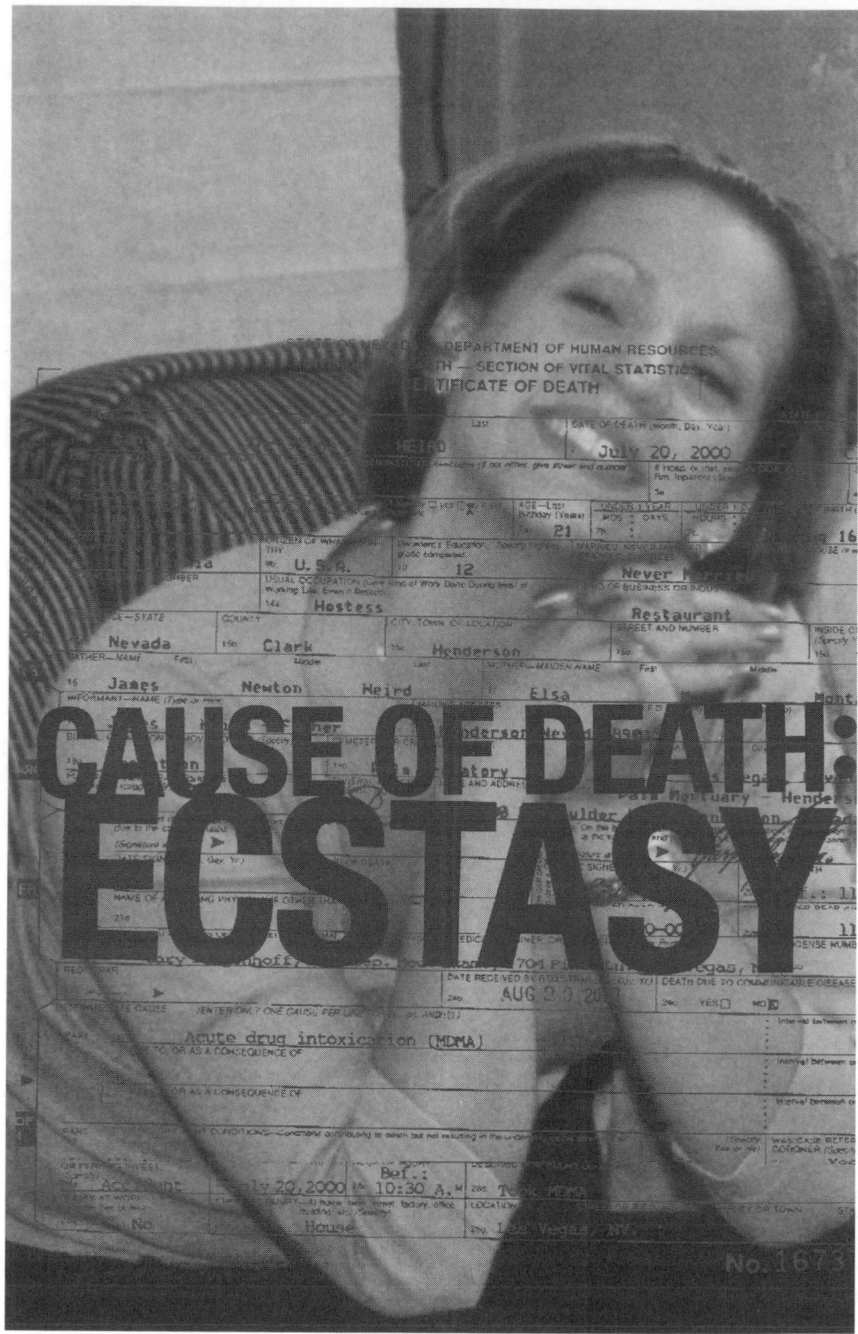

Fig. 7.2. National Youth Anti-Drug Media Campaign advertisement. *Source:* Public service announcement provided courtesy of the Partnership for a Drug-Free America.

I don't smoke weed
Respect, goals, and motivation are not things I want to lose over drugs.
Pop Singer: Jessica Simpson
Office of National Drug Control Policy
Partnership for a Drug-Free America

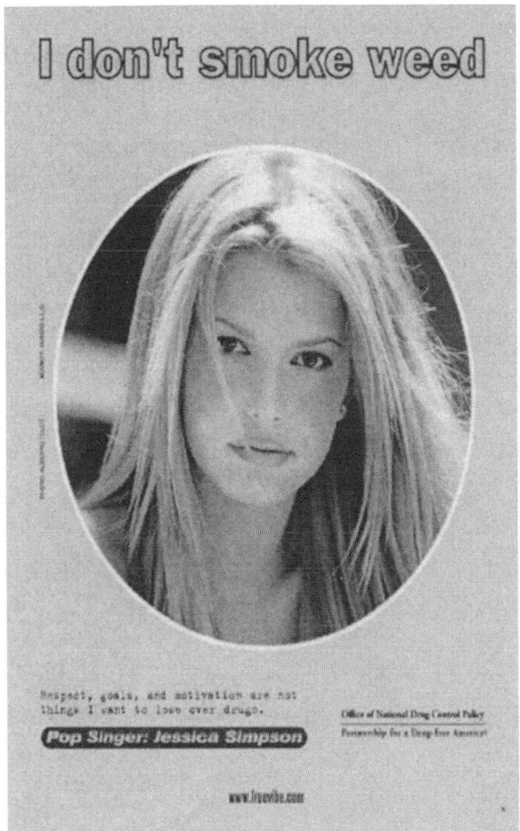

Fig. 7.3. Partnership for a Drug-Free America advertisement. *Source:* Public service announcement provided courtesy of the Partnership for a Drug-Free America.

Researchers

Although there have been marked changes since the 1970s, failure to include women in most research on substance use and abuse has left health care and public health professionals, policy makers, and women themselves without the knowledge they need to prevent or treat the problem. Researchers need to investigate remaining questions about the consequences of tobacco, alcohol, and drug use for women of all ages. Failure to explore key gender differences results in prevention efforts that at best are not optimally effective and at worst are completely ineffective or even harmful.

RESEARCH ON PREVENTION FOR GIRLS AND YOUNG WOMEN. One reason effective programming for girls is so limited is that girls and young women have been largely neglected by researchers who, more often than not, either focus only on boys or lump girls and boys together in their studies of the pathways to substance abuse, the consequences of such abuse, and how to prevent and treat it.

RESEARCH ON SUBSTANCE USE AND ABUSE IN COLLEGE STUDENTS AND YOUNG ADULT WOMEN. Preliminary research among college students supports the efficacy of brief parental interventions, particularly between high school and college, but more information is needed on precisely how these conversations and lessons should be delivered and how effective they are with daughters particularly. Additionally, research must be conducted to examine how universities, particularly university health centers, can reach out to campus women and engage them in substance-abuse prevention efforts, as well as how to reach out to high-risk college women for whom the need for timely intervention is more acute. Research in the area of young adult female substance abuse prevention is nearly nonexistent and sorely needed. Topics that should be addressed include determining the venues through which women in this age group might best be reached, the experiences and life circumstances that might be markers for substance use or abuse, and who is best equipped and qualified to identify and prevent substance abuse in these women.

RESEARCH ON SUBSTANCE USE AND ABUSE IN OLDER WOMEN. Gerontology is a growing field, and its leaders need to pay greater attention to the substance abuse problems of older adults.[82] Particularly needed is clinical and epidemiological research on the extent of alcohol abuse and alcoholism and the extent, correlates, causes, and consequences of psychoactive prescription and over-the-counter drug abuse and addiction among older women. Opening these doors of knowledge will inform efforts to assure that every older woman uses the drugs she needs safely and effectively.

Research on the role of race/ethnicity and income in the development of substance abuse and addiction among older women also is needed, as is further study of smoking and alcohol and prescription drug abuse in active retirement communities. With so little known about these problems, such communities may inadvertently aggravate the problem with social events that encourage heavy drinking and staff physicians who look the other way. But the evidence is largely anecdotal. We need solid research to inform prevention and treatment efforts that are effective in these settings.

Policy Makers

The preceding sections have described what various individuals and institutions can do to identify and circumvent risk from developing into actual substance use and abuse among girls and women. Policy makers have the opportunity to help achieve these goals and the responsibility to encourage the advancement of prevention efforts designed specifically to meet the needs of women. Research supports the notion that at each stage of life women use substances and experience consequences from that use differently from men, and policy efforts to prevent substance abuse in girls and women need to reflect those differences. In many areas, policy efforts may need to focus on providing the funding necessary to more fully explore and address gender differences.

REGULATION. One of the keys to preventing substance abuse has been and will continue to be regulation. Efforts to protect children, pregnant women, and nonsmokers over the last forty years have had an immensely beneficial effect on the lives of millions of Americans, but there's still work to be done.

Because of its enormous power in shaping public perception and reaching a wide audience of girls and women, the advertising industry and entertainment media can serve as a positive force in substance abuse education. While parents have a responsibility to instill in their daughters media literacy that will allow them to judge such advertisements and depictions of substance use with the suspicion that they deserve, the mass media as a whole also has a responsibility to American girls. If advertisers and television and movie producers will not supply positive messages on their own, advertising and media reform should be implemented so that public health trumps profits, and parent and school messages about the dangers of substance use are not undermined by the media.

In 2001, tobacco companies spent $11.2 billion, or more than $30 million per day, on advertising and promotion. This expenditure amounted to more than $39 for each person in the United States, or $241 for each adult smoker, and was a 17 percent increase over the previous year.[83] In 2002, the alcohol industry spent $409 million—nearly one-quarter of its $2 billion in advertising monies—on magazine advertising alone.[84] Hundreds of magazines in which cigarettes and alcohol are promoted reach young readers. Magazines with high proportions of young female readers should refuse advertisements from cigarette and alcohol companies and include more articles discussing the dangers of smoking, drinking, and excessive dieting. It is doable. For example, currently, magazines such as *Good Housekeeping* and newspapers such as the *Boston Globe,* the *New York Times,* the *San José Mercury News,* the *Seattle Times* and the *Honolulu Star-Bulletin* do not run tobacco ads.[85] However, because they reach a more mature audience, their effect on young potential users is minimal.

In 2002, the alcohol industry spent $58 million on 6,251 television ads for college sports programming.[86] Recently, the Center for Science in the Public Interest launched a campaign to end television alcohol advertising during college sports. They found that

7 in 10 Americans believe that beer companies know that their ads appeal to underage drinkers, and two-thirds believe that beer companies advertise during sporting events to reach underage drinkers. In addition, 71 percent of Americans are in favor of a ban on all alcohol advertising during televised college games.[87] In a national survey conducted by CASA, almost three-quarters of respondents (74%) supported some version of a policy that would restrict alcohol advertising. Support was stronger among females (80%) than among males (69%). The alcohol industry has a significant financial interest in underage and adult excessive drinking in the amount of 48.9 percent of consumer expenditures for alcohol. Because of this conflict of interest with the public health, high drinking rates among underage drinkers, and the association between alcohol and violence—particularly sexual violence against women—policy makers should institute regulatory controls to protect underage youth from exposure to industry sales and advertising practices, require prominent warning labels on all alcohol advertisements, and require the inclusion of federal dietary guidelines regarding consumption on all product labels, including the caloric content of the product.[88]

The Internet also plays a significant role in the fastest growing drug problem in the United States—prescription drug abuse. Many Web sites not only sell them but also offer online prescribing services—a risky practice according to the Food and Drug Administration. Hundreds of other Web sites *illegally* sell prescription drugs without requiring any prescriptions or offering prescription services.[89]

This is such a new phenomenon that laws have not yet kept pace with the problem, and there is little, if any, regulation. A recent CASA study found that during a one-week period in 2004, 495 Web sites directly or indirectly offered customers controlled—abusable and addictive—prescription drugs. The most commonly sold on the Internet were CNS depressants—sedatives and tranquilizers such as Valium and Xanax—followed by opioid pain killers such as Vicodin and Percocet, and stimulants such as Ritalin and Adderall. Most of these Web sites (68%) were "portal" sites and did not directly sell these drugs but linked the potential buyers to other sites that did. But almost one-third of these sites were "anchor" sites that directly sold these controlled drugs. Most (94%) of these sites did not require a prescription; 49 percent offered an "online consultation."[90] A replication of this analysis one year later found that illegal Internet drug availability had not decreased; rather, there appeared to be even greater availability of opioids online.

With 85 percent of teenagers and young adults regularly surfing the Web, the Internet poses a tremendous challenge to those interested in preventing substance abuse.[91] And the ranks of the technologically savvy are expanding. An estimated eight million U.S. senior citizens (65 years and over) use the Internet.[92] For older Americans who may be living in isolation or are incapacitated, the Internet provides an open window to the outside world, an instant means of communication and an easy way to shop without leaving home. Once online, they can order discounted prescription drugs without having to see their doctors for a prescription or go to a drug store. While this can be tremendously beneficial, it also has the potential to create or exacerbate problems of drug misuse and abuse. Research has shown that there is a strong connection between the availability of drugs and subsequent drug abuse and addiction.[93] Policy makers must regulate the Internet industry more effectively and give law enforcement the funding and support they need to address the problem.

The Internet also provides an easy way to obtain cheaper, untaxed cigarettes and alcohol. One study found that children who tried to buy cigarettes online without a valid I.D. were successful 94 percent of the time.[94] The purchase of alcohol over the Internet also is a tremendous problem. Buying alcohol over the Internet and ordering alcohol for home delivery presently can occur without the purchaser presenting proof of age. Few studies have documented the prevalence of these methods of acquiring alcohol among children, but one study found that 10 percent of twelfth graders and 7.3 percent of 18 to 20 year olds reported using these services.[95]

As with cigarettes, proposed methods for regulating home delivery of alcohol include having deliverers obtain and record the purchaser's identification information, such as a driver's license, and having a purchaser sign a statement affirming that he or she is age 21 or older.[96]

TAXATION. "Sin" taxes on alcohol and tobacco are used by states to raise revenue, but they also have a tremendous impact on smoking and drinking. For example, alcohol consumption among the general population appears to decline as the price of alcohol goes up.[97] Particularly for younger drinkers with less ready cash, increases in the purchase price of alcohol limits its accessibility. Also, a study of pregnant women found that they reacted more strongly than the larger adult population to increases in cigarette taxes. For every 10 percent increase in the price of cigarettes, smoking rates among pregnant women fall by 7 percent. Smoking among pregnant white women, older women, and highly educated women was influenced most by a tax increase.[98]

BANS. The fundamental commercial strategy to limit underage drinking is to ban commercial sales and gifts of alcohol to minors, including prohibiting the sale of alcohol to minors even if accompanied by an adult. Currently, commercial sales of alcohol to minors are banned in all states, but exceptions are made in certain states when a minor is accompanied by an adult or when a minor has written authorization from a parent. A complete ban on sales and gifts to minors would help eliminate these disparities and eliminate the incentive for teens to cross state lines to obtain alcohol (and possibly drive home while under the influence). Another approach is to restrict minors' access to establishments that sell alcohol.[99]

BARRING SMOKING IN BARS

New York City's Mayor Michael Bloomberg succeeded in banning all indoor smoking, including in bars. The previous law, passed in 1995, banned smoking in restaurants with more than 35 seats, but bar areas and stand-alone bars were exempt. The new law does not offer these exemptions. According to the mayor's office, working for eight hours in a smoke-filled bar is equivalent to smoking a half a pack of cigarettes a day. Bloomberg believes that bartenders, waitresses, and waiters should have the same opportunity of working in a smoke-free environment as other employees have. Bloomberg posed the following to the New York City Council, "Does your desire to smoke anywhere, at any time trump the right of others to breathe clean air in the workplace? Common sense and common decency demand the following answer: The need to breathe clean air is more important than the license to pollute it."

Source: New York City Office of the Mayor. (2002). *Mayor Michael R. Bloomberg testifies before City Council in favor of 2002 Smoke-free Air Act.* [Press release, October 2002]. New York: New York City Office of the Mayor.

The recent increase in state- and local-level bans on smoking in public places has proven controversial; however, the immediate outcries of the potential for these bans to ruin local businesses—particularly bars—appears to have been somewhat overblown. Furthermore, small studies of the health benefits of these bans are providing increasing evidence of their dramatic effects, even in the short term.

For example, in Helena, Montana, a six-month smoking ban allowed for a simple investigation of its effects. Researchers were able to document the rate of hospital admissions for heart attacks before and after the ban was in effect and found a 40 percent reduction in heart attacks during the ban compared to the average number of heart attacks recorded for the same six-month period in the four years before the ban and in the year after it (from 40 to 24). No similar decline in heart attacks was found for people living outside Helena, where the ban was not in effect.[100] Although this study has limitations—it is not a randomized controlled study, it is based on a small sample, and it did not measure patients' exposure to tobacco smoke—it does provide preliminary evidence for the potential health benefits of smoking bans. Further evidence comes from a recent survey of tobacco use in New York City, where large tobacco tax increases, bans on smoking in bars and other public areas, and improved smoking cessation resources have been credited with a decline in the number of smokers over the course of one year from 22 percent of adults to 19 percent, representing 100,000 fewer smokers in all parts of the city, across both genders, and in all ages and ethnic groups.[101]

Perhaps once more concrete evidence of this nature accumulates in those areas where bans have been put into effect, policy makers will begin to face less resistance to efforts to improve public health by protecting people from the immediate and long-term dangers of exposure to secondhand smoke. Such bans also may reduce the amount and frequency of tobacco use among smokers, providing further health benefits even to those who choose not to quit.

LAW ENFORCEMENT. There are many strategies to limit underage drinkers' and smokers' access to cigarettes and alcohol. Law enforcement plays an important role on the street. Various undercover strategies may be used to test retailers' compliance with laws regarding the sale of alcohol to minors ("compliance checks"), to catch minors asking strangers to purchase alcohol for them ("shoulder tap"), or to catch minors who try to purchase alcohol ("cops in shops").[102]

Another proposed method for deterring teen possession is to strictly enforce bans on the possession and use of false identification. One study found that over one-third (36%) of underage high school and college students have used some form of false identification.[103] Local policy makers and college administrations should work together to ensure a strong law enforcement presence in and around universities and colleges, especially during sporting events when underage alcohol use rates are particularly high.

EDUCATION AND ANTI-SUBSTANCE-USE CAMPAIGNS. Comprehensive substance-control programs have been shown to be effective in reducing substance abuse. For example, Arizona, California, Florida, Maine, Massachusetts, and Oregon have created science-based tobacco control programs that include such strategies as interventions targeted at children and teens in hospitals and other health care facilities; referrals to treatment specialists with childcare and transportation provided; media campaigns, hotlines, Web sites, and educational materials; and partnerships among local, state, and regional government and community agencies.[104] These programs have effectively reduced smoking rates among girls and women.[105] From 1988 to 1997, lung cancer rates among women declined by 5 percent in California but increased by 13 percent elsewhere in the United States.[106] However, 44 states still lack such programs. Policy makers should push for greater funding and support for programs that address smoking and drinking and that target the needs of girls and women at the state level.

One program that has been enormously successful but is in danger of losing its funding is the *Truth* antismoking media campaign of the American Legacy Foundation. Currently, the tobacco companies are no longer required to make payments to the fund that supports this campaign because their market share dropped just below the threshold required by the Master Settlement Agreement. In March 2004, all the living former U.S. Secretaries of Health, U.S. Surgeons General, and Directors of the Centers for Disease Control and Prevention formed the Citizens' Commission to Protect the Truth with the goal of collecting one million petition signatures in support of its effort to demand that the funding continue. The commission is filing amicus briefs in appropriate tobacco litigation and asking courts to order tobacco companies to provide funds for the *Truth* campaign as one of the remedies for tobacco company misconduct. Policy makers should back this effort and find a way to ensure continued funding for the one of few evidence-based anti-substance-use campaigns that works.

Finally, educating the public remains critical. States with bold prevention programs show greater reductions in tobacco consumption than states that have not adequately funded tobacco prevention. A 2003 report found that only Maine, Maryland, Minnesota, and Mississippi funded tobacco prevention annually within the Centers for Disease Control's recommended range for funding. Michigan, Missouri, Tennessee, and the District of Columbia had not committed any annual funds to tobacco prevention. In fact, most states are not on track to meet the U.S. Department of Health and Human Services' Healthy People 2010 prevention agenda as it relates to women and smoking.[107]

TRAINING. Policy makers should encourage organizations like the American Medical Association (AMA), the American Dental Association (ADA), and the American Pharmacists Association (APA) to help develop federal screening guidelines and instruments for doctors, dentists, and pharmacists that target substance use and abuse, particularly prescription drug abuse, in girls and women. Despite an increase in educational initiatives about prescription drug abuse, there remains a need to educate health care professionals to better understand and address this problem with their patients. Physician, nursing, and pharmacy licensing and certifying boards—including residency training, postgraduate fellowship, and continuing medical education—should create strong requirements regarding substance abuse and addiction education. These requirements should include training in knowledge, attitudes, and skills, training on how to deal with the problem in male and female individuals of all ages, and training on all types of substances of abuse. Questions about substance abuse should be on every exam for licensing, license renewal, or registration for physicians, nurses, and other health professionals.

In addition, training people who distribute cigarettes and alcohol to deal with underage drinkers and smokers is very important. Program curriculum requirements of this nature may include staff notification and acknowledgment of legal responsibility and consequences of violation, identification check procedures for individuals who appear to be underage, and checks by store management to ensure compliance with regulations. In certain states, retailers who participate in these types of programs avoid legal responsibility for harm to underage patrons who are served alcohol illegally.[108] Although evaluations of the effectiveness of responsible beverage service training have been inconclusive, there has been strong evidence that they are effective in curbing sales to minors when properly enforced.[109]

FINANCIAL SUPPORT AND INCENTIVES. Often overlooked is the necessity of financial support and incentives for policy change. The government can make the efforts of health professionals more effective by reimbursing them to perform screenings for substance abuse and other health risk behaviors that affect girls and young women and mandating that insurance companies do so. Medicare, Medicaid, private insurers, and managed care organizations should pay physicians to talk to patients about substance abuse and reimburse patients for the cost of treatment. Without institutional support to address the lack of money to compensate physicians for their efforts, physician training alone will be insufficient. Unless Medicare, managed care organizations, and other insurers pay for treatment, older adults with alcohol and drug problems will continue to be recognized only when they need to be hospitalized for the costly consequences—the heart attacks, cancer, and hip fractures—that disable women and take their lives.

To ensure that all colleges and universities commit to making alcohol control a priority, federal and state governments should consider making some portion of funding for public institutions contingent on their implementation of an effective alcohol control program; holding colleges and universities legally liable for consequences of student drinking (e.g., property damage, accidents, sex crimes, death); and requiring institutions to notify parents of underage students who have violated school alcohol policies.

Finally, the government should increase its support of research that focuses on women, particularly girls and older women. The National Institutes of Health and other funders should expand research on alcohol, psychoactive prescription drug, and over-the-counter drug use and abuse among older women, as well as substance abuse treatment and smoking cessation strategies for them.

Not only would women benefit from policy makers' efforts to curb substance abuse but a national survey of adults indicates that women consistently are more supportive than males of various actual and proposed alcohol control policies and efforts.[110] This is not too surprising if one considers how substance abuse adversely affects women and casts a pall over their own and their family members' health, financial resources, and well-being. Policy makers should capitalize on this enormous base of support and rally mothers, daughters, wives, and sisters to the cause of curbing smoking, excessive drinking, and drug use in their own and in others' families across the nation.

Conclusion

Six million girls and women (ages 12 and older) abuse or are addicted to alcohol, 15 million use illicit drugs (including the misuse of prescription drugs), and 32 million smoke cigarettes.[111] Unless America recognizes substance abuse and addiction as public health problems that can be prevented and treated, these numbers will continue to climb. We have the means and the intellectual and community resources to eliminate this immense problem, saving millions of lives and improving the quality of life for millions more girls, women, and their families. What we need is the will to do so.

nowledgments acknowledgments

The National Center on Addiction and Substance Abuse (CASA) at Columbia University expresses its appreciation to the Bristol-Myers Squibb Foundation, Inc., and particularly to CASA board member Peter Dolan, the company's chief executive officer, and John Damonti, president of the foundation, who had the insight and courage to fund all three of CASA's studies on substance abuse and women and to make this book possible. This research is an important part of the foundation's larger commitment to women's health in our nation and the world. We also greatly appreciate the help of our distinguished advisory panels for each of CASA's three reports on substance abuse and women.

This book, and the policy research on which it is based, was prepared under the direction of Susan E. Foster, M.S.W., CASA's vice president and director of policy research and analysis. She was assisted by Linda Richter, Ph.D., senior research manager; Jeanne Reid, former senior research associate; Joan Liebmann-Smith, Ph.D., writer; Sally Mays and Rachel Adams, research assistants; Heather Horowitz, research associate; and Tisha Hooks, editor. Other CASA staff who contributed were David Man, Ph.D., librarian; Ivy Truong, library research associate; Barbara Kurzweil, library research specialist; Alex Greenshields, bibliographic database manager; and Jane Carlson and Jennie Hauser, who handled the administrative responsibilities.

Although many individuals and institutions contributed to this effort, the findings and opinions expressed herein are the sole responsibility of CASA.

appendix appendix appendix appendix appendix

Resources

Finding Treatment

Addiction Resource Guide
www.addictionresourceguide.com

This site lists substance abuse treatment facilities that provide individualized care and cater to women only or address problems that may be particularly relevant for women, including domestic violence, pregnancy, overeating, anorexia, or bulimia.

American Society of Addiction Medicine (ASAM)
www.asam.org

ASAM is the nation's medical specialty society dedicated to educating physicians and improving the treatment of individuals suffering from alcoholism and other addictions. The Web site is geared to health professionals; however, it also contains helpful consumer information, including links to an extensive list of recovery and treatment centers.

SAMHSA Substance Abuse Treatment Facility Locator
http://findtreatment.samhsa.gov

This Substance Abuse and Mental Health Services Administration (SAMHSA) site allows visitors to search for substance abuse treatment facilities by location and then to narrow the field further to facilities just for women or that offer free assistance.

Self-Help Recovery Programs

Alcoholics Anonymous (AA)
www.alcoholics-anonymous.org

Alcoholics Anonymous is a fellowship of men and women who share their experience, strength, and hope with each other that they may solve their common problem and help others to recover from alcoholism. This site provides information about the AA program.

Al-Anon/Alateen Family Groups
www.al-anon.alateen.org

This fellowship is for people who have been affected by someone else's drinking—parents, children, spouses, partners, brothers, sisters, other family members, friends, employers, employees, and co-workers of alcoholics. The site provides information about the programs and how to locate a meeting in your area.

Narcotics Anonymous (NA)
www.na.org

Modeled after Alcoholics Anonymous, Narcotics Anonymous is a nonprofit fellowship of men and women who are recovering addicts who meet regularly to help each other stay clean. NA is open to any drug addict who wishes to become drug-free, regardless of the particular drug or combination of drugs used. This site contains information on meeting locations.

Nicotine Anonymous
www.nicotine-anonymous.org

Nicotine Anonymous is a nonprofit fellowship of men and women helping each other live nicotine-free lives. Nicotine Anonymous welcomes all those seeking freedom from nicotine addiction, including those using cessation programs and nicotine withdrawal aids. The primary purpose of Nicotine Anonymous is to help all those who would like to cease using tobacco and nicotine products in any form.

Prescription Anonymous, Inc.
www.prescriptionanonymous.org

Rx Anonymous is a voluntary fellowship of men and women who have taken a pledge to carry a message of hope to the millions of people who suffer from addiction to prescription drug and/or other mood-altering substances. The Web site offers online support, news, and information.

Women for Sobriety
www.womenforsobriety.org

Women for Sobriety is a nonprofit self-help organization of women dedicated to helping other women overcome alcoholism and other addictions. This Web site helps women locate a New Life Program meeting close to them.

Information—General

American Cancer Society
www.cancer.org

Homepage of the American Cancer Society, this site provides information about the links between addiction and cancer.

American Council for Drug Education
www.drughelp.org

DrugHelp is a private, nonprofit information and referral network providing information on specific drugs and treatment options and referrals to public and private treatment programs, self-help groups, family support groups, and crisis centers throughout the United States. DrugHelp is a service of the American Council for Drug Education, an affiliate of Phoenix House.

Drug Abuse and Chemical Dependency Resources Guide
http://open-mind.org

This site is intended to help those in or seeking recovery from various addictions, obsessions, and compulsions, such as drugs, alcohol, sex, and food, as well as helping family, friends, anxiety sufferers, and abuse survivors find information, support, and resources. This site offers a comprehensive lists of drug abuse–related links.

Girl Power
www.girlpower.gov

This site, sponsored by the U.S. Department of Health and Human Services, is aimed at teaching 9- to 13-year old girls and their parents how to stay alcohol-, tobacco-, and drug-free.

March of Dimes
www.modimes.org

The March of Dimes homepage offers information on the effects of substance abuse on pregnancy and children.

National Association of Addiction Treatment Providers (NAATP)
www.naatp.org

The mission of NAATP, a membership organization of treatment providers, is to promote, assist, and enhance the delivery of ethical, effective, research-based treatment for alcoholism and other drug addictions. It provides treatment-related information to its members and the public and advocates for increased access to and availability of quality treatment for those who suffer from alcoholism and other drug addictions.

National Council on Alcoholism and Drug Dependence
www.ncadd.org/

National Council on Alcoholism and Drug Dependence provides education and information to the public and advocates for prevention, intervention, and treatment through offices in New York and Washington and a nationwide network of affiliates. The site includes information on women, alcohol, and drugs.

National Council on Patient Information and Education (NCPIE)
www.talkaboutrx.org

NCPIE is a coalition of organizations whose mission is to stimulate and improve communication of information on appropriate medicine use to consumers and health care professionals. NCPIE develops programs and provides educational resources.

National Women's Health Resource Center, Inc. (NWHRC)
www.healthywomen.org

NWHRC helps women educate themselves about health topics important to women, including substance abuse. The nonprofit organization, dedicated to helping women make informed decisions about their health, encourages women to embrace healthy lifestyles to promote wellness and prevent disease.

Prevention Online (Prevline)
www.health.org

SAMHSA's National Clearinghouse for Alcohol and Drug Information (NCADI) is a comprehensive source of information about substance abuse prevention and addiction treatment. The site allows the user to search for publications specific to women and substance abuse.

The National Center on Addiction and Substance Abuse (CASA) at Columbia University
www.casacolumbia.org

CASA's missions are to inform Americans of the economic and social costs of substance abuse and its impact on their lives; to assess what works in prevention, treatment, and law enforcement; to encourage every individual and institution to take responsibility to combat substance abuse and addiction; to provide those on the front lines with the tools they need to succeed; and to remove the stigma of abuse and replace shame and despair with hope. This

Web site offers reports issued by the center that can be downloaded free, including three major reports on substance abuse and women on which this book is based. It also includes the complete bibliography for this publication.

Women's Addiction Foundation
www.womenfdn.org/default.htm

This Web site of the Canadian organization Women's Addiction Foundation contains a large variety of fact sheets on the relationship of addiction to alcohol, tobacco, and drugs and on topics ranging from depression to relationship violence to disordered eating. Another section provides links to other sites for special populations, such as young women, older women, and lesbians, as well as sites that deal with specific substances such as benzodiazepines.

Information—Tobacco

American Legacy Foundation
www.americanlegacy.org

The Web site for the American Legacy Foundation, and a partner site, www.quitnet.com offer practical tips for quitting smoking.

American Lung Association
www.lungusa.org

Homepage of the American Lung Association, this site provides information on smoking, its links to lung cancer, and tobacco control.

American Medical Women's Association
www.amwa-doc.org

This site of the American Medical Women's Association provides information on the health risks of smoking to women and describes techniques for quitting smoking.

Centers for Disease Control and Prevention
www.cdc.gov

The Centers for Disease Control and Prevention Web site provides information on the health risks of smoking and provides facts on quitting and health consequences of smoking.

Smoke Free Families
www.smokefreefamilies.org

The Smoke-Free Families program is sponsored by the Robert Wood Johnson Foundation. Their Web site offers reasons to quit, tips for quitting, and resources to help quit, with a special emphasis on the importance of quitting while pregnant.

Information—Alcohol

Join Together

www.alcoholscreening.org

A service of Join Together to determine "how much is too much."

National Institute on Alcohol Abuse and Alcoholism

www.niaaa.nih.gov/publications/brochurewomen/women.htm

This National Institute on Alcohol Abuse and Alcoholism publication, *Alcohol: A Women's Health Issue,* describes safe vs. problem drinking for women and indicates areas for future research. From the NIAAA homepage, the reader can search for extensive information on women and alcohol.

Women and Alcohol

http://alcoholism.about.com/cs/women

This site covers a variety of topics relating to women and alcohol, summarizing government reports, academic research, and information from other Web sites.

Information—Drugs

National Institute on Drug Abuse

www.nida.nih.gov

From the National Institute on Drug Abuse homepage, the reader can search for extensive listings on women and drugs. The site provides links to a collection of notes describing research on women's health and gender differences relating to drug abuse.

Prescription Drug Abuse

www.prescriptionabuse.org

This Web site offers information, news, and research about addiction to prescription drugs. The site posts stories of recovery from addicts and family members; it also features a discussion forum, lists of commonly abused drugs, and an "Ask the Doctor" page.

Sources: Adapted from Colvin, R. (2002). *Prescription drug addiction. The hidden epidemic. A guide to coping and understanding.* Omaha, NE: Addicus Books, and information from the World Wide Web.

notesnotesnotesnotes

Chapter 1. Pathways to Substance Abuse among Girls and Women

1. Cullen, K. W., Koehly, L. A., Anderson, C., Baranowski, T., Prokhorov, A., Basen-Engquist, K., et al. (1999). Gender differences in chronic disease risk behaviors through the transition out of high school. *American Journal of Preventive Medicine, 17*(1), 1–7; Petersen, A. C., & Hamburg, B. A. (1986). Adolescence: A developmental approach to problems and psychopathology. *Behavior Therapy, 17*(5), 480–499; The National Center on Addiction and Substance Abuse (CASA) at Columbia University. (2003). *The formative years: Pathways to substance abuse among girls and young women ages 8–22.* New York: CASA.
2. Johnson, N. G., Roberts, M. C., & Worell, J. (1999). *Beyond appearance: A new look at adolescent girls.* Washington, DC: American Psychological Association; Straussner, S. L. A., & Brown, S. (Eds.). (2002). *The handbook of addiction treatment for women.* San Francisco: Jossey-Bass; Golombek, H., Marton, P., Stein, B., & Korenblum, M. (1986). A study of disturbed and non-disturbed adolescents: The Toronto Adolescent Longitudinal Study. *Canadian Journal of Psychiatry, 31*(6), 532–535; Schave, D., & Schave, B. (1989). *Early adolescence and the search for self.* New York: Praeger.
3. Johnson, N. G., Roberts, M. C., & Worell, J. (1999); Golombek, H., Marton, P., Stein, B., & Korenblum, M. (1986); Pipher, M. B. (1994). *Reviving Ophelia: Saving the selves of adolescent girls.* New York: Putnam; Straussner, S. L. A., & Brown, S. (2002); Schave, D., & Schave, B. (1989).
4. Johnson, N. G., Roberts, M. C., & Worell, J. (1999); López, R. I. (2002). *The teen health book: A parent's guide to adolescent health and well-being.* New York: W. W. Norton.
5. Johnson, N. G., Roberts, M. C., & Worell, J. (1999).
6. Jones, D. C. (2001). Social comparison and body image: Attractiveness comparisons to models and peers among adolescent girls and boys. *Sex Roles, 45*(9–10), 645–664.
7. Johnson, N. G., Roberts, M. C., & Worell, J. (1999).

8. Straussner, S. L. A., & Brown, S. (2002); Golombek, H., Marton, P., Stein, B., & Korenblum, M. (1986); Schave, D., & Schave, B. (1989).
9. Durkin, K. (1995). *Developmental social psychology: From infancy to old age.* Cambridge, MA: Blackwell; Nolen-Hoeksema, S. (2001). Gender differences in depression. *Current Directions in Psychological Science, 10*(5), 173–176; Petersen, A. C., & Hamburg, B. A. (1986).
10. Taylor, J. M., Gilligan, C., & Sullivan, A. M. (1995). *Between voice and silence: Women and girls, race and relationship.* Cambridge, MA: Harvard University Press; Pipher, M. B. (1994).
11. Durkin, K. (1995).
12. Erikson, E. H. (1963). *Childhood and society.* New York: W. W. Norton.
13. Dweck, C. S., & Licht, B. G. (1980). Learned helplessness and intellectual achievement. In J. Garber & M. E. P. Seligman (Eds.), *Human helplessness: Theory and applications* (pp. 197–221). New York: Academic Press; Johnson, N. G., Roberts, M. C., & Worell, J. (1999); Read, C. R. (1991). Gender distribution in programs for the gifted. *Roeper Review, 13*(4), 188–193.
14. Straussner, S. L. A., & Brown, S. (2002); Golombek, H., Marton, P., Stein, B., & Korenblum, M. (1986); Schave, D., & Schave, B. (1989).
15. Ibid.
16. Ibid.
17. Durkin, K. (1995).
18. Straussner, S. L. A., & Brown, S. (2002); Golombek, H., Marton, P., Stein, B., & Korenblum, M. (1986); Schave, D., & Schave, B. (1989).
19. López, R. I. (2002).
20. Straussner, S. L. A., & Brown, S. (2002).
21. Brennan, P. L., & Moos, R. H. (1996). Late-life drinking behavior: The influence of personal characteristics, life context and treatment. *Alcohol Health and Research World, 20*(3), 197–204; Glass, T. A., Prigerson, H., Kasl, S. V., & Mendes de Leon, C. F. (1995). The effects of negative life events on alcohol consumption among older men and women. *Journal of Gerontology, 50B*(4), 205–216; Richardson, V. E., & Kilty, K. M. (1995). Gender differences in mental health: Before and after retirement: A longitudinal analysis. *Journal of Women and Aging, 7*(1/2), 19–35; Breslin, F. C., O'Keefe, M. K., Burrell, L., Ratliff-Crain, J., & Baum, A. (1995). The effects of stress and coping on daily alcohol use in women. *Addictive Behaviors, 20*(2), 141–147; Gomberg, E. S. L. (1994). Risk factors for drinking over a woman's life span. *Alcohol Health and Research World, 18*(3), 220–227; Jennison, K. M. (1992). Impact of stressful life events and social support on drinking among older adults: A general population survey. *International Journal of Aging and Human Development, 35*(2), 99–123; Gomberg, E. S. L. (1991). Women and alcohol: Psychosocial aspects. In D. J. Pittman & H. R. White (Eds.), *Society, culture and drinking patterns reexamined* (pp. 263–284). New Brunswick, NJ: Alcohol Research Documentation, Rutgers Center of Alcohol Studies; Finlayson, R. E., Hurt, R. D., Davis, L. J., & Morse, R. M. (1988). Alcoholism in elderly persons: A study of the psychiatric and psychosocial features of 216 inpatients. *Mayo Clinic Proceedings, 63*(8), 761–768; Malcolm, M. T. (1984). Alcohol and drug use in the elderly visited at home. *International Journal of the Addictions, 19*(4), 411–418; Graham, K., Saunders, S. J., Flower, M. C., Timney, C. B., White-

Campbell, M., & Pietropaolo, A. Z. (1995). *Addictions treatment for older adults: Evaluation of an innovative client-centered approach.* New York: Haworth Press; Zisook, S., & Shuchter, S. R. (1991). Depression through the first year after the death of a spouse. *American Journal of Psychiatry, 148*(10), 1346–1352.

22. Samuels, S. C. (1997). Midlife crisis: Helping patients cope with stress, anxiety, and depression. *Geriatrics, 52*(7), 55–56; Danello, M. A. (1987). Women's health: A course of action: Health concerns of older women. *Public Health Reports, Suppl.*, 14–18.
23. Straussner, S. L. A., & Brown, S. (2002).
24. Finlayson, R. E., Hurt, R. D., Davis, L. J., & Morse, R. M. (1988); Kunz, J. L., & Graham, K. (1996). Life course changes in alcohol consumption in leisure activities of men and women. *Journal of Drug Issues, 26*(4), 805–829.
25. Jinks, M. J., & Raschko, R. R. (1990). A profile of alcohol and prescription drug abuse in a high-risk community-based elderly population. *Annals of Pharmacotherapy, 24*(10), 971–975; Atkinson, R. M., Ganzini, L., & Bernstein, M. J. (1992). Alcohol and substance-use disorders in the elderly. In J. E. Birren, R. B. Sloane, & G. D. Cohen (Eds.), *Handbook of mental health and aging* (pp. 516–555). New York: Academic Press.
26. The National Center on Addiction and Substance Abuse (CASA) at Columbia University. (1998). *Under the rug: Substance abuse and the mature woman.* New York: CASA.
27. Han, C., McGue, M. K., & Iacono, W. G. (1999). Lifetime tobacco, alcohol and other substance use in adolescent Minnesota twins: Univariate and multivariate behavioral genetic analyses. *Addiction, 94*(7), 981–993; Maes, H. H., Woodard, C. E., Murrelle, L., Meyer, J. M., Silberg, J. L., Hewitt, J. K., et al. (1999). Tobacco, alcohol and drug use in eight-to-sixteen year-old twins: The Virginia Twin Study of Adolescent Behavioral Development. *Journal of Studies on Alcohol, 60*(3), 293–305; Rose, R. J. (1998). A developmental behavior-genetic perspective on alcoholism risk. *Alcohol Health and Research World, 22*(2), 131–143; van den Bree, M. B. M., Johnson, E. O., Neale, M. C., & Pickens, R. W. (1998). Genetic and environmental influences on drug use and abuse/dependence in male and female twins. *Drug and Alcohol Dependence, 52*(3), 231–241.
28. Han, C., McGue, M. K., & Iacono, W. G. (1999); Kendler, K. S., Neale, M. C., Heath, A. C., Kessler, R. C., & Eaves, L. J. (1994). A twin-family study of alcoholism in women. *American Journal of Psychiatry, 151*(5), 707–715; Maes, H. H., Woodard, C. E., Murrelle, L., Meyer, J. M., Silberg, J. L., Hewitt, J. K., et al. (1999); Meller, W. H., Rinehart, R., Cadoret, R. J., & Troughton, E. (1988). Specific familial transmission in substance abuse. *International Journal of the Addictions, 23*(10), 1029–1039; Rose, R. J. (1998); van den Bree, M. B. M., Johnson, E. O., Neale, M. C., & Pickens, R. W. (1998).
29. Bierut, L. J., Dinwiddie, S. H., Begleiter, H., Crowe, R. R., Hesselbrock, V., Nurnberger, J. I., et al. (1998). Familial transmission of substance dependence: Alcohol, marijuana, cocaine, and habitual smoking: A report from the Collaborative Study on the Genetics of Alcoholism. *Archives of General Psychiatry, 55*(11), 982–988; Han, C., McGue, M. K., & Iacono, W. G. (1999); Heath, A. C., Bucholz, K. K., Madden, P. A. F., Dinwiddie, S. H., Slutske, W. S., Bierut, L. J., et al. (1997). Genetic and environmental contributions to alcohol dependence

risk in a national twin sample: Consistency of findings in women and men. *Psychological Medicine, 27*(6), 1381–1396; Kendler, K. S., Neale, M. C., Heath, A. C., Kessler, R. C., & Eaves, L. J. (1994); Kendler, K., Neale, M. C., Sullivan, P., Corey, L. A., Gardner, C. O., & Prescott, C. A. (1999). A population-based twin study in women of smoking initiation and nicotine dependence. *Psychological Medicine, 29*(2), 299–308; Maes, H. H., Woodard, C. E., Murrelle, L., Meyer, J. M., Silberg, J. L., Hewitt, J. K., et al. (1999); Merikangas, K. R., Stolar, M., Stevens, D. E., Goulet, J., Presig, M. A., Fenton, B., et al. (1998). Familial transmission of substance use disorders. *Archives of General Psychiatry, 55*(11), 973–979; Prescott, C. A., Aggen, S. H., & Kendler, K. S. (1999). Sex differences in the sources of genetic liability to alcohol abuse and dependence in a population-based sample of U.S. twins. *Alcoholism: Clinical and Experimental Research, 23*(7), 1136–1144; van den Bree, M. B. M., Johnson, E. O., Neale, M. C., & Pickens, R. W. (1998); Zickler, P. (2000). Evidence builds that genes influence cigarette smoking. *NIDA Notes, 15*(2), 1, 5.

30. Heath, A. C., Slutske, W. S., & Madden, P. A. F. (1997). Gender differences in the genetic contribution to alcoholism risk and to alcohol consumption patterns. In R. W. Wilsnack & S. C. Wilsnack (Eds.), *Gender and alcohol: Individual and social perspectives* (pp. 114–149). New Brunswick, NJ: Rutgers Center of Alcohol Studies; Schuckit, M. A., Smith, T. L., Kalmijn, J., Tsuang, J., Hesselbrock, V., & Bucholz, K. (2000). Response to alcohol in daughters of alcoholics: A pilot study and a comparison with sons of alcoholics. *Alcohol and Alcoholism, 35*(3), 242–248.
31. Schuckit, M. A., Smith, T. L., Kalmijn, J., Tsuang, J., Hesselbrock, V., & Bucholz, K. (2000).
32. Lundahl, L. H., & Lukas, S. E. (2001). The impact of familial alcoholism on alcohol reactivity in female social drinkers. *Experimental and Clinical Psychopharmacology, 9*(1), 101–109.
33. Ellis, B. J., McFadyen-Ketchum, S., Dodge, K. A., Pettit, G. S., & Bates, J. E. (1999). Quality of early family relationships and individual differences in the timing of pubertal maturation in girls: A longitudinal test of an evolutionary model. *Journal of Personality and Social Psychology, 77*(2), 387–401; Tarter, R., Vanyukov, M., Giancola, P., Dawes, M., Blackson, T., Mezzich, A., et al. (1999). Etiology of early age onset substance use disorder: A maturational perspective. *Development and Psychopathology, 11*(4), 657–683; Tschann, J. M., Adler, N. E., Irwin Jr., C. E., Millstein, S. G., Turner, R. A., & Kegeles, S. M. (1994). Initiation of substance use in early adolescence: The roles of pubertal timing and emotional distress. *Health Psychology, 13*(4), 326–333.
34. Dick, D. M., Rose, R. J., Viken, R. J., & Kaprio, J. (2000). Pubertal timing and substance use: Associations between and within families across late adolescence. *Developmental Psychology, 36*(2), 180–189; Harrell, J. S., Bangdiwala, S. I., Deng, S., Webb, J. P., & Bradley, C. (1998). Smoking initiation in youth: The roles of gender, race, socioeconomics, and developmental status. *Journal of Adolescent Health, 23*(5), 271–279; Martin, C., Logan, T. K., Leukefeld, C., Milich, R., Omar, H., & Clayton, R. (2001). Adolescent and young adult substance use: Associated with sensation seeking, self-esteem and retrospective report of early pubertal onset: A preliminary examination. *International Journal of Adolescent Medicine and Health, 13*(3), 211–219; Prokopcáková, A. (1998). Drug experimenting and pubertal maturation in

girls. *Studia Psychologica, 40*(4), 287–290; Tarter, R., Vanyukov, M., Giancola, P., Dawes, M., Blackson, T., Mezzich, A., et al. (1999); Tschann, J. M., Adler, N. E., Irwin Jr., C. E., Millstein, S. G., Turner, R. A., & Kegeles, S. M. (1994); Wichstrøm, L. (2001). The impact of pubertal timing on adolescents' alcohol use. *Journal of Research on Adolescence, 11*(2), 131–150; Wiesner, M., & Ittel, A. (2002). Relations of pubertal timing and depressive symptoms to substance use in early adolescence. *Journal of Early Adolescence, 22*(1), 5–23; Wilson, D. M., Killen, J. D., Hayward, C., Robinson, T. N., Hammer, L. D., Kraemer, H. C., et al. (1994). Timing and rate of sexual maturation and the onset of cigarette and alcohol use among teenage girls. *Archives of Pediatrics and Adolescent Medicine, 148*(8), 789–795.

35. Ellis, B. J., McFadyen-Ketchum, S., Dodge, K. A., Pettit, G. S., & Bates, J. E. (1999); Treloar, S. A., & Martin, N. G. (1990). Age at menarche as a fitness trait: Nonadditive genetic variance detected in a large twin sample. *American Journal of Human Genetics, 47*(1), 137–148.

36. Bauman, K. E., Foshee, V. A., Koch, G. G., Haley, N. J., & Downtown, M. I. (1989). Testosterone and cigarette smoking in early adolescence. *Journal of Behavioral Medicine, 12*(5), 425–433; Kandel, D. B., & Udry, J. R. (1999). Prenatal effects of maternal smoking on daughters' smoking: Nicotine or testosterone exposure? *American Journal of Public Health, 89*(9), 1377–1383; Martin, C. A., Logan, T. K., Portis, C., Leukefeld, C. G., Lynam, D., Staton, M., et al. (2001). The association of testosterone with nicotine use in young adult females. *Addictive Behaviors, 26*(2), 279–283.

37. Caspi, A., Lynam, D., Moffit, T. E., & Silva, P. A. (1993). Unraveling girls' delinquency: Biological, dispositional, and contextual contributions to adolescent misbehavior. *Developmental Psychology, 29*(1), 19–30; Dick, D. M., Rose, R. J., Viken, R. J., & Kaprio, J. (2000); Prokopcáková, A. (1998); Stice, E., Presness, K., & Bearman, S. K. (2001). Relation of early menarche to depression, eating disorders, substance abuse, and comorbid psychopathology among adolescent girls. *Developmental Psychology, 37*(5), 608–619; Tarter, R., Vanyukov, M., Giancola, P., Dawes, M., Blackson, T., Mezzich, A., et al. (1999); Tschann, J. M., Adler, N. E., Irwin Jr., C. E., Millstein, S. G., Turner, R. A., & Kegeles, S. M. (1994).

38. Crisp, A., Sedgwick, P., Halek, C., Joughin, N., & Humphrey, H. (1999). Why may teenage girls persist in smoking? *Journal of Adolescence, 22*(5), 657–672; Dawes, M. A., Antelman, S. M., Vanyukov, M. M., Giancola, P., Tarter, R. E., Susman, E. J., et al. (2000). Developmental sources of variation in liability to adolescent substance use disorders. *Drug and Alcohol Dependence, 61*(1), 3–14; Prokopcáková, A. (1998).

39. Atkinson, R. M., Ganzini, L., & Bernstein, M. J. (1992); Barry, P. P. (1986). Gender as a factor in treating the elderly. In B. A. Ray & M. C. Braude (Eds.), *Women and drugs: A new era for research. NIDA research monograph 65* (DHHS Pub. No. [ADM] 86-1447, pp. 65–69). Rockville, MD: U.S. Department of Health and Human Services, Public Health Service, Alcohol, Drug Abuse, and Mental Health Administration, National Institute on Drug Abuse; Braude, M. C. (1986). Drugs and drug interactions in elderly women. In B. A. Ray & M. C. Braude (Eds.), *Women and drugs: A new era for research: NIDA research monograph 65*; Dufour, M. C., Archer, L., & Gordis, E. (1992). Alcohol and the elderly. *Clinics in Geriatric Medicine, 8*(1), 127–141; Gambert, S. R. (1992). Substance abuse in the elderly. In J. Lowinson, P. Ruiz, R. B.

Millman, & J. G. Langrod (Eds.), *Substance abuse: A comprehensive textbook* (pp. 843–851). Baltimore, MD: Williams and Wilkins; Gear, R. W., Miaskowski, C., Gordon, N. C., Paul, S. M., Heller, P. H., & Levine, J. D. (1996). Kappa-opioids produce significantly greater analgesia in women than in men. *Nature Medicine, 2*(11), 1248–1250; Greenblatt, D. J., Sellers, E. M., & Shader, R. I. (1982). Drug therapy in old age. *New England Journal of Medicine, 306*(18), 1081–1088; Leung, J., Boisse, N. R., & Amitay, O. (1995). Sex differences in spontaneous withdrawal following acute benzodiazepine dependence induction. In L. S. Harris (Ed.), *Problems of drug dependence, 1994: Proceedings of the 56th Annual Scientific Meeting: Volume 2: Abstracts: NIDA research monograph no. 153* (NIH Pub. No. 95-3883, p. 237). Rockville, MD: U.S. Department of Health and Human Services, National Institutes of Health, National Institute on Drug Abuse; Vestal, R. E., McGuire, E. A., Tobin, J. D., Andres, R., Norris, A. H., & Mezey, E. (1977). Aging and ethanol metabolism. *Clinical Pharmacology and Therapeutics, 21*(3), 343–354; Vogel-Sprott, M., & Barrett, P. (1984). Age, drinking habits and the effects of alcohol. *Journal of Studies on Alcohol, 45*(6), 517–521.

40. Barry, P. P. (1986); Braude, M. C. (1986); Lamy, P. P. (1988). Actions of alcohol and drugs in older people. *Generations, 12*(4), 9–13; Montamat, S. C., Cusack, B. J., & Vestal, R. E. (1989). Management of drug therapy in the elderly. *New England Journal of Medicine, 321*(5), 303–309.
41. Barry, P. P. (1986); Braude, M. C. (1986).
42. Barry, P. P. (1986); German, P. S., & Burton, L. C. (1989). Clinicians, the elderly and drugs. *Journal of Drug Issues, 19*(2), 221–243.
43. Atkinson, R. M., Ganzini, L., & Bernstein, M. J. (1992).
44. Giancola, P. R., & Mezzich, A. C. (2000). Neuropsychological deficits in female adolescents with a substance use disorder: Better accounted for by conduct disorder? *Journal of Studies on Alcohol, 61*(6), 809–817; Heath, A. C., Slutske, W. S., & Madden, P. A. F. (1997); Slutske, W. S., Heath, A. C., Dinwiddie, S. H., Madden, P. A. F., Bucholz, K. K., Dunne, M. P., et al. (1998). Common genetic risk factors for conduct disorder and alcohol dependence. *Journal of Abnormal Psychology, 107*(3), 363–374.
45. Heath, A. C., Bucholz, K. K., Madden, P. A. F., Dinwiddie, S. H., Slutske, W. S., Bierut, L. J., et al. (1997); Miles, D. R., van den Bree, M. B. M., & Pickens, R. W. (2002). Sex differences in shared genetic and environmental influences between conduct disorder symptoms and marijuana use in adolescents. *American Journal of Medical Genetics, 114*(2), 159–168; Slutske, W. S., Heath, A. C., Dinwiddie, S. H., Madden, P. A. F., Bucholz, K. K., Dunne, M. P., et al. (1998).
46. Disney, E. R., Elkins, I. J., McGue, M., & Iacono, W. G. (1999). Effects of ADHD, conduct disorder, and gender on substance use and abuse in adolescence. *American Journal of Psychiatry, 156*(10), 1515–1521.
47. Kendler, K. S., Heath, A. C., Neale, M. C., Kessler, R. C., & Eaves, L. J. (1993). Alcoholism and major depression in women: A twin study of the causes of comorbidity. *Archives of General Psychiatry, 50*(9), 690–698; Kendler, K. S., Neale, M. C., MacLean, C. J., Health, A. C., Eaves, L. J., & Kessler, R. C. (1993). Smoking and major depression: A causal analysis.

Archives of General Psychiatry, 50(1), 36–43; Prescott, C. A., Aggen, S. H., & Kendler, K. S. (2000). Sex-specific genetic influences on the comorbidity of alcoholism and major depression in a population-based sample of US twins. *Archives of General Psychiatry, 57*(8), 803–811.

48. Kendler, K. S., Heath, A. C., Neale, M. C., Kessler, R. C., & Eaves, L. J. (1993).

49. Substance Abuse and Mental Health Services Administration, Office of Applied Studies. (2003). *Overview of findings from the 2002 National Survey on Drug Use and Health: National findings* (DHHS Pub. No. [SMA] 03-3774). Rockville, MD: U.S. Department of Health and Human Services; Substance Abuse and Mental Health Services Administration, Office of Applied Studies. (2004). *Women with co-occurring serious mental illness and a substance use disorder: The NSDUH report.* Rockville, MD: U.S. Department of Health and Human Services.

50. Block, J., Block, J. H., & Keyes, S. (1988). Longitudinally foretelling drug usage in adolescence: Early childhood personality and environmental precursors. *Child Development, 59*(2), 336–355; Friedman, A. S., Granick, S., Bransfield, S., Kreisher, C., & Khalsa, J. (1995). Gender differences in early life risk factors for substance use/abuse: A study of an African-American sample. *American Journal of Drug and Alcohol Abuse, 21*(4), 511–531; Shedler, J., & Block, J. (1990). Adolescent drug use and psychological health: A longitudinal inquiry. *American Psychologist, 45*(5), 612–630; Tarter, R. E. (1988). Are there inherited behavioral traits that predispose to substance abuse? *Journal of Consulting and Clinical Psychology, 56*(2), 189–196; Windle, M. (1991). The difficult temperament in adolescence: Associations with substance use, family support, and problem behaviors. *Journal of Clinical Psychology, 47*(2), 310–315.

51. Kumpulainen, K. (2000). Psychiatric symptoms and deviance in early adolescence predict heavy alcohol use 3 years later. *Addiction, 95*(12), 1847–1857; Lerner, J. V., & Vicary, J. R. (1984). Difficult temperament and drug use: Analyses from the New York Longitudinal Study. *Journal of Drug Education, 14*(1), 1–8; Reinherz, H. Z., Giaconia, R. M., Hauf, A. M. C., Wasserman, M. S., & Paradis, A. D. (2000). General and specific childhood risk factors for depression and drug disorders by early adulthood. *Journal of the American Academy of Child and Adolescent Psychiatry, 39*(2), 223–231; Shedler, J., & Block, J. (1990); Windle, M. (1991).

52. Burt, R., Dinh, K., Peterson, A., & Sarason, I. (2000). Predicting adolescent smoking: A prospective study of personality variables. *Preventive Medicine, 30*(2), 115–125; Cicchetti, D., & Rogosch, F. A. (1999). Psychopathology as risk for adolescent substance use disorders: A developmental psychopathology perspective. *Journal of Clinical Child Psychology, 28*(3), 355–365; Parent, E. C., & Newman, D. L. (1999). The role of sensation-seeking in alcohol use and risk-taking behavior among college women. *Journal of Alcohol and Drug Education, 44*(2), 12–28.

53. Johnson, N. G., Roberts, M. C., & Worell, J. (1999).

54. Schoen, C., Davis, K., Collins, K. S., Greenberg, L., Des Roches, C., & Abrams, M. (1997). *The Commonwealth fund survey of the health of adolescent girls.* New York: Commonwealth Fund.

55. Ibid.

56. Ludwig, K. B., & Pittman, J. F. (1999). Adolescent prosocial values and self-efficacy in relation to delinquency, risky sexual behavior, and drug use. *Youth and Society, 30*(4), 461–482.

57. CASA. (2003). *The formative years.*

58. Ibid.

59. Centers for Disease Control and Prevention, Grunbaum, J. A., Kann, L., Kinchen, S. A., Williams, B., Ross, J. G., et al. (2002). Youth risk behavior surveillance: United States, 2001. *Morbidity and Mortality Weekly Report: Surveillance Summaries, 51*(SS–4).

60. Ibid.

61. The National Center on Addiction and Substance Abuse (CASA) at Columbia University. (2003). *Food for thought: Substance abuse and eating disorders.* New York: CASA.

62. Bellafante, G. (2003, March 9). When midlife seems just an empty plate. *New York Times,* 9. 1.

63. Aneshensel, C. S., Rutter, C. M., & Lachenbruch, P. A. (1991). Social structure, stress, and mental health: Competing conceptual and analytic models. *American Sociological Review, 56*(2), 166–178.

64. Byrne, D., Byrne, A., & Reinhart, M. (1995). Personality, stress and the decision to commence cigarette smoking in adolescence. *Journal of Psychosomatic Research, 39*(1), 53–62.

65. Hoffmann, J. P., & Su, S. S. (1998). Stressful life events and adolescent substance use and depression: Conditional and gender differentiated effects. *Substance Use and Misuse, 33*(11), 2219–2262.

66. Whalen, C. K., Jamner, L. D., Henker, B., & Delfino, R. J. (2001). Smoking and moods in adolescents with depressive and aggressive dispositions: Evidence from surveys and electronic diaries. *Health Psychology, 20*(2), 99–111.

67. Schoen, C., Davis, K., Collins, K. S., Greenberg, L., Des Roches, C., & Abrams, M. (1997).

68. (CASA). (2003). *The formative years.*

69. Ibid.

70. Ibid.

71. Ibid.

72. Ibid.

73. Ibid.

74. (CASA). (1998). *Under the rug.*

75. Kennedy, G. J., Kelman, H. R., & Thomas, C. (1990). The emergence of depressive symptoms in late life: The importance of declining health and increasing disability. *Journal of Community Health, 15*(2), 93–104; Blazer, D., Hughes, D. C., & George, L. K. (1987). The epidemiology of depression in an elderly community population. *Gerontologist, 27*(3), 281–287; Wolk, S. I., & Weissman, M. M. (1995). Women and depression: An update. In American Psychiatric Press (Ed.), *Review of psychiatry: Volume 14* (pp. 227–259). Washington, DC: American Psychiatric Press; Stallones, L., Marx, M. B., & Garrity, T. F. (1990). Prevalence and correlates of depressive symptoms among older U.S. adults. *American Journal of Preventive Medicine, 6*(5), 295–303; Harlow, S. D., Goldberg, E. L., & Comstock, G. W. (1991). A longitudinal study of risk factors for depressive symptomatology in elderly widowed and married women. *American Journal of Epidemiology, 134*(5), 526–538.

76. Robbins, C. A. (1991). Social roles and alcohol abuse among older men and women. *Family and Community Health, 13*(4), 37–48; Wilsnack, R. W., & Cheloha, R. (1987). Women's roles and problem drinking across the lifespan. *Social Problems, 34*(3), 231–248.

77. Green, B. H., Copeland, J. R. M., Dewey, M. E., Sharma, V., Saunders, P. A., Davidson, I. A., et al. (1992). Risk factors for depression in elderly people: A prospective study. *Acta Psychiatrica Scandinavica, 86*(3), 213–217.

78. Ibid.; Zisook, S., & Shuchter, S. R. (1991); Harlow, S. D., Goldberg, E. L., & Comstock, G. W. (1991). A longitudinal study of the prevalence of depressive symptomatology in elderly widowed and married women. *Archives of General Psychiatry, 48*(12), 1065–1068; Harlow, S. D., Goldberg, E. L., & Comstock, G. W. (1991). A longitudinal study of risk factors for depressive symptomatology.

79. Helzer, J. E., & Pryzbeck, T. R. (1988). The co-occurrence of alcoholism with other psychiatric disorders in the general population and its impact on treatment. *Journal of Studies on Alcohol, 49*(3), 219–224; Brennan, P. L., Moos, R. H., & Kim, J. Y. (1993). Gender differences in the individual characteristics and life contexts of late-middle-aged and older problem drinkers. *Addiction, 88*(6), 781–790.

80. Agency for Health Care Policy and Research. (1996). *Smoking cessation: Clinical practice guidelines no. 18.* Atlanta, GA: U.S. Department of Health and Human Services, Centers for Disease Control and Prevention; Giovino, G. A., Henningfield, J. E., Tomar, S. L., Escobedo, L. G., & Slade, J. (1995). Epidemiology of tobacco use and dependence. *Epidemiological Reviews, 17*(1), 48–65; Glassman, A. H., Helzer, J. E., Covey, L. S., Cottler, L. B., Stetner, F., Tipp, J. E., et al. (1990). Smoking, smoking cessation and major depression. *JAMA, 264*(12), 1546–1549; Kendler, K. S., Neale, M. C., MacLean, C. J., Health, A. C., Eaves, L. J., & Kessler, R. C. (1993).

81. Felitti, V. (2002). The relation between adverse childhood experience and adult health: Turning gold into lead. *Permanente Journal, 6*(1), 44–47; Felitti, V. J., Anda, R. F., Nordenberg, D., Williamson, D. F., Spitz, A. M., Edwards, V., et al. (1998). Relationship of childhood abuse and household dysfunction to many of the leading causes of death in adults: The Adverse Childhood Experiences (ACE) Study. *American Journal of Preventive Medicine, 14*(4), 245–258.

82. Schoen, C., Davis, K., Collins, K. S., Greenberg, L., Des Roches, C., & Abrams, M. (1997).

83. Ibid.

84. Widom, C. S., Weiler, B. L., & Cottler, L. B. (1999). Childhood victimization and drug abuse: A comparison of prospective and retrospective findings. *Journal of Consulting and Clinical Psychology, 67*(6), 867–880.

85. Garnefski, N., & Arends, E. (1998). Sexual abuse and adolescent maladjustment: Differences between male and female victims. *Journal of Adolescence, 21*(1), 99–107.

86. Flanigan, B. J., Potrykus, P. A., & Marti, D. (1988). Alcohol and marijuana use among female adolescent incest victims. *Alcoholism Treatment Quarterly, 5*(1–2), 231–248; Harrison, P. A., Hoffman, N. G., & Edwall, G. E. (1989). Differential drug use patterns among sexually

abused adolescent girls in treatment for chemical dependency. *International Journal of the Addictions, 24*(6), 499–514; Pedersen, W., & Skrondal, A. (1996). Alcohol and sexual victimization: A longitudinal study of Norwegian girls. *Addiction, 91*(4), 565–581; Singer, M. I., Petchers, M. K., & Hussey, D. (1989). The relationship between sexual abuse and substance abuse among psychiatrically hospitalized adolescents. *Child Abuse and Neglect, 13*(3), 319–325.

87. Rounds-Bryant, J. L., Kristiansen, P. L., Fairbank, J. A., & Hubbard, R. L. (1998). Substance use, mental disorders, abuse, and crime: Gender comparisons among a national sample of adolescent drug treatment clients. *Journal of Child and Adolescent Substance Abuse, 7*(4), 19–34.
88. Harrison, P. A., Hoffman, N. G., & Edwall, G. E. (1989).
89. Galaif, E. R., Stein, J. A., Newcomb, M. D., & Bernstein, D. P. (2001). Gender differences in the prediction of problem alcohol use in adulthood: Exploring the influence of family factors and childhood maltreatment. *Journal of Studies on Alcohol, 62*(4), 486–493; Jasinski, J. L., Williams, L. M., & Siegel, J. (2000). Childhood physical and sexual abuse as risk factors for heavy drinking among African-American women: A prospective study. *Child Abuse and Neglect, 24*(8), 1061–1071; Widom, C. S., Weiler, B. L., & Cottler, L. B. (1999); Wilsnack, S. C., Vogeltanz, N., Klassen, A. D., & Harris, T. R. (1997). Childhood sexual abuse and women's substance abuse: National survey findings. *Journal of Studies on Alcohol, 58*(3), 264–271.
90. Johnson, P. B., & Johnson, H. L. (2000). Reaffirming the power of parental influence on adolescent smoking and drinking decisions. *Adolescent and Family Health, 1*(1), 37–43; Richter, L., & Richter, D. M. (2001). Exposure to parental tobacco and alcohol use: Effects on children's health and development. *American Journal of Orthopsychiatry, 71*(2), 182–203; The National Center on Addiction and Substance Abuse (CASA) at Columbia University. (2001). *National survey of American attitudes on substance abuse VI: Teens.* New York: CASA.
91. Block, J., Block, J. H., & Keyes, S. (1988); Kandel, D. B. (1985). On processes of peer influences in adolescent drug use: A developmental perspective. *Advances in Alcohol and Substance Abuse, 4*(3–4), 139–163.
92. CASA. (2003). *The formative years.*
93. Ibid.
94. Brody, G. H., Flor, D. L., Hollet-Wright, N., McCoy, J. K., & Donovan, J. (1999). Parent-child relationships, child temperament profiles and children's alcohol use norms. *Journal of Studies on Alcohol, Suppl. 13,* 45–51; McMaster, L. E., & Wintre, M. (1996). The relations between perceived parental reciprocity, perceived parental approval, and adolescent substance use. *Journal of Adolescent Research, 11*(4), 440–460.
95. The National Center on Addiction and Substance Abuse (CASA) at Columbia University. (2005). *CASA's analysis of the National Survey on Drug Use and Health (NSDUH), 2003* [Data file]. Rockville, MD: U.S. Department of Health and Human Services, Substance Abuse and Mental Health Services Administration.
96. Fletcher, A. C., & Jefferies, B. C. (1999). Parental mediators of associations between per-

ceived authoritative parenting and early adolescent substance use. *Journal of Early Adolescence, 19*(4), 465–487.

97. Andrews, J. A., Hops, H., Ary, D., Tildesley, E., & Harris, J. (1993). Parental influence on early adolescent substance use: Specific and non-specific effects. *Journal of Early Adolescence, 13*(3), 285–310; Jackson, C., Henriksen, L., & Dickinson, D. (1999). Alcohol-specific socialization, parenting behaviors and alcohol use by children. *Journal of Studies on Alcohol, 60*(3), 362–367; Kandel, D. B., & Andrews, K. (1987). Processes of adolescent socialization by parents and peers. *International Journal of the Addictions, 22*(4), 319–342; Peterson, P. L., Hawkins, J. D., Abbott, R. D., & Catalano, R. F. (1994). Disentangling the effects of parental drinking, family management, and parental alcohol norms on current drinking by black and white adolescents. *Journal of Research on Adolescence, 4*(2), 203–227.
98. Adlaf, E. M., & Ivis, F. J. (1996). Structure and relations: The influence of familial factors on adolescent substance use and delinquency. *Journal of Child and Adolescent Substance Abuse, 5*(3), 1–19; Barnes, G. M., & Farrell, A. D. (1992). Parental support and control as predictors of adolescent drinking, delinquency, and related behavior problems. *Journal of Marriage and the Family, 54*(4), 763–776; Chilcoat, H. D., Dishion, T. J., & Anthony, J. C. (1995). Parent monitoring and the incidence of drug sampling in urban elementary school children. *American Journal of Epidemiology, 141*(1), 25–31; Li, X., Feigelman, S., & Stanton, B. (2000). Perceived parental monitoring and health risk behaviors among urban low-income African-American children and adolescents. *Journal of Adolescent Health, 27*(1), 43–48; Rodgers-Farmer, A. Y. (2000). Parental monitoring and peer group association: Their influence on adolescent substance use. *Journal of Social Service Research, 27*(2), 1–18; Steinberg, L., Fletcher, A., & Darling, N. (1994). Parental monitoring and peer influences on adolescent substance use. *Pediatrics, 93*(6, Pt. 2), 1060–1064; Vakalahi, H. F., Harrison, R. S., & Janzen, F. V. (2000). The influence of family-based risk and protective factors on adolescent substance use. *Journal of Family Social Work, 4*(1), 21–34.
99. Catalano, R. F., Morrison, D. M., Wells, E. A., Gillmore, M. R., Iritani, B., & Hawkins, J. D. (1992). Ethnic differences in family factors related to early drug initiation. *Journal of Studies on Alcohol, 53*(3), 208–217.
100. Ibid.
101. Adlaf, E. M., & Smart, R. G. (1985). Drug use and religious affiliation, feelings and behaviour. *British Journal of Addiction, 80*(2), 163–171; Brown, T. L., Parks, G. S., Zimmerman, R. S., & Phillips, C. M. (2001). The role of religion in predicting adolescent alcohol use and problem drinking. *Journal of Studies on Alcohol, 62*(5), 696–705; CASA. (2003). *The formative years.*
102. CASA. (2003). *The formative years.*
103. Forthun, L. F., Bell, N. J., Peek, C. W., & Sun, S.-W. (1999). Religiosity, sensation seeking, and alcohol/drug use in denominational and gender contexts. *Journal of Drug Issues, 29*(1), 75–90; Levin, J. S., & Taylor, R. J. (1993). Gender and age differences in religiosity among black Americans. *Gerontologist, 33*(1), 16–23; Miller, A. S., & Hoffmann, J. P. (1995). Risk and religion: An explanation of gender differences in religiosity. *Journal for the Scientific Study of Religion, 34*(1), 63–75.

104. Adlaf, E. M., & Smart, R. G. (1985); Brown, T. L., Parks, G. S., Zimmerman, R. S., & Phillips, C. M. (2001).
105. Templin, D. P., & Martin, M. J. (1999). The relationship between religious orientation, gender, and drinking patterns among Catholic college students. *College Student Journal, 33*(4), 488–495.
106. Graham, K., Carver, V., & Brett, P. J. (1995). Alcohol and drug use by older women: Results of a national survey. *Canadian Journal on Aging, 14*(4), 769–791.
107. The National Center on Addiction and Substance Abuse (CASA) at Columbia University. (2004). *CASA analysis of the Health and Retirement Study, wave 1 data 1992* [Data file]. Ann Arbor, MI: Survey Research Center.
108. Allison, K. W., Crawford, I., Leone, P. E., Trickett, E., Perez-Febles, A., Burton, L. M., et al. (1999). Adolescent substance use: Preliminary examinations of school and neighborhood context. *American Journal of Community Psychology, 27*(2), 111–141; The National Center on Addiction and Substance Abuse (CASA) at Columbia University. (2001). *Malignant neglect: Substance abuse and America's schools.* New York: CASA.
109. Benard, B. (1991). *Fostering resiliency in kids: Protective factors in family, school, and community.* Portland, OR: Northwest Regional Educational Laboratory; Resnick, M. D., Bearman, P. S., Blum, R. W., Bauman, K. E., Harris, K. M., Jones, J., et al. (1997). Protecting adolescents from harm: Findings from the National Longitudinal Study on Adolescent Health. *JAMA, 278*(10), 823–832; Rhodes, J. E., & Jason, L. (1988). *Preventing substance abuse among children and adolescents.* New York: Pergamon.
110. Wallace, J. M. (1999). The social ecology of addiction: Race, risk, and resilience. *Pediatrics, 103*(5), 1122–1127.
111. The National Center on Addiction and Substance Abuse (CASA) at Columbia University. (2002). *CASA analysis of the National Household Survey on Drug Abuse (NHSDA), 1999* [Data file]. Rockville, MD: U.S. Department of Health and Human Services, Substance Abuse and Mental Health Services Administration.
112. Hops, H., Davis, B., & Lewin, L. M. (1999). The development of alcohol and other substance use: A gender study of family and peer context. *Journal of Studies on Alcohol, Suppl. 13*, 22–31.
113. Pulkkinen, L., & Pitkanen, T. (1994). A prospective study of the precursors to problem drinking in young adulthood. *Journal of Studies on Alcohol, 55*(5), 578–587.
114. CASA. (2002).
115. The National Center on Addiction and Substance Abuse (CASA) at Columbia University. (2003). *CASA analysis of the National Survey on Drug Use and Health, 2002* [Data file]. Rockville, MD: U.S. Department of Health and Human Services, Substance Abuse and Mental Health Services Administration, Office of Applied Studies.
116. Luthar, S. S., & D'Avanzo, K. (1999). Contextual factors in substance use: A study of suburban and inner-city adolescents. *Development and Psychopathology, 11*(4), 845–867.
117. Ibid.
118. Luthar, S. S., & Becker, B. E. (2002). Privileged but pressured? A study of affluent youth. *Child Development, 73*(5), 1593–1610.

119. CASA. (2002); CASA. (2003). *The formative years.*

120. Barber, J. G., Bolitho, F., & Bertrand, L. D. (1999). Intrapersonal versus peer group predictors of adolescent drug use. *Children and Youth Services Review, 21*(7), 565–579; Borsari, B., & Carey, K. B. (2001). Peer influences on college drinking: A review of the research. *Journal of Substance Abuse, 13*(4), 391–424; Simons-Morton, B., Haynie, D. L., Crump, A. D., & Saylor, K. E. (2001). Peer and parent influences on smoking and drinking among early adolescents. *Health Education and Behavior, 28*(1), 95–107.

121. Hu, F. B., Flay, B. R., Hedeker, D., Siddiqui, O., & Day, L. E. (1995). The influences of friends' and parental smoking on adolescent smoking behavior: The effects of time and prior smoking. *Journal of Applied Social Psychology, 25*(22), 2018–2047.

122. Belle, D. (1989). Gender differences in children's social networks and supports. In D. Belle (Ed.), *Children's social network and social supports* (pp. 173–188). New York: John Wiley and Sons.

123. Ibid.

124. Cauce, A. M., Felner, R. D., & Primavera, J. (1982). Social support in high-risk adolescents: Structural components and adaptive impact. *American Journal of Community Psychology, 10*(4), 417–428.

125. Borsari, B., & Carey, K. B. (2001); Chassin, L., Presson, C. C., Montello, D., McGrew, J., & Sherman, S. J. (1986). Changes in peer and parent influence during adolescence: Longitudinal versus cross-sectional perspectives on smoking initiation. *Developmental Psychology, 22*(3), 327–334; Reifman, A., Barnes, G. M., Dintcheff, B. A., Farrell, M. P., & Uhteg, L. (1998). Parental and peer influences on the onset of heavier drinking among adolescents. *Journal of Studies on Alcohol, 59*(3), 311–317.

126. CASA. (2003). *The formative years.*

127. Simons-Morton, B., Haynie, D. L., Crump, A. D., & Saylor, K. E. (2001).

128. Santor, D. A., Messervey, D., & Kusumaker, V. (2000). Measuring peer pressure, popularity, and conformity in adolescent boys and girls: Predicting school performance, sexual attitudes, and substance abuse. *Journal of Youth and Adolescence, 29*(2), 163–182; Simons-Morton, B., Haynie, D. L., Crump, A. D., & Saylor, K. E. (2001).

129. CASA. (2003). *The formative years.*

130. Ibid.

131. Seguire, M., & Chalmers, K. I. (2000). Late adolescent female smoking. *Journal of Advanced Nursing, 31*(6), 1422–1429.

132. Michell, L., & Amos, A. (1997). Girls, pecking order and smoking. *Social Science and Medicine, 44*(12), 1861–1869.

133. Ibid.

134. Farrell, A. D., & White, K. S. (1998). Peer influences and drug use among urban adolescents: Family structure and parent-adolescent relationship as protective factors. *Journal of Counseling and Clinical Psychology, 66*(2), 248–258; Simons-Morton, B., Haynie, D. L., Crump, A. D., & Saylor, K. E. (2001).

135. Simons-Morton, B., Haynie, D. L., Crump, A. D., & Saylor, K. E. (2001).

136. Crum, R. M., Lillie-Blanton, M., & Anthony, J. C. (1996). Neighborhood environment and opportunity to use cocaine and other drugs in late childhood and early adolescence. *Drug and Alcohol Dependence, 43*(3), 155–161; Moon, D. G., Hecht, M. L., Jackson, K. M., & Spellers, R. E. (1999). Ethnic and gender differences and similarities in adolescent drug use and refusals of drug offers. *Substance Use and Misuse, 34*(8), 1059–1083; Robinson, L. A., & Klesges, R. C. (1997). Ethnic and gender differences in risk factors for smoking onset. *Health Psychology, 16*(6), 499–505.

137. Van Etten, M. L., Neumark, Y. D., & Anthony, J. C. (1999). Male-female differences in the earliest stages of drug involvement. *Addiction, 94*(9), 1413–1419.

138. Centers for Disease Control and Prevention, Grunbaum, J. A., Kann, L., Kinchen, S. A., Williams, B., Ross, J. G., et al. (2004). Youth risk behavior surveillance: United States, 2003. *Morbidity and Mortality Weekly Report, 53*(SS-2).

139. Centers for Disease Control and Prevention, Grunbaum, J. A., Kann, L., Kinchen, S. A., Williams, B., Ross, J. G., et al. (2002). Youth risk behavior surveillance: United States, 2001. *Morbidity and Mortality Weekly Report, 51*(SS-4).

140. Castrucci, B. C., Gerlach, K. K., Kaufman, N. J., & Orleans, C. J. (2002). Adolescents' acquisition of cigarettes through noncommercial sources. *Journal of Adolescent Health, 31*(4), 322–326.

141. CASA. (2005).

142. Ibid.

143. Moon, D. G., Hecht, M. L., Jackson, K. M., & Spellers, R. E. (1999). Ethnic and gender differences and similarities in adolescent drug use and refusals of drug offers. *Substance Use and Misuse, 34*(8), 1059–1083.

144. Greene, S. M. (1992). *Alcohol, tobacco campaigns frequently aim at women, children, minorities: Marketers target "vulnerable" consumers.* www.drugs.indiana.edu (accessed June 11, 2002).

145. Center on Alcohol Marketing and Youth. (2002). *Television: Alcohol's vast adland.* Washington, DC: Georgetown University, Center on Alcohol Marketing and Youth.

146. American Medical Association. (2002). *Underage drinkers at higher risk of brain damage than adults, American Medical Association report reveals* [Press release]. Chicago: American Medical Association.

147. Bonnie, R. J., & O'Connell, M. E. (Eds.). (2004). *Reducing underage drinking: A collective responsibility.* Washington, DC: National Academy Press.

Chapter 2. Women and Smoking

1. Centers for Disease Control and Prevention. (2004). Cigarette smoking among adults: United States, 2002. *Morbidity and Mortality Weekly Report, 53*(20), 427–430.

2. Grunbaum, J. A., Kann, L., Kinchen, S., Ross, J., Hawkins, J., Lowry, R., et al. (2004). Youth Risk Behavior Surveillance: United States, 2003. *Morbidity and Mortality Weekly Report: Surveillance Summaries, 53*(SS-2).

3. Office of the Surgeon General. (2001). *Women and smoking: A report of the Surgeon General* (GPO Item No. 0483-L-06). Washington, DC: U.S. Government Printing Office.
4. U.S. Department of Health and Human Services. (2004). *Reducing tobacco use: A report of the Surgeon General* (GPO Item No. 0494-H-04). Washington, DC: U.S. Government Printing Office; Office of the Surgeon General. (2001). *Women and smoking.*
5. The National Center on Addiction and Substance Abuse (CASA) at Columbia University. (2005). *CASA's analysis of the National Survey on Drug Use and Health (NSDUH), 2003* [Data file]. Rockville, MD: U.S. Department of Health and Human Services, Substance Abuse and Mental Health Services Administration.
6. Centers for Disease Control and Prevention. (2002). Annual smoking-attributable mortality, years of potential life lost, and economic costs: United States 1995–1999. *Morbidity and Mortality Weekly Report, 51*(14), 300–303.
7. Office of the Surgeon General. (2001). *Women and smoking.*
8. Patel, J. D., Bach, P. B., & Kris, M. G. (2004). Lung cancer in US women: A contemporary epidemic. *JAMA, 291*(14), 1763–1768.
9. Centers for Disease Control and Prevention. (2002). Annual smoking-attributable mortality.
10. Ibid.
11. CASA. (2005).
12. Centers for Disease Control and Prevention. (2002). Annual smoking-attributable mortality.
13. Casper, M. L., Barnett, E., Halverson, J. A., Elmes, G. A., Braham, V. E., Majeed, Z. A., et al. (2002). *Women and heart disease: An atlas of racial and ethnic disparities in mortality* (2nd ed.). Atlanta, GA: Centers for Disease Control and Prevention.
14. Rich-Edwards, J. W., Manson, J. E., Hennekens, C. H., & Buring, J. E. (1995). The primary prevention of coronary heart disease in women. *New England Journal of Medicine, 332*(26), 1758–1766; Rosenberg, L., Palmer, J. R., & Shapiro, S. (1990). Decline in the risk of myocardial infarction among women who stop smoking. *New England Journal of Medicine, 322*(4), 213–217.
15. Patel, J. D., Bach, P. B., & Kris, M. G. (2004).
16. Office of the Surgeon General. (2001). *Women and smoking.*
17. Patel, J. D., Bach, P. B., & Kris, M. G. (2004).
18. Ibid.
19. Wyckoff, E. (1997). *Dry drunk: The culture of tobacco in the 17th and 18th century Europe.* www.nypl.org/research (accessed January 2, 2002).
20. Kluger, R. (1996). *Ashes to ashes.* New York: Knopf.
21. Office of the Surgeon General. (2001). *Women and smoking.*
22. CigarWoman.com. (1998). *A look at women and cigars: From the 19th century to the 1990's.* www.cigarwoman.com (accessed January 3, 2002).
23. Jensen, P. M. (1994). A history of women and smoking. *Canadian Woman Studies/Les Cahiers De La Femme, 14*(3), 29–32.
24. Hirschfelder, A. B. (1999). *Encyclopedia of smoking and tobacco.* Phoenix, AZ: Oryx.

25. Kluger, R. (1996).
26. Hirschfelder, A. B. (1999).
27. Kluger, R. (1996).
28. Ibid.
29. Office of the Surgeon General. (2001). *Women and smoking.*
30. Jensen, P. M. (1994).
31. Kluger, R. (1996).
32. Pierce, J. P., & Gilpin, E. A. (1995). A historical analysis of tobacco marketing and the uptake of smoking by youth in the United States: 1890–1977. *Health Psychology, 14*(6), 500–508.
33. Community Outreach Health Information System (COHIS). (2002). *COHIS: The ashtray: Smoking and tobacco abuse: The history of tobacco.* www.bu.edu (accessed December 28, 2001).
34. Pierce, J. P., & Gilpin, E. A. (1995).
35. Office of the Surgeon General. (2001). *Women and smoking.*
36. Ibid.
37. Moyer, D. (2000). *The tobacco reference guide.* www.tobaccoprogram.org (accessed February 24, 2004).
38. Office of the Surgeon General. (2001). *Women and smoking.*
39. Husten, C. G., Chrismon, J. H., & Reddy, M. N. (1996). Trends and effects of cigarette smoking among girls and women in the United States, 1965–1993. *Journal of the American Medical Women's Association, 51*(1), 11–18.
40. Office of the Surgeon General. (2001). *Women and smoking.*
41. Pierce, J. P., & Gilpin, E. A. (1995).
42. Office of the Surgeon General. (2001). *Women and smoking.*
43. Pierce, J. P., & Gilpin, E. A. (1995).
44. Pierce, J. P., Lee, L., & Gilpin, E. A. (1994). Smoking initiation by adolescent girls, 1944 through 1988. *JAMA, 271*(8), 608–611.
45. Kaufman, N. J., & Nichter, M. (2001). The marketing of tobacco to women: Global perspective. In J. M. Samet & S.-Y. Yoon (Eds.), *Women and the tobacco epidemic: Challenges for the 21st century* (pp. 69–98). Geneva, Switzerland: World Health Organization.
46. Wynder, E. L., & Graham, E. (1950). Tobacco smoking as a possible etiologic factor in bronchiogenic carcinoma: A study of 684 proven cases. *JAMA, 143*(4), 329–336.
47. Centers for Disease Control and Prevention, Office of Smoking and Health. (1999). Achievements in public health, 1900–1999: Tobacco use, United States, 1900–1999. *Morbidity and Mortality Weekly Report, 48*(43), 986–993.
48. Surgeon General's Advisory Committee on Smoking and Health. (1964). *Smoking and health: Report of the advisory committee to the Surgeon General of the Public Health Service* (Public Health Service Pub. No. 1103). Washington, DC: U.S. Government Printing Office.
49. Centers for Disease Control and Prevention, Office of Smoking and Health. (1999); Surgeon General's Advisory Committee on Smoking and Health. (1964).
50. Centers for Disease Control and Prevention. (2002). Cigarette smoking among adults: United States, 2000. *Morbidity and Mortality Weekly Report, 51*(29), 642–645; Centers for Dis-

ease Control and Prevention, National Center for Chronic Disease Prevention and Health Promotion. (2002). *Smoking prevalence among U.S. adults.* www.cdc.gov/tobacco (accessed April 12, 2004); Office of the Surgeon General. (2001). *Women and smoking.*

51. Substance Abuse and Mental Health Services Administration, Office of Applied Studies. (2002). *Results from the 2001 National Household Survey on Drug Abuse: Volume 1: Summary of national findings* (DHHS Pub. No. [SMA] 02-3758). Rockville, MD: U.S. Department of Health and Human Services.
52. Giovino, G. A., Henningfield, J. E., Tomar, S. L., Escobedo, L. G., & Slade, J. (1995). Epidemiology of tobacco use and dependence. *Epidemiological Reviews, 17*(1), 48–65.
53. Husten, C. G., Chrismon, J. H., & Reddy, M. N. (1996); Husten, C. (personal communication, May 20, 1998).
54. CASA. (2005).
55. The National Center on Addiction and Substance Abuse (CASA) at Columbia University. (1998). *Under the rug: Substance abuse and the mature woman.* New York: CASA.
56. CASA. (1998); King, A. C., Taylor, C. B., & Haskell, W. L. (1990). Smoking in older women: Is being female a "risk factor" for continued cigarette use? *Archives of Internal Medicine, 150*(9), 1841–1846.
57. Kandel, D. B., & Chen, K. (2000). Extent of smoking and nicotine dependence in the United States: 1991–1993. *Nicotine and Tobacco Research, 2*(3), 263–274.
58. Pierce, J. P., Lee, L., & Gilpin, E. A. (1994).
59. Johnston, L. D., O'Malley, P. M., & Bachman, J. G. (2001). *Monitoring the future: National survey results on drug use, 1975–2000: Volume 1: Secondary school students* (NIH Pub. No. 01-4924). Bethesda, MD: U.S. Department of Health and Human Services, National Institutes of Health, National Institute on Drug Abuse.
60. Johnston, L. D., O'Malley, P. M., & Bachman, J. G. (2001); Grunbaum, J. A., Kann, L., Kinchen, S., Ross, J., Hawkins, J., Lowry, R., et al. (2004).
61. American Legacy Foundation. (2000). *Legacy first look report: Cigarette smoking among youth: Results from the 1999 National Youth Tobacco Survey.* Washington, DC: American Legacy Foundation.
62. Grunbaum, J. A., Kann, L., Kinchen, S., Ross, J., Hawkins, J., Lowry, R., et al. (2004).
63. Ibid.; Wagner, E. F., & Atkins, J. H. (2000). Smoking among teenage girls. *Journal of Child and Adolescent Substance Abuse, 9*(4), 93–110.
64. Wallace, J. M., & Bachman, J. G. (1991). Explaining racial/ethnic differences in adolescent drug use: The impact of background and lifestyle. *Social Problems, 38*(3), 333–357.
65. Grunbaum, J. A., Kann, L., Kinchen, S., Ross, J., Hawkins, J., Lowry, R., et al. (2004); Wallace, J. M., Bachman, J. G., O'Malley, P. M., Schulenberg, J. E., Cooper, S. M., & Johnston, L. D. (2002). Gender and ethnic differences in smoking, drinking and illicit drug use among American 8th, 10th and 12th grade students, 1976–2000. *Addiction, 98*(2), 225–234.
66. Catalano, R. F., Morrison, D. M., Wells, E. A., Gillmore, M. R., Iritani, B., & Hawkins, J. D. (1992). Ethnic differences in family factors related to early drug initiation. *Journal of Studies on Alcohol, 53*(3), 208–217; Grunbaum, J. A., Kann, L., Kinchen, S., Ross, J., Hawkins, J.,

Lowry, R., et al. (2004); Johnson, R. A., & Hoffmann, J. P. (2000). Adolescent cigarette smoking in U.S. racial/ethnic subgroups: Findings from the National Education Longitudinal Study. *Journal of Health and Social Behavior, 41*(4), 392–407.

67. Grunbaum, J. A., Kann, L., Kinchen, S., Ross, J., Hawkins, J., Lowry, R., et al. (2004).
68. Johnston, L. D., O'Malley, P. M., & Bachman, J. G. (2003). *Monitoring the future: National survey results on drug use, 1975–2002: Volume 2, college students and adults ages 19–40* (NIH Pub. No. 03-5376). Bethesda, MD: U.S. Department of Health and Human Services, National Institutes of Health, National Institute on Drug Abuse.
69. Rigotti, N. A., Lee, J. E., & Wechsler, H. (2000). US College students' use of tobacco products: Results of a national survey. *JAMA, 284*(6), 699–705.
70. Johnston, L. D., O'Malley, P. M., & Bachman, J. G. (2000). *Monitoring the future: National survey results on drug use, 1975–1999: Volume 2: College students and adults ages 19–40* (NIH Pub. No. 00-4803). Bethesda, MD: U.S. Department of Health and Human Services, National Institutes of Health, National Institute on Drug Abuse.
71. Office of the Surgeon General. (2001). *Women and smoking.*
72. Johnston, L. D., O'Malley, P. M., & Bachman, J. G. (2000).
73. Office of the Surgeon General. (2001). *Women and smoking.*
74. Rigotti, N. A., Lee, J. E., & Wechsler, H. (2000).
75. Farrell, E. F. (2005, March 18). The battle for hearts and lungs. *Chronicle of Higher Education.*
76. Ibid.
77. The National Center on Addiction and Substance Abuse (CASA) at Columbia University. (2003). *The formative years: Pathways to substance abuse among girls and young women ages 8–22.* New York: CASA.
78. Wechsler, H., Rigotti, N. A., Gledhill-Hoyt, J., & Lee, H. (1998). Increased levels of cigarette use among college students: A cause for national concern. *JAMA, 280*(19), 1673–1678.
79. Brecher, E. M., & Editors of Consumer Reports Magazine. (1972). *Consumers Union report on licit and illicit drugs.* www.druglibrary.org (accessed December 28, 2001).
80. Hirschfelder, A. B. (1999).
81. Hampl, J. S., & Betts, N. M. (1999). Cigarette use during adolescence: Effects on nutritional status. *Nutrition Reviews, 57*(7), 215–221.
82. Zickler, P. (2003). Nicotine's multiple effects on the brain's reward system drive addiction. *NIDA Notes, 17*(6).
83. Mansvelder, H. D., & McGehee, D. S. (2000). Long-term potentiation of excitatory inputs to brain reward areas by nicotine. *Neuron, 27*(2), 349–357.
84. Hampl, J. S., & Betts, N. M. (1999).
85. Hunter, S. M. (2001). Quitting. In J. M. Samet & S.-Y. Yoon (Eds.), *Women and the tobacco epidemic: Challenges for the 21st century* (pp. 121–146). Geneva, Switzerland: World Health Organization.
86. Kandel, D. B., & Chen, K. (2000).
87. Ibid.

88. DiFranza, J. R., Savageau, J. A., Rigotti, N. A. F. K., Ockene, J. K., McNeill, A. D., Coleman, M., et al. (2002). Development of symptoms of tobacco dependence in youths: 30 month follow up data from the DANDY study. *Tobacco Control, 11*(3), 228–235.
89. Breslau, N., & Peterson, E. L. (1996). Smoking cessation in young adults: Age at initiation of cigarette smoking and other suspected influences. *American Journal of Public Health, 86*(2), 214–220; Lando, H. A., Thai, D. T., Murray, D. M., Robinson, L. A., Jeffery, R. W., Sherwood, N. E., et al. (1999). Age of initiation, smoking patterns, and risk in a population of working adults. *Preventive Medicine, 29*(6, Pt. 1), 590–598.
90. Pierce, J. P., & Gilpin, E. A. (1995).
91. Office of the Surgeon General. (1980). *The health consequences of smoking for women: A report of the Surgeon General.* Washington, DC: U.S. Department of Health and Human Services, Public Health Service, Office of the Assistant Secretary for Health, Office on Smoking and Health.
92. Office of the Surgeon General. (2001). *Women and smoking.*
93. Centers for Disease Control and Prevention. (2002). Annual smoking-attributable mortality.
94. Ramirez, A. G., & Gallion, K. J. (1993). Nicotine dependence among blacks and Hispanics. In C. T. Orleans & J. Slade (Eds.), *Nicotine addiction: Principles and management* (pp. 350–364). New York: Oxford University Press; Solomon, L. J., & Flynn, B. S. (1993). Women who smoke. In C. T. Orleans & J. Slade (Eds.), *Nicotine addiction: Principles and management* (pp. 339–349).
95. English, P. B., Eskenazi, B., & Christianson, R. E. (1994). Black-white differences in serum cotinine levels among pregnant women and subsequent effects on infant birthweight. *American Journal of Public Health, 84*(9), 1439–1443.
96. Royce, J. M., Hymowitz, N., Corbett, K., Hartwell, T. D., & Orlandi, M. A. (1993). Smoking cessation factors among African Americans and whites. *American Journal of Public Health, 83*(2), 220–226; Solomon, L. J., & Flynn, B. S. (1993). But see Ahijevych, K., Gillespie, J., Demirci, M., & Jagadeesh, J. (1996). Menthol and nonmenthol cigarettes and smoke exposure in black and white women. *Pharmacology, Biochemistry and Behavior, 53*(2), 355–360.
97. DeNavas, C., & U.S. Bureau of the Census. (1995). *Income, poverty, and valuation of noncash benefits, 1993* (GPO Item No. 0142-C-07). Washington, DC: U.S. Government Printing Office.
98. Husten, C. G., Chrismon, J. H., & Reddy, M. N. (1996); National Center for Chronic Disease Prevention and Health Promotion. (2001). *Cigarette smoking-related mortality.* www.cdc.gov/tobacco.
99. American Cancer Society. (2003). *Cigarette smoking.* www.cancer.org (accessed March 31, 2004).
100. American College of Chest Physicians. (2004). *Smoking trends and health issues: Women and girls.* http://speakerskit.chestnet.org (accessed January 3, 2002).
101. Zang, E., & Wynder, E. (1996). Differences in lung cancer risk between men and women. *Journal of the National Cancer Institute, 88*(3–4), 183–192.
102. Dresler, C. M. (1998). The lung cancer epidemic in women: Why female smokers are at much greater risk than men. *Women's Health in Primary Care, 1*(1), 85–92.

103. Mason, J. O., Tolsma, D. O., Peterson, H. B., & Rowland Hogue, C. J. (1988). Health promotion for women: Reduction of smoking in primary care settings. *Clinical Obstetrics and Gynecology, 31*(4), 989–1002.

104. Thun, M. J., Day-Lally, C. A., Calle, E. E., Flanders, W. D., & Heath, C. W. (1995). Excess mortality among cigarette smokers: Changes in a 20-year interval. *American Journal of Public Health, 85*(9), 1223–1230.

105. Office of the Surgeon General. (2001). *Women and smoking.*

106. American Lung Association. (2003). *Facts about lung cancer.* www.lungusa.org (accessed March 31, 2004).

107. Ernster, V. L. (1996). Female lung cancer. *Annual Review of Public Health, 17,* 97–114.

108. Office of the Surgeon General. (1989). *Reducing the health consequences of smoking: 25 years of progress: A report of the Surgeon General* (DHHS Pub. No. [CDC] 89-8411). Washington, DC: U.S. Government Printing Office.

109. Holt, V. L., Daling, J. R., McKnight, B., Moore, D. E., Stergachis, A., & Weiss, N. S. (1994). Cigarette smoking and functional ovarian cysts. *American Journal of Epidemiology, 139*(8), 781–786; Licciardone, J. C., Brownson, R. C., Chang, J. C., & Wilkens, J. R. (1990). Uterine cervical cancer risk in cigarette smokers: A meta-analytic study. *American Journal of Preventive Medicine, 6*(5), 274–281; Office of the Surgeon General. (2001). *Women and smoking*; Sood, A. K. (1991). Cigarette smoking and cervical cancer: Meta-analysis and critical review of recent studies. *American Journal of Preventive Medicine, 7*(4), 208–213; Winkelstein, W. (1990). Smoking and cervical cancer, current status: A review. *American Journal of Epidemiology, 131*(6), 945–957.

110. Dobson, R. (2002). Risk of breast cancer increases with numbers of years' smoking. *British Medical Journal, 325*(7359), 298.

111. Office of the Surgeon General. (1989).

112. American Heart Association. (2004). *Heart disease and stroke statistics: 2004 update.* Dallas, TX: American Heart Association; Gardner, P., & Hudson, B. L. (1996). Advance report of final mortality statistics, 1993. *Monthly Vital Statistics Report, 44*(7).

113. Rich-Edwards, J. W., Manson, J. E., Hennekens, C. H., & Buring, J. E. (1995).

114. Centers for Disease Control and Prevention. (1993). Cigarette smoking-attributable mortality and years of potential life lost: United States, 1990. *Morbidity and Mortality Weekly Report, 42*(33), 645–649; Office of the Surgeon General. (1989).

115. American Heart Association. (2004). *Risk factors and coronary heart disease.* www. americanheart.org (accessed February 27, 2004).

116. Office of the Surgeon General. (1989).

117. American Heart Association. (2004). *Risk factors and coronary heart disease.*

118. Rich-Edwards, J. W., Manson, J. E., Hennekens, C. H., & Buring, J. E. (1995); Rosenberg, L., Palmer, J. R., & Shapiro, S. (1990).

119. Willett, W. C., Green, A., Stampfer, M. J., Speizer, F. E., Colditz, G. A., Rosner, B., et al. (1987). Relative and absolute excess risks of coronary heart disease among women who smoke cigarettes. *New England Journal of Medicine, 317*(21), 1303–1309.

120. Shopland, D. R., & Office of the Surgeon General. (1983). *The health consequences of smoking: Cardiovascular disease: A report of the Surgeon General* (DHHS Pub. No. [PHS] 84-50204). Washington, DC: U.S. Government Printing Office.
121. Aronow, W. S., Ahn, C., & Gutstein, H. (1996). Risk factors for new atherothrombotic brain infarction in 664 older men and 1,488 older women. *American Journal of Cardiology, 77*(15), 1381–1383; Office of the Surgeon General. (1989).
122. Office of the Surgeon General. (2001). *Women and smoking.*
123. Chapman, K. R., Tashkin, D. P., & Pye, D. J. (2001). Gender bias in the diagnosis of COPD. *Chest, 119*(6), 1691–1695.
124. Langhammer, A., Holmen, J., Johnsen, R., Bjermer, L., & Gulsvik, A. (2000). Cigarette smoking gives more respiratory symptoms among women than among men: The Nørd-Trøndelag Health Study (HUNT). *Journal of Epidemiology and Community Health, 54*(12), 917–922.
125. Straten, M. V., Carrasco, D., Paterson, M. S., McCrary, M. L., Meyer, D. J., & Tyring, S. K. (2001). Tobacco use and skin disease. *Southern Medical Journal, 94*(6), 621–634.
126. Hart, G. T., Brown, D. M., & Mincer, H. (1995). Tobacco use and dental disease. *Journal of the Tennessee Dental Association, 75*(2), 25–27.
127. Axelsson, P., Paulander, J., & Lindhe, J. (1998). Relationship between smoking and dental status in 35-, 50-, 65-, and 75-year-old individuals. *Journal of Clinical Periodontology, 25*(4), 297–305; Haber, J., Wattles, J., Crowley, M., Mandell, R., Joshipura, K., & Kent, R. L. (1993). Evidence for cigarette smoking as a major risk factor for periodontitis. *Journal of Periodontology, 64*(1), 16–23.
128. American Lung Association. (2002). *Secondhand smoke* [Fact sheet]. www.lungusa.org (accessed February 24, 2004).
129. Centers for Disease Control and Prevention. (2002). Annual smoking-attributable mortality.
130. Fontham, E. T. H., Correa, P., Reynolds, P., Wu-Williams, A., Buffler, P. A., Greenberg, R. S., et al. (1994). Environmental tobacco smoke and lung cancer in nonsmoking women: A multicenter study. *JAMA, 271*(22), 1752–1759.
131. Farkas, A. J., Gilpin, E. A., Distefan, J. M., & Pierce, J. P. (1999). The effects of household and workplace smoking restrictions on quitting behaviours. *Tobacco Control, 8*(3), 261–265.
132. American Lung Association. (2003). *When you smoke, your family smokes!* www.lungusa.org (accessed March 22, 2004).
133. Ensrud, K. E., Nevitt, M. C., Yunis, C., Cauley, J. A., Seeley, D. G., Fox, K. M., et al. (1994). Correlates of impaired function in older women. *Journal of the American Geriatrics Society, 42*(5), 481–489; Nelson, H. D., Nevitt, M. C., Scott, J. C., Stone, K. L., & Cummings, S. R. (1994). Smoking, alcohol, and neuromuscular and physical function of older women. *JAMA, 272*(23), 1825–1832.
134. Nelson, H. D., Nevitt, M. C., Scott, J. C., Stone, K. L., & Cummings, S. R. (1994).
135. Seddon, J. M., Willett, W. C., Speizer, F. E., & Hankinson, S. E. (1996). A prospective study of cigarette smoking and age-related macular degeneration in women. *JAMA, 276*(14), 1141–1146.

136. Baron, J. A., La Vecchia, C., & Levi, F. (1990). The antiestrogenic effect of cigarette smoking in women. *American Journal of Obstetrics and Gynecology, 162*(2), 502–514; Hopper, J. L., & Seeman, E. (1994). The bone density of female twins discordant for tobacco use. *New England Journal of Medicine, 330*(6), 387–392; Slemenda, C. W. (1994). Cigarettes and the skeleton. *New England Journal of Medicine, 330*(6), 430.
137. Hopper, J. L., & Seeman, E. (1994).
138. Baron, J. A., La Vecchia, C., & Levi, F. (1990); Hopper, J. L., & Seeman, E. (1994); Jensen, J., Christiansen, C., & Rodbro, P. (1985). Cigarette smoking, serum estrogens and bone loss during hormone-replacement therapy after early menopause. *New England Journal of Medicine, 313*(16), 973–975; Slemenda, C. W. (1994).
139. Franceschi, S., Schinella, D., Bidoli, E., Dal Maso, L., La Vecchia, C., Parazzini, F., et al. (1996). The influence of body size, smoking and diet on bone density in pre- and postmenopausal women. *Epidemiology, 7*(4), 411–414; Longcope, C., & Johnston, C. C. (1988). Androgen and estrogen dynamics in pre- and postmenopausal women: A comparison between smokers and nonsmokers. *Journal of Clinical Endocrinology and Metabolism, 76*(2), 379–383; Williams, A. R., Weiss, N. S., Ure, C. L., Ballard, J., & Daling, J. R. (1982). Effect of weight, smoking and estrogen use on the risk of hip and forearm fractures in postmenopausal women. *Journal of Obstetrics and Gynecology, 60*(6), 695–699.
140. Slemenda, C. W. (1994); Willett, W., Stampfer, M. J., Bain, C., Lipnick, R., Speizer, F. E., Rosner, B., et al. (1983). Cigarette smoking, relative weight, and menopause. *American Journal of Epidemiology, 117*(6), 651–658.
141. Office of the Surgeon General. (2001). *Women and smoking.*
142. Slemenda, C. W. (1994); Willett, W., Stampfer, M. J., Bain, C., Lipnick, R., Speizer, F. E., Rosner, B., et al. (1983).
143. Hopper, J. L., & Seeman, E. (1994); Looker, A. C., Johnston, C. C., Wahner, H. W., Dunn, W. L., Calvo, M. S., Harris, T. B., et al. (1995). Prevalence of low femoral bone density in older U.S. women from NHANES III. *Journal of Bone and Mineral Research, 10*(5), 796–802; Slemenda, C. W. (1994).
144. Slemenda, C. W. (1994).
145. Vogt, M. T., Cauley, J. A., Scott, J. C., Kuller, L. H., & Browner, W. S. (1996). Smoking and mortality among older women. *Archives of Internal Medicine, 156*(6), 630–636.
146. Fried, L. P., Kronmal, R. A., Newman, A. B., Bild, D. E., Mittelmark, M. B., Polak, J. F., et al. (1998). Risk factors for 5-year mortality in older adults: The cardiovascular health study. *JAMA, 279*(8), 585–592.
147. Office of the Surgeon General. (1994). *Preventing tobacco use among young people: A report of the Surgeon General.* Washington, DC: U.S. Government Printing Office.
148. Gold, D. R., Wang, X., Wypij, D., Speizer, F. E., Ware, J. H., & Dockery, D. W. (1996). Effects of cigarette smoking on lung function in adolescent boys and girls. *New England Journal of Medicine, 335*(13), 931–937.
149. Holmen, T. L., Barrett-Connor, E., Holmen, J., & Bjermer, L. (2000). Health problems in

teenage daily smokers versus nonsmokers, Norway, 1995–1997: The Nørd-Trøndelag health study. *American Journal of Epidemiology, 151*(2), 148–155.

150. Johnson, P. B., & Richter, L. (2002). The relationship between smoking, drinking, and adolescents' self-perceived health and frequency of hospitalization: Analyses from the 1997 National Household Survey on Drug Abuse. *Journal of Adolescent Health, 30*(3), 175–183.
151. Paulus, D., Saint-Remy, A., & Jeanjean, M. (2000). Oral contraception and cardiovascular risk factors during adolescence. *Contraception, 62*(3), 113–116.
152. Office of the Surgeon General. (2001). *Women and smoking.*
153. Arday, D. R., Govino, G. A., Schulman, J., Nelson, D. E., Mowery, P., & Samet, J. M. (1995). Cigarette smoking and self-reported health problems among US high school seniors, 1982–1989. *American Journal of Health Promotion, 10*(2), 111–116.
154. Wu, L.-T., & Anthony, J. C. (1999). Tobacco smoking and depressed mood in late childhood and early adolescence. *American Journal of Public Health, 89*(12), 1837–1840.
155. Goodman, E., & Capitman, J. (2000). Depressive symptoms and cigarette smoking among teens. *Pediatrics, 106*(4), 748–755; CASA. (2003). *The formative years*; Wu, L.-T., & Anthony, J. C. (1999).
156. CASA. (2003). *The formative years.*
157. Goodman, E., & Capitman, J. (2000).
158. Breslau, N., & Klein, D. F. (1999). Smoking and panic attacks: An epidemiologic investigation. *Archives of General Psychiatry, 56*(12), 1141–1147.
159. Abdelrahman, A. I., Rodriguez, G., Ryan, J. A., French, J. F., & Weinbaum, D. (1998). The epidemiology of substance use among middle school students: The impact of school, familial, community and individual risk factors. *Journal of Child and Adolescent Substance Abuse, 8*(1), 55–75.
160. French, S. A., & Perry, C. L. (1996). Smoking among adolescent girls: Prevalence and etiology. *Journal of the American Medical Women's Association, 51*(1–2), 25–28.
161. CASA. (2003). *The formative years.*
162. Kandel, D. B., Yamaguchi, K., & Chen, K. (1992). Stages of progression in drug involvement from adolescence to adulthood: Further evidence for the gateway theory. *Journal of Studies on Alcohol, 53*(5), 447–457.
163. Substance Abuse and Mental Health Services Administration, Office of Applied Studies. (2002). *Results,* vol. 1.
164. Pomerleau, O. F., Collins, A. C., Shiffman, S., & Pomerleau, C. S. (1993). Why some people smoke and others do not: New perspectives. *Journal of Consulting and Clinical Psychology, 61*(5), 723–731.
165. Office of the Surgeon General. (2001). *Women and smoking.*
166. Richter, L., & Richter, D. M. (2001). Exposure to parental tobacco and alcohol use: Effects on children's health and development. *American Journal of Orthopsychiatry, 71*(2), 182–203; Vakalahi, H. F. (2001). Adolescent substance use and family-based risk and protective factors: A literature review. *Journal of Drug Education, 31*(1), 29–46.

167. Clayton, S. (1991). Gender differences in psychosocial determinants of adolescent smoking. *Journal of School Health, 61*(3), 115–120; Conrad, K. M., Flay, B. R., & Hill, D. (1992). Why children start smoking cigarettes: Predictors of onset. *British Journal of Addiction, 87*(12), 1711–1724.
168. Chassin, L., Presson, C. C., Montello, D., McGrew, J., & Sherman, S. J. (1986). Changes in peer and parent influence during adolescence: Longitudinal versus cross-sectional perspectives on smoking initiation. *Developmental Psychology, 22*(3), 327–334; Kandel, D. B., Wu, P., & Davies, M. (1994). Maternal smoking during pregnancy and smoking by adolescent daughters. *American Journal of Public Health, 84*(9), 1407–1413; Hu, F. B., Flay, B. R., Hedeker, D., Siddiqui, O., & Day, L. E. (1995). The influences of friends' and parental smoking on adolescent smoking behavior: The effects of time and prior smoking. *Journal of Applied Social Psychology, 25*(22), 2018–2047.
169. Bauman, K. E., Foshee, V. A., & Haley, N. J. (1992). The interaction of sociological and biological factors in adolescent cigarette smoking. *Addictive Behaviors, 17*(5), 459–467; Kandel, D. B., Wu, P., & Davies, M. (1994).
170. Andrews, J. A., Hops, H., Ary, D., Tildesley, E., & Harris, J. (1993). Parental influence on early adolescent substance use: Specific and non-specific effects. *Journal of Early Adolescence, 13*(3), 285–310; Males, M. (1995). The influence of parental smoking on youth smoking: Is the recent downplaying justified? *Journal of School Health, 65*(6), 228–221.
171. Clayton, S. (1991).
172. Kandel, D. B., Wu, P., & Davies, M. (1994).
173. Ibid.
174. Hall, W., Madden, P., & Lynskey, M. (2002). The genetics of tobacco use: Methods, findings and policy implications. *Tobacco Control, 11*(2), 119–124.
175. Ibid.
176. Ibid.
177. Burt, R., Dinh, K., Peterson, A., & Sarason, I. (2000). Predicting adolescent smoking: A prospective study of personality variables. *Preventive Medicine, 30*(2), 115–125.
178. Stein, J., Newcomb, M., & Bentler, P. (1996). Initiation and maintenance of tobacco smoking: Changing personality correlates in adolescence and young adulthood. *Journal of Applied Social Psychology, 26*(2), 160–187.
179. Amos, A., Gray, D., Currie, C., & Elton, R. (1997). Healthy or druggy? Self-image, ideal image and smoking behaviour among young people. *Social Science and Medicine, 45*(6), 847–858.
180. Aloise-Young, P. A., & Hennigan, K. M. (1996). Self-image, the smoker stereotype and cigarette smoking: Developmental patterns from fifth through eighth grade. *Journal of Adolescence, 19*(2), 163–177; Seguire, M., & Chalmers, K. I. (2000). Late adolescent female smoking. *Journal of Advanced Nursing, 31*(6), 1422–1429.
181. Seguire, M., & Chalmers, K. I. (2000).
182. Michell, L., & Amos, A. (1997). Girls, pecking order and smoking. *Social Science and Medicine, 44*(12), 1861–1869.

183. Abdelrahman, A. I., Rodriguez, G., Ryan, J. A., French, J. F., & Weinbaum, D. (1998).
184. Hu, F. B., Flay, B. R., Hedeker, D., Siddiqui, O., & Day, L. E. (1995).
185. Chassin, L., Presson, C. C., Montello, D., McGrew, J., & Sherman, S. J. (1986).
186. Wang, M. Q., Fitzhugh, E. C., Westerfield, R. C., & Eddy, J. M. (1995). Family and peer influences on smoking behavior among American adolescents: An age trend. *Journal of Adolescent Health, 16*(3), 200–203.
187. Simons-Morton, B., Haynie, D. L., Crump, A. D., & Saylor, K. E. (2001). Peer and parent influences on smoking and drinking among early adolescents. *Health Education and Behavior, 28*(1), 95–107.
188. CASA. (2003). *The formative years.*
189. Seguire, M., & Chalmers, K. I. (2000).
190. Wills, T., Sandy, J., Shinar, O., & Yaeger, A. (1999). Contributions of positive and negative affect to adolescent substance use: Test of bidimensional model in a longitudinal study. *Psychology of Addictive Behaviors, 13*(4), 327–338.
191. Simantov, E., Schoen, C., & Klein, J. (2000). Health-compromising behaviors: Why do adolescents smoke or drink? *Archives of Pediatrics and Adolescent Medicine, 154*(10), 1025–1033.
192. Bray, R. M., Fairbank, J. A., & Marsden, M. E. (1999). Stress and substance use among military women and men. *American Journal of Drug and Alcohol Abuse, 25*(2), 239–256; CASA. (2003). *The formative years.*
193. CASA. (2003). *The formative years.*
194. Byrne, D., Byrne, A., & Reinhart, M. (1995). Personality, stress and the decision to commence cigarette smoking in adolescence. *Journal of Psychosomatic Research, 39*(1), 53–62.
195. National Center for Health Statistics. (1994). *Teenage Attitudes and Practices Survey 2, 1993.* Ann Arbor, MI: Inter-university Consortium for Political and Social Research.
196. Commonwealth Fund. (1997). *Facts on risky behaviors: The Commonwealth Fund survey of the health of adolescent girls.* www.cmwf.org (accessed March 8, 2004).
197. Guthrie, B. J., Young, A. M., Boyd, C. J., & Kintner, E. K. (2001). Dealing with daily hassles: Smoking and African-American adolescent girls. *Journal of Adolescent Health, 29*(2), 109–115.
198. Guthrie, B. J., Young, A. M., Williams, D. R., Boyd, C. J., & Kintner, E. K. (2002). African American girls' smoking habits and day to day experiences with racial discrimination. *Nursing Research, 51*(3), 183–190.
199. Johnson, J. G., Cohen, P., Pine, D. S., Klein, D. F., Kasen, S., & Brook, J. S. (2000). Association between cigarette smoking and anxiety disorders during adolescence and early adulthood. *JAMA, 284*(18), 2348–2351.
200. Grunberg, N. E., & Klein, L. C. (1998). The relevance of stress and eating to the study of gender and drug use. In C. L. Wetherington & A. B. Roman (Eds.), *Drug addiction research and the health of women* (NIH Pub. No. 98-4290, pp. 173–186). Rockville, MD: U.S. Department of Health and Human Services, National Institutes of Health, National Institute on Drug Abuse.
201. Pomerleau, C. C., Berman, B. A., Gritz, E. R., Marks, J. L., & Goeters, S. (1994). Why women smoke. In R. R. Watson (Ed.), *Addictive behaviors in women* (pp. 39–70). Totowa, NJ: Humana Press.

202. Austin, S. B., & Gortmaker, S. L. (2001). Dieting and smoking initiation in early adolescent girls and boys: A prospective study. *American Journal of Public Health, 91*(3), 446–450.

203. Maine, M. (2000). *Body wars: Making peace with women's bodies: An activist's guide.* Carlsbad, CA: Gürze Books.

204. Grunbaum, J. A., Kann, L., Kinchen, S., Ross, J., Hawkins, J., Lowry, R., et al. (2004).

205. Austin, S. B., & Gortmaker, S. L. (2001); Voorhees, C. C., Schreiber, G. B., Schumann, B. C., Biro, F., & Crawford, P. B. (2002). Early predictors of daily smoking in young women: The National Heart, Lung, and Blood Institute Growth and Health Study. *Preventive Medicine, 34*(6), 616–624.

206. French, S. A., Perry, C. L., Leon, G. R., & Fulkerson, J. A. (1994). Weight concerns, dieting behavior, and smoking initiation among adolescents: A prospective study. *American Journal of Public Health, 84*(11), 1818–1820; Granner, M. L., Black, D. R., & Abood, D. A. (2002). Levels of cigarette and alcohol use related to eating-disorder attitudes. *American Journal of Health Behavior, 26*(1), 43–55; Pomerleau, C. C., Berman, B. A., Gritz, E. R., Marks, J. L., & Goeters, S. (1994).

207. Camp, D. E., Klesges, R. C., & Relyea, G. (1993). The relationship between body weight concerns and adolescent smoking. *Health Psychology, 12*(1), 24–32; Klesges, R. C., & Meyers, A. W. (1989). Smoking, body weight, and their effects on smoking behavior: A comprehensive review of the literature. *Psychological Bulletin, 106*(2), 204–230.

208. Austin, S. B., & Gortmaker, S. L. (2001).

209. Grunberg, N. E., & Klein, L. C. (1998); Bryant, A. (2000, March 20). In tobacco's face. *Newsweek, 135*(12), 40–41.

210. Gross, J., Stitzer, M. L., & Maldonado, J. (1989). Nicotine replacement: Effects of postcessation weight gain. *Journal of Consulting and Clinical Psychology, 57*(1), 87–92.

211. Wyckoff, E. (1997).

212. Tobaccoads.org. (2004). *Misty: Slim 'n sassy tobacco advertisement.* www.tobaccoads.org (accessed November 5, 2004).

213. *Capri advertising.* (1998). www.geocities.com/SouthBeach/Palms/2120/capriads.htm (accessed January 29, 2003).

214. Office of the Surgeon General. (2001). *Marketing cigarettes to women* [Fact sheet]. www.cdc.gov (accessed February 27, 2004).

215. Landers, S. J. (2002). *Antitobacco activists lift smokescreen behind teen smoking.* www.ama-assn.org (accessed February 27, 2004).

216. Johnston, L. D., O'Malley, P. M., Bachman, J. G., & Schulenberg, J. E. (2005). *Monitoring the future: National results on adolescent drug use: Overview of key findings, 2004* (NIH Pub. No. 05-5726). Bethesda, MD: U.S. Department of Health and Human Services, National Institutes of Health, National Institute on Drug Abuse.

217. DiFranza, J. R., Savageau, J. A., & Aisquith, B. F. (1996). Youth access to tobacco: The effects of age, gender, vending machine locks, and "It's the Law" programs. *American Journal of Public Health, 86*(2), 221–224.

218. American College of Chest Physicians. (2004).

219. DiFranza, J. R., Savageau, J. A., & Aisquith, B. F. (1996).
220. Centers for Disease Control and Prevention, Grunbaum, J. A., Kann, L., Kinchen, S. A., Williams, B., Ross, J. G., et al. (2002). Youth risk behavior surveillance: United States, 2001. *Morbidity and Mortality Weekly Report: Surveillance Summaries, 51*(SS-4).
221. Campaign for Tobacco-free Kids. (2004). *Women and girls and tobacco.* http://tobaccofreekids.org (accessed February 27, 2004).
222. Chung, P. J., Garfield, C. F., Rathouz, P. J., & Lauderdale, D. (2002). Youth targeting by tobacco manufacturers since the master settlement agreement. *Health Affairs, 21*(2), 254–263.
223. Campaign for Tobacco-free Kids. (2000). *New study shows tobacco advertising impacts kids more than adults: Three-quarters of teens also say it is easy for minors to buy cigarettes: Study released on Kick Butts Day as kids call on next president to protect them from tobacco* [Press release]. www.tobaccofreekids.org (accessed March 18, 2004).
224. Office of the Surgeon General. (2000). *Tobacco advertising and promotion: The Surgeon General's report on reducing tobacco use* [Fact sheet]. www.cdc.gov/tobacco/sgr (accessed March 29, 2004); Campaign for Tobacco-free Kids. (2004). *Tobacco marketing to kids* [Fact sheet]. www.tobaccofreekids.org (accessed March 26, 2004).
225. Whelan, E. M. (1998). *Health advice in women's magazines: Up in smoke.* www.acsh.org (accessed February 27, 2004).
226. Pierce, J. P., Choi, W. S., Gilpin, E. A., Farkas, A. J., & Berry, C. C. (1998). Tobacco industry promotion of cigarettes and adolescent smoking. *JAMA, 279*(7), 511–515.
227. Biener, L., & Siegel, M. (2000). Tobacco marketing and adolescent smoking: More support for a causal inference. *American Journal of Public Health, 90*(3), 407–411.
228. Campaign for Tobacco-free Kids. (2000).
229. Centers for Disease Control and Prevention. (1996). Projected smoking-related deaths among youth: United States. *Morbidity and Mortality Weekly Report, 45*(44), 971–974.
230. American Lung Association. (2002). *Teenage girls as the target of the tobacco industry* [Fact sheet]. www.lungusa.org (accessed March 26, 2004).
231. Samet, J. M., & Yoon, S.-Y. (Eds.). (2001). *Women and the tobacco epidemic: Challenges for the 21st century.* Geneva, Switzerland: World Health Organization, Johns Hopkins School of Health, Institute for Global Tobacco Control; Hammond, R., Rowell, A., Campaign for Tobacco-free Kids, & Action on Smoking and Health. (2001). *Trust us: We're the tobacco industry.* www.ash.org.uk (accessed March 18, 2004).
232. Patel, J. D., Bach, P. B., & Kris, M. G. (2004).
233. Glantz, S. A. (2001). Smoking in teenagers and watching films showing smoking: Hollywood needs to stop promoting smoking worldwide [Editorial]. *British Medical Journal, 323*(7326), 1378–1379.
234. Sargent, J. D., Beach, M. L., Dalton, M. A., Mott, L. A., Tickle, J. J., Ahrens, M. B., et al. (2001). Effect of seeing tobacco use in films on trying smoking among adolescents: Cross sectional study. *British Medical Journal, 323*(7326), 1394–1397.
235. Ibid.

236. Everett, S. A., Schnuth, R. L., & Tribble, J. L. (1998). Tobacco and alcohol use in top-grossing American films. *Journal of Community Health, 23*(4), 317–324.
237. Sargent, J. D., Beach, M. L., Dalton, M. A., Mott, L. A., Tickle, J. J., Ahrens, M. B., et al. (2001).
238. Escamilla, G., Cradock, A. L., & Kawachi, I. (2000). Women and smoking in Hollywood movies: A content analysis. *American Journal of Public Health, 90*(3), 412–414.
239. Roberts, D. F., & Christenson, P. G. (2000). *"Here's looking at you, kid": Alcohol, drugs and tobacco in the entertainment media: A literature review prepared by the National Center on Addiction and Substance Abuse at Columbia University.* Menlo Park, CA: Henry J. Kaiser Family Foundation.
240. Escamilla, G., Cradock, A. L., & Kawachi, I. (2000).
241. Office of National Drug Control Policy, & Substance Abuse and Mental Health Services Administration. (1999). *Substance use in popular movies and music.* www.mediacampaign.org (accessed December 4, 2001).
242. Goldstein, A. O., Sobel, R. A., & Newman, G. R. (1999). Tobacco and alcohol use in G-rated children's animated films. *JAMA, 281*(12), 1131–1136.
243. Ng, C., & Dakake, B. (2002). *Tobacco at the movies: Tobacco use in PG–13 films.* http: / /masspirg.org (accessed October 31, 2002).
244. Martin, G., & Elkin, E. J. (1995). *Aficionadas: Women and their cigars.* www.cigaraficionado .com (accessed January 31, 2002).
245. Federal Trade Commission. (1999). *Cigar sales and advertising and promotional expenditures for calendar years 1996 and 1997.* Washington, DC: U.S. Federal Trade Commission.
246. Substance Abuse and Mental Health Services Administration, Office of Applied Studies. (2002). *Results,* vol. 1; Substance Abuse and Mental Health Services Administration, Office of Applied Studies. (2002). *Results from the 2001 National Household Survey on Drug Abuse: Volume 2: Technical appendices and selected data tables* (DHHS Pub. No. [SMA] 02-3759). Rockville, MD: U.S. Department of Health and Human Services, Substance Abuse and Mental Health Services Administration, Office of Applied Studies.
247. Federal Trade Commission. (1999).
248. Office of the Surgeon General. (2001). *Women and smoking.*
249. Federal Trade Commission. (1999).
250. Office of the Surgeon General. (2001). *Women and smoking.*
251. Grunbaum, J. A., Kann, L., Kinchen, S., Ross, J., Hawkins, J., Lowry, R., et al. (2004).
252. Rigotti, N. A., Lee, J. E., & Wechsler, H. (2000).
253. Office of the Surgeon General. (2001). *Women and smoking.*
254. Johnston, L. D., O'Malley, P. M., & Bachman, J. G. (2003). *Monitoring the future: National survey results on drug use, 1975–2002: Volume 1, secondary school students* (NIH Pub. No. 03-5375). Bethesda, MD: U.S. Department of Health and Human Services, National Institutes of Health, National Institute on Drug Abuse.
255. Office of the Surgeon General. (2001). *Women and smoking.*
256. Johnston, L. D., O'Malley, P. M., & Bachman, J. G. (2003). *Monitoring the future,* vol. 1.
257. Office of the Surgeon General. (2001). *Marketing cigarettes to women.*

258. Sepe, E., Ling, P. M., & Glantz, S. A. (2002). Smooth moves: Bar and nightclub tobacco promotions that target young adults. *American Journal of Public Health, 92*(3), 414–419.

259. Ibid.

260. Smokefree.net. (2003). www.smokefree.net (accessed February 27, 2004).

261. Loose, C. (2004). *Public smoking ban spreads around world.* www.philly.com (accessed April 12, 2004).

Chapter 3. Women and Alcohol

1. The National Center on Addiction and Substance Abuse (CASA) at Columbia University. (2005). *CASA's analysis of the National Survey on Drug Use and Health (NSDUH), 2003* [Data file]. Rockville, MD: U.S. Department of Health and Human Services, Substance Abuse and Mental Health Services Administration.

2. Grunbaum, J. A., Kann, L., Kinchen, S., Ross, J., Hawkins, J., Lowry, R., et al. (2004). Youth Risk Behavior Surveillance: United States, 2003. *Morbidity and Mortality Weekly Report: Surveillance Summaries, 53*(SS-2).

3. Ibid.

4. The National Center on Addiction and Substance Abuse (CASA) at Columbia University. (1996). *Substance abuse and the American woman.* New York: CASA.

5. Wechsler, H., Lee, J. E., Kuo, M., Seibring, M., Nelson, T. F., & Lee, H. (2002). Trends in college binge drinking during a period of increased prevention efforts: Findings from 4 Harvard School of Public Health College Alcohol Study surveys: 1993–2001. *Journal of American College Health, 50*(5), 203–217.

6. Collins, J. J., & Messerschmidt, P. M. (1993). Epidemiology of alcohol-related violence. *Alcohol Health and Research World, 17*(2), 93–100; Koss, M. P. (1988). Hidden rape: Sexual aggression and victimization in a national sample of students in higher education. In A. W. Burgess (Ed.), *Rape and sexual assault: Volume 2* (pp. 3–25). New York: Garland; Rada, R. T. (1975). Alcoholism and forcible rape. *American Journal of Psychiatry, 132*(4), 444–446.

7. National Institute on Alcohol Abuse and Alcoholism. (1999). Are women more vulnerable to alcohol's effects? *Alcohol Alert, 46*; CASA. (1996).

8. National Institute on Alcohol Abuse and Alcoholism. (1999). Are women more vulnerable?; CASA. (1996).

9. CASA. (1996).

10. National Institute on Alcohol Abuse and Alcoholism. (2003). *FAQ's on alcohol abuse and alcoholism.* www.niaaa.nih.gov (accessed February 6, 2004).

11. National Institute on Alcohol Abuse and Alcoholism. (2003). *Alcohol: A women's health issue* (NIH Pub. No. 03-4956). Bethesda, MD: U.S. Department of Health and Human Services, National Institutes of Health, National Institute on Alcohol Abuse and Alcoholism.

12. CASA. (2005).

13. Ibid.

14. Ibid.

15. Schoenborn, C. A., & Adams, P. F. (2002). *Alcohol use among adults: United States, 1997–98: Advance data no. 324* (DHHS Pub. No. [PHS] 2001–1250). Hyattsville, MD: U.S. Department of Health and Human Services, Centers for Disease Control and Prevention, National Center for Health Statistics.
16. Dooley, D., & Prause, J. (1998). Underemployment and alcohol misuse in the National Longitudinal Survey of Youth. *Journal of Studies on Alcohol, 59*(6), 669–680; Terza, J. V. (2002). Alcohol abuse and employment: A second look. *Journal of Applied Econometrics, 17*(4), 393–404.
17. Schoenborn, C. A., & Adams, P. F. (2002).
18. Centers for Disease Control and Prevention. (2002). Alcohol use among women of childbearing age: United States, 1991–1999. *Morbidity and Mortality Weekly Report, 51*(13), 273–276.
19. Substance Abuse and Mental Health Services Administration, Office of Applied Studies. (2002). *Results from the 2001 National Household Survey on Drug Abuse: Volume 1: Summary of national findings* (DHHS Pub. No. [SMA] 02-3758). Rockville, MD: U.S. Department of Health and Human Services; The National Center on Addiction and Substance Abuse (CASA) at Columbia University. (2003). *The formative years: Pathways to substance abuse among girls and young women ages 8–22.* New York: CASA.
20. Johnston, L. D., O'Malley, P. M., Bachman, J. G., & Schulenberg, J. E. (2004). *Monitoring the future: National survey results on drug use, 1975–2003: Volume 1, secondary school students* (NIH Pub. No. 04-5507). Bethesda, MD: U.S. Department of Health and Human Services, National Institutes of Health, National Institute on Drug Abuse.
21. Ibid.; CASA. (2003). *The formative years.*
22. Grunbaum, J. A., Kann, L., Kinchen, S., Ross, J., Hawkins, J., Lowry, R., et al. (2004).
23. Ibid.
24. The National Center on Addiction and Substance Abuse (CASA) at Columbia University. (2002). *Teen tipplers: America's underage drinking epidemic.* New York: CASA.
25. Substance Abuse and Mental Health Services Administration. (2002). *Alcohol use among girls.* www.health.org (accessed April 10, 2002).
26. Grunbaum, J. A., Kann, L., Kinchen, S., Ross, J., Hawkins, J., Lowry, R., et al. (2004).
27. Grant, B. F., & Dawson, D. A. (1997). Age at onset of alcohol use and its association with DSM-IV alcohol abuse and dependence: Results from the National Longitudinal Alcohol Epidemiologic Survey. *Journal of Substance Abuse, 9,* 103–110.
28. Grunbaum, J. A., Kann, L., Kinchen, S., Ross, J., Hawkins, J., Lowry, R., et al. (2004).
29. Ibid.
30. Substance Abuse and Mental Health Services Administration, Office of Applied Studies. (2002). *Low rates of alcohol use among Asian youths: The NHSDA report* [Fact sheet]. Rockville, MD: U.S. Department of Health and Human Services.
31. Johnston, L. D., O'Malley, P. M., & Bachman, J. G. (2003). *Monitoring the future: National survey results on drug use, 1975–2002: Volume 2, college students and adults ages 19–40* (NIH Pub. No. 03-5376). Bethesda, MD: U.S. Department of Health and Human Services, National Institutes of Health, National Institute on Drug Abuse.

32. Johnston, L. D., O'Malley, P. M., Bachman, J. G., & Schulenberg, J. E. (2004). *Monitoring the future: National survey results on drug use, 1975–2003: Volume 2, College students and adults ages 19–45* (NIH Pub. No. 04-5508). Bethesda, MD: U.S. Department of Health and Human Services, National Institutes of Health, National Institute on Drug Abuse.
33. Wechsler, H., Lee, J. E., Kuo, M., Seibring, M., Nelson, T. F., & Lee, H. (2002).
34. McCabe, S. E. (2002). Gender differences in collegiate risk factors for heavy episodic drinking. *Journal of Studies on Alcohol, 63*(1), 49–56.
35. Ozegovic, J. J., Bikos, L. H., & Szymanski, D. M. (2001). Trends and predictors of alcohol use among undergraduate female students. *Journal of College Student Development, 42*(5), 447–455; Wechsler, H. (1996). Alcohol and the American college campus: A report from the Harvard School of Public Health. *Change, 28*(4), 20–26.
36. Wechsler, H., Lee, J. E., Kuo, M., Seibring, M., Nelson, T. F., & Lee, H. (2002).
37. Knight, J. R., Wechsler, H., Kuo, M., Seibring, M., Weitzman, E. R., & Schuckit, M. A. (2002). Alcohol abuse and dependence among U.S. college students. *Journal of Studies on Alcohol, 63*(3), 263–270.
38. CASA. (2005).
39. Ibid.
40. Liberto, J. G., & Oslin, D. W. (1997). Early versus late onset of alcoholism in the elderly. In A. M. Gurnack (Ed.), *Older adults' misuse of alcohol, medicines, and other drugs: Research and practice issues* (pp. 94–112). New York: Springer.
41. Atkinson, R. M. (1994). Late onset problem drinking in older adults. *International Journal of Geriatric Psychiatry, 9*(4), 321–326; Brennan, P. L., Moos, R. H., & Kim, J. Y. (1993). Gender differences in the individual characteristics and life contexts of late-middle-aged and older problem drinkers. *Addiction, 88*(6), 781–790; Gomberg, E. S. L. (1995). Older women and alcohol: Use and abuse. In M. Galanter (Ed.), *Recent developments in alcoholism: Women and alcoholism: Volume 12* (pp. 61–79). New York: Plenum; Holzer, C. E., Robins, L. E., Myers, J. K., Weissman, M. M., Tischler, G. L., Leaf, P. J., et al. (1984). Antecedents and correlates of alcohol abuse and dependence in the elderly. In G. Maddox, L. N. Robins, & N. Rosenberg (Eds.), *Nature and extent of alcohol problems among the elderly: Proceedings of a workshop November 3–4, 1983: NIAAA research monograph no. 14* (DHHS Pub. No. [ADM] 84-1321, pp. 217–244). Rockville, MD: U.S. Department of Health and Human Services, Public Health Service, Alcohol, Drug Abuse, and Mental Health Administration, National Institute on Alcohol Abuse and Alcoholism; Welte, J. W., & Mirand, A. L. (1994). Lifetime drinking patterns of elders from a general population survey. *Drug and Alcohol Dependence, 35*(2), 133–140.
42. The National Center on Addiction and Substance Abuse (CASA) at Columbia University. (1998). *Under the rug: Substance abuse and the mature woman*. New York: CASA.
43. Straussner, S. L. A., & Attia, P. R. (2002). Women's addiction and treatment through a historical lens. In S. L. A. Straussner & S. Brown (Eds.), *The handbook of addiction treatment for women* (pp. 3–25). San Francisco: Jossey-Bass.
44. Sandmaier, M. (1992). *The invisible alcoholics: Women and alcohol* (2nd ed.). Blue Ridge Summit, PA: TAB Books.

45. Straussner, S. L. A., & Attia, P. R. (2002).
46. Blume, S. B. (1991). Sexuality and stigma: The alcoholic woman. *Alcohol Health and Research World, 15*(2), 139–146; Leigh, B. C. (1995). A thing so fallen, and so vile: Images of drinking and sexuality in women. *Contemporary Drug Problems, 22*(3), 415–434; Sandmaier, M. (1992).
47. Straussner, S. L. A., & Attia, P. R. (2002).
48. Sandmaier, M. (1992).
49. Sparks, A. (1897). Alcoholism in women. *Medico-Legal Journal, 15,* 219. In Sandmaier, M. (1992).
50. Straussner, S. L. A., & Attia, P. R. (2002).
51. Sandmaier, M. (1992).
52. Ibid.
53. Straussner, S. L. A., & Attia, P. R. (2002).
54. Gallup Organization. (2004). *Percent who drink beverage alcohol, by gender, 1939–2003.* www.niaaa.nih.gov (accessed November 9, 2004).
55. Substance Abuse and Mental Health Services Administration, Office of Applied Studies. (2003). *Overview of findings from the 2002 National Survey on Drug Use and Health: National findings* (DHHS Pub. No. [SMA] 03-3774). Rockville, MD: U.S. Department of Health and Human Services; Substance Abuse and Mental Health Services Administration, Office of Applied Studies. (2004). Women with co-occuring serious mental illness and a substance use disorder: The NSDUH report. Rockville, MD: U.S. Department of Health and Human Services.
56. Wilsnack, S. C., & Wilsnack, R. W. (1995). Drinking and problem drinking in US women: Patterns and recent trends. In M. Galanter (Ed.), *Recent developments in alcoholism, volume 12: Women and alcoholism* (pp. 29–60). New York: Plenum.
57. Griesler, P. C., & Kandel, D. B. (1998). The impact of maternal drinking during and after pregnancy on the drinking of adolescent offspring. *Journal of Studies on Alcohol, 59*(3), 292–304.
58. Prescott, C. A., Caldwell, C. B., Carey, G., Vogler, G. P., Trumbetta, S. L., & Gottesman, I. I. (2005). The Washington twin study of alcoholism. *American Journal of Medical Genetics. Part B, Neuropsychiatric Genetics, 134*(1), 48–55.
59. Heath, A. C., Bucholz, K. K., Madden, P. A. F., Dinwiddie, S. H., Slutske, W. S., Bierut, L. J., et al. (1997). Genetic and environmental contributions to alcohol dependence risk in a national twin sample: Consistency of findings in women and men. *Psychological Medicine, 27*(6), 1381–1396; Prescott, C. A., Aggen, S. H., & Kendler, K. S. (1999). Sex differences in the sources of genetic liability to alcohol abuse and dependence in a population-based sample of U.S. twins. *Alcoholism: Clinical and Experimental Research, 23*(7), 1136–1144.
60. Han, C., McGue, M. K., & Iacono, W. G. (1999). Lifetime tobacco, alcohol and other substance use in adolescent Minnesota twins: Univariate and multivariate behavioral genetic analyses. *Addiction, 94*(7), 981–993; Heath, A. C., Bucholz, K. K., Madden, P. A. F., Dinwiddie, S. H., Slutske, W. S., Bierut, L. J., et al. (1997).
61. Heath, A. C., Bucholz, K. K., Madden, P. A. F., Dinwiddie, S. H., Slutske, W. S., Bierut, L. J., et al. (1997).
62. Schuckit, M. A., Smith, T. L., Kalmijn, J., Tsuang, J., Hesselbrock, V., & Bucholz, K. (2000). Response to alcohol in daughters of alcoholics: A pilot study and a comparison with sons of alcoholics. *Alcohol and Alcoholism, 35*(3), 242–248.

63. Lundahl, L. H., & Lukas, S. E. (2001). The impact of familial alcoholism on alcohol reactivity in female social drinkers. *Experimental and Clinical Psychopharmacology, 9*(1), 101–109.
64. CASA. (1996).
65. Curran, G. M., Stoltenberg, S. F., Hill, E. M., Mudd, S. A., Blow, F. C., & Zucker, R. A. (1999). Gender differences in the relationships among SES, family history of alcohol disorders and alcohol dependence. *Journal of Studies on Alcohol, 60*(6), 825–832.
66. The National Center on Addiction and Substance Abuse (CASA) at Columbia University. (1997). *Back to school 1997: National survey of American attitudes on substance abuse III: Teens and their parents, teachers and principals.* New York: CASA.
67. CASA. (2005).
68. Heath, A. C., Bucholz, K. K., Madden, P. A. F., Dinwiddie, S. H., Slutske, W. S., Bierut, L. J., et al. (1997).
69. Pedersen, W., Mastekaasa, A., & Wichstrøm, L. (2001). Conduct problems and early cannabis initiation: A longitudinal study of gender differences. *Addiction, 96*(3), 415–431.
70. Walitzer, K. S., & Sher, K. J. (1996). A prospective study of self-esteem and alcohol use disorders in early adulthood: Evidence for gender differences. *Alcoholism: Clinical and Experimental Research, 20*(6), 1118–1124.
71. Schoen, C., Davis, K., Collins, K. S., Greenberg, L., Des Roches, C., & Abrams, M. (1997). *The Commonwealth Fund survey of the health of adolescent girls.* New York: Commonwealth Fund.
72. Kumpulainen, K., & Roine, S. (2002). Depressive symptoms at the age of 12 years and future heavy alcohol use. *Addictive Behaviors, 27*(3), 425–436.
73. Walitzer, K. S., & Sher, K. J. (1996).
74. Wright, L. S. (1983). Correlates of reported drinking problems among male and female college students. *Journal of Alcohol and Drug Education, 28*(3), 47–57.
75. Galaif, E. R., Stein, J. A., Newcomb, M. D., & Bernstein, D. P. (2001). Gender differences in the prediction of problem alcohol use in adulthood: Exploring the influence of family factors and childhood maltreatment. *Journal of Studies on Alcohol, 62*(4), 486–493; Jasinski, J. L., Williams, L. M., & Siegel, J. (2000). Childhood physical and sexual abuse as risk factors for heavy drinking among African American women: A prospective study. *Child Abuse and Neglect, 24*(8), 1061–1071; Miller, B. A., Downs, W. R., & Testa, M. (1993). Interrelationships between victimization experiences and women's alcohol use. *Journal of Studies on Alcohol, Suppl. 11*, 109–117; Wilsnack, S. C., Vogeltanz, N., Klassen, A. D., & Harris, T. R. (1997). Childhood sexual abuse and women's substance abuse: National survey findings. *Journal of Studies on Alcohol, 58*(3), 264–271.
76. CASA. (1996).
77. Miller, B. A., Downs, W. R., & Testa, M. (1993).
78. Felitti, V. J., Anda, R. F., Nordenberg, D., Williamson, D. F., Spitz, A. M., Edwards, V., et al. (1998). Relationship of childhood abuse and household dysfunction to many of the leading causes of death in adults: The Adverse Childhood Experiences (ACE) Study. *American Journal of Preventive Medicine, 14*(4), 245–258.

79. Schoen, C., Davis, K., Collins, K. S., Greenberg, L., Des Roches, C., & Abrams, M. (1997).
80. Donovan, J. E. (2002). Gender differences in alcohol involvement in children and adolescents: A review of the literature. In J. M. Howard, S. E. Martin, P. D. Mail, M. E. Hilton, & E. D. Taylor (Eds.), *Women and alcohol: Issues for prevention research: NIAAA research monograph no. 32* (NIH Pub. No. 96-3817, pp. 133–162). Bethesda, MD: U.S. Department of Health and Human Services, Public Health Service, National Institutes of Health, National Institute on Alcohol Abuse and Alcoholism.
81. Simons-Morton, B., Haynie, D. L., Crump, A. D., & Saylor, K. E. (2001). Peer and parent influences on smoking and drinking among early adolescents. *Health Education and Behavior, 28*(1), 95–107.
82. Barber, J. G., Bolitho, F., & Bertrand, L. D. (1999). Intrapersonal versus peer group predictors of adolescent drug use. *Children and Youth Services Review, 21*(7), 565–579; Simons-Morton, B., Haynie, D. L., Crump, A. D., & Saylor, K. E. (2001).
83. Ozegovic, J. J., Bikos, L. H., & Szymanski, D. M. (2001).
84. Wechsler, H. (1996).
85. Borsari, B., & Carey, K. B. (2001). Peer influences on college drinking: A review of the research. *Journal of Substance Abuse, 13*(4), 391–424.
86. Wilsnack, R. W., & Cheloha, R. (1987). Women's roles and problem drinking across the lifespan. *Social Problems, 34*(3), 231–248.
87. Alexander, F., & Duff, R. W. (1988). Drinking in retirement communities. *Generations, 12*(4), 58–62; Caracci, G., & Miller, N. S. (1991). Epidemiology and diagnosis of alcoholism in the elderly (A review). *International Journal of Geriatric Psychiatry, 6*(7), 511–515.
88. Alexander, F., & Duff, R. W. (1988).
89. CASA. (2003). *The formative years.*
90. Liberto, J. G., & Oslin, D. W. (1997).
91. Atkinson, R. M. (1994); Brennan, P. L., Moos, R. H., & Kim, J. Y. (1993); Gomberg, E. S. L. (1995); Holzer, C. E., Robins, L. E., Myers, J. K., Weissman, M. M., Tischler, G. L., Leaf, P. J., et al. (1984); Welte, J. W., & Mirand, A. L. (1994).
92. Liberto, J. G., & Oslin, D. W. (1997); Schonfeld, L., & Dupree, L. W. (1991). Antecedents of drinking for early- and late-onset elderly alcohol abusers. *Journal of Studies on Alcohol, 52*(6), 587–592.
93. Dupree, L. W., Broskowski, H., & Schonfeld, L. (1984). The gerontology alcohol project: A behavioral treatment program for elderly alcohol abusers. *Gerontologist, 24*(5), 510–516; Liberto, J. G., & Oslin, D. W. (1997).
94. Breslin, F. C., O'Keefe, M. K., Burrell, L., Ratliff-Crain, J., & Baum, A. (1995). The effects of stress and coping on daily alcohol use in women. *Addictive Behaviors, 20*(2), 141–147; Brennan, P. L., & Moos, R. H. (1996). Late-life drinking behavior: The influence of personal characteristics, life context and treatment. *Alcohol Health and Research World, 20*(3), 197–204; Glass, T. A., Prigerson, H., Kasl, S. V., & Mendes de Leon, C. F. (1995). The effects of negative life events on alcohol consumption among older men and women. *Journal of Gerontol-*

ogy, *50B*(4), 205–216; Gomberg, E. S. L. (1994). Risk factors for drinking over a woman's life span. *Alcohol Health and Research World, 18*(3), 220–227; Jennison, K. M. (1992). Impact of stressful life events and social support on drinking among older adults: A general population survey. *International Journal of Aging and Human Development, 35*(2), 99–123.

95. CASA. (1996).
96. Finlayson, R. E., Hurt, R. D., Davis, L. J., & Morse, R. M. (1988). Alcoholism in elderly persons: A study of the psychiatric and psychosocial features of 216 inpatients. *Mayo Clinic Proceedings, 63*(8), 761–768; Kunz, J. L., & Graham, K. (1996). Life course changes in alcohol consumption in leisure activities of men and women. *Journal of Drug Issues, 26*(4), 805–829.
97. Alexander, F., & Duff, R. W. (1988); Brennan, P. L., & Moos, R. H. (1996); Wilsnack, R. W., & Cheloha, R. (1987).
98. CASA. (2003). *The formative years.*
99. Ibid.
100. Johnson, H. L., & Johnson, P. B. (1998). Possible precursors of gender drinking differences. *Journal of Addictive Diseases, 17*(3), 1–12.
101. Donovan, J. E. (2002).
102. Beck, K. H., Thombs, D. L., Mahoney, C. A., & Fingar, K. M. (1995). Social context and sensation seeking: Gender differences in college student drinking motivations. *International Journal of the Addictions, 30*(9), 1101–1115; Noel, N. E., & Lisman, S. A. (1980). Alcohol consumption by college women following exposure to unsolvable problems: Learning helplessness or stress-induced drinking. *Behavior Research and Therapy, 18*(5), 429–440; Wright, L. S. (1983).
103. Borjesson, W., & Dunn, M. (2001). Alcohol expectancies of women and men in relation to alcohol use and perceptions of the effects of alcohol on the opposite sex. *Addictive Behaviors, 26*(5), 707–719.
104. Beck, K. H., Thombs, D. L., Mahoney, C. A., & Fingar, K. M. (1995).
105. Wilsnack, S. C. (1996). Patterns and trends in women's drinking: Recent findings and some implications for prevention. In J. Howard (Ed.), *Women and alcohol: Issues for prevention research: NIAAA research monograph #32* (NIH Pub. No. 96-3817, pp. 19–63). Bethesda, MD: U.S. Department of Health and Human Services, Public Health Service, National Institutes of Health, National Institute on Alcohol Abuse and Alcoholism.
106. Klassen, A. D., & Wilsnack, S. C. (1986). Sexual experience and drinking among women in a U.S. national survey. *Archives of Sexual Behavior, 15*(5), 363–392.
107. The National Center on Addiction and Substance Abuse (CASA) at Columbia University. (1999). *Dangerous liaisons: Substance abuse and sex.* New York: CASA.
108. CASA. (1999).
109. Wilsnack, S. C., & Wilsnack, R. W. (1995).
110. CASA. (1999); Wilsnack, S. C., & Wilsnack, R. W. (1995).
111. Johnston, L. D., O'Malley, P. M., Bachman, J. G., & Schulenberg, J. E. (2004). *Monitoring the future,* vol. 1.

112. Office of Inspector General. (1991). *Youth and alcohol: A national survey, drinking habits, access, attitudes, and knowledge.* Washington, DC: U.S. Department of Health and Human Services.
113. Harrison, P. A., Fulkerson, J. A., & Park, E. (2000). The relative importance of social versus commercial sources in youth access to tobacco, alcohol, and other drugs. *Preventive Medicine, 31*(1), 39–48; Jones-Webb, R., Toomey, T. L., Miner, K., Wagenaar, A. C., Wolfson, M., & Poon, R. (1997). Why and in what context adolescents obtain alcohol from adults: A pilot study. *Substance Use and Misuse, 32*(2), 218–228; Wagenaar, A. C., Toomey, T. L., Murray, D. M., Short, B. J., Wolfson, M., & Jones-Webb, R. (1996). Sources of alcohol for underage drinkers. *Journal of Studies on Alcohol, 57*(3), 325–333.
114. Mayer, R. R., Forster, J. L., Murray, D. M., & Wagenaar, A. C. (1998). Social settings and situations of underage drinking. *Journal on Studies of Alcohol, 59*(2), 207–215.
115. Harrison, P. A., Fulkerson, J. A., & Park, E. (2000).
116. Wagenaar, A. C., Toomey, T. L., Murray, D. M., Short, B. J., Wolfson, M., & Jones-Webb, R. (1996).
117. Forster, J. L., McGovern, P. G., Wagenaar, A. C., Wolfson, M., Perry, C. L., & Anstine, P. S. (1994). The ability of young people to purchase alcohol without age identification in northeastern Minnesota, USA. *Addiction, 89*(6), 699–705; Preusser, D., & Williams, A. (1992). Sales of alcohol to underage purchasers in three New York counties and Washington, D.C. *Journal of Public Health Policy, 13*(3), 306–317.
118. Office of Inspector General. (1991).
119. Chaloupka, F. J., & Wechsler, H. (1996). Binge drinking in college: The impact of price, availability, and alcohol control policies. *Contemporary Economic Policy, 14*(4), 112–124.
120. Kilbourne, J. (1999). *Can't buy me love: How advertising changes the way we think and feel.* New York: Touchstone.
121. Sandmaier, M. (1992).
122. Straussner, S. L. A., & Attia, P. R. (2002).
123. Sandmaier, M. (1992).
124. Jacobson, M., Atkins, R., & Hacker, G. (1983). *The booze merchants: The inebriating of America.* Washington, DC: Center for Science in the Public Interest.
125. Kilbourne, J. (1999); Straussner, S. L. A., & Attia, P. R. (2002).
126. Center on Alcohol Marketing and Youth. (2003). *Marketing gallery: Bacardi Rum.* http://camy.org (accessed March 22, 2004).
127. Elliott, S. (1993, September 13). The media business: Advertising: In a whiskey patch to Generation X members, Leo Burnett tries to prove it is not their fathers' agency. *New York Times,* D7.
128. Center for Science in the Public Interest. (2001). *National poll shows "alcopops" drinks lure teens: Groups demand government investigate "starter suds"* [Press release]. Washington, DC: Center for Science in the Public Interest.
129. Join Together. (2002). *Parents warned about gelatin "Zippers."* www.jointogether.org (accessed February 12, 2004).

130. The National Center on Addiction and Substance Abuse (CASA) at Columbia University. (2003). *The economic value of underage drinking and excessive drinking to the alcohol industry: A CASA white paper.* New York: CASA.
131. Substance Abuse and Mental Health Services Administration, Office of Applied Studies. (2003). *2002 National Survey on Drug Use and Health: Detailed tables.* http://oas.samsha.gov (accessed October 27, 2004).
132. Cozens, C. (2003). *Laddish beer ads accused of alienating women.* http://media.guardian.co.uk (accessed February 12, 2004).
133. Realbeer.com. (2003). *Interbrew wants more women drinkers: Meanwhile, Molson extends "twins" ads approach.* http://realbeer.com (accessed February 12, 2004).
134. Mumenthaler, M. S., Taylor, J. L., O'Hara, R., & Yesavage, J. A. (1999). Gender differences in moderate drinking effects. *Alcohol Research and Health, 23*(1), 55–64.
135. Ely, M., Hardy, R., Longford, N. T., & Wadsworth, M. E. J. (1999). Gender differences in the relationship between alcohol consumption and drink problems are largely accounted for by body water. *Alcohol and Alcoholism, 34*(6), 894–902; Frezza, M., di Padova, C., Pozzato, G., Terpin, M., Baraona, E., & Lieber, C. S. (1990). High blood alcohol levels in women: The role of decreased gastric alcohol dehydrogenase activity and first-pass metabolism. *New England Journal of Medicine, 322*(2), 95–99; National Institute on Alcohol Abuse and Alcoholism. (1999). Are women more vulnerable?; Slutske, W. S., Piasecki, T. M., & Hunt-Carter, E. E. (2003). Development and initial validation of the Hangover Symptoms Scale: Prevalence and correlates of hangover symptoms in college students. *Alcoholism: Clinical and Experimental Research, 27*(9), 1442–1450; CASA. (1996).
136. Gavaler, J. S. (1998). Alcoholic beverages as a source of estrogens. *Alcohol Health and Research World, 22*(3), 220–227.
137. Mumenthaler, M. S., Taylor, J. L., O'Hara, R., & Yesavage, J. A. (1999).
138. DeWit, D. J., Adlaf, E. M., Offord, D. R., & Ogborne, A. C. (2000). Age at first alcohol use: A risk factor for the development of alcohol disorders. *American Journal of Psychiatry, 157*(5), 745–750; Grant, B. F., & Dawson, D. A. (1997).
139. CASA. (2005).
140. Grant, B. F., & Dawson, D. A. (1997).
141. DeWit, D. J., Adlaf, E. M., Offord, D. R., & Ogborne, A. C. (2000).
142. CASA. (1998).
143. Dees, W. L., Hiney, J. K., & Srivastava, V. (1998). Alcohol's effects on female puberty. *Alcohol Health and Research World, 22*(3), 165–169.
144. National Institute on Alcohol Abuse and Alcoholism. (1990). Alcohol and women. *Alcohol Alert, 10.*
145. Grodstein, F., Goldman, M. B., & Cramer, D. W. (1994). Infertility in women and moderate alcohol use. *American Journal of Public Health, 84*(9), 1429–1432.
146. National Institute on Alcohol Abuse and Alcoholism. (1994). Alcohol and hormones. *Alcohol Alert, 26.*
147. National Institute on Alcohol Abuse and Alcoholism. (1990).

148. National Center for Health Statistics. (1998). *Ten leading causes of death, United States: 1998, all races, both sexes.* www.webapp.cdc.gov (accessed March 19, 2001); Substance Abuse and Mental Health Services Administration. (2001). *SAMHSA fact sheet: Consequences of underage alcohol use.* www.health.org (accessed February 16, 2001).
149. Pacific Institute for Research and Evaluation, Levy, D. T., Miller, T. R., & Cox, K. C. (1999). *Costs of underage drinking: Updated edition.* Calverton, MD: Pacific Institute for Research and Evaluation.
150. Greenblatt, J. C. (1999). *Patterns of alcohol use among adolescents and associations with emotional and behavioral problems: OAS working paper.* Rockville, MD: U.S. Department of Health and Human Services, Substance Abuse and Mental Health Services Administration, Office of Applied Studies.
151. Jersild, D. (2002, May 31). Alcohol in the vulnerable lives of college women. *Chronicle of Higher Education, 48*(38), B10.
152. Kelly, T. M., Lynch, K. G., Donovan, J. E., & Clark, D. B. (2001). Alcohol use disorders and risk factor interactions for adolescent suicidal ideation and attempts. *Suicide and Life-Threatening Behavior, 31*(2), 181–193.
153. Grabbe, L., Demi, A., Camann, M. A., & Potter, L. (1997). The health status of elderly persons in the last year of life: A comparison of deaths by suicide, injury, and natural causes. *American Journal of Public Health, 87*(3), 434–437.
154. Light, J. M., Grube, J. W., Madden, P. A., & Gover, J. (2003). Adolescent alcohol use and suicidal ideation: A nonrecursive model. *Addictive Behaviors, 28*(4), 705–724.
155. Ibid.
156. Centers for Disease Control and Prevention, National Center for Injury Prevention and Control. (2004). *Water-related injuries.* www.cdc.gov/ncipc (accessed February 12, 2004).
157. Centers for Disease Control and Prevention. (2002). Involvement by young drivers in fatal alcohol-related motor-vehicle crashes: United States, 1982–2001. *Morbidity and Mortality Weekly Report, 51*(48), 1089–1091.
158. National Highway Traffic Safety Administration, National Center for Statistics and Analysis. (2002). *Traffic safety facts 2001: Alcohol* [Fact sheet] (DOT Pub. No. HS 809 470). Washington, DC: U.S. Department of Transportation, National Highway Traffic Safety Administration, National Center for Statistics and Analysis.
159. Yi, H., Williams, G. D., & Dufour, M. C. (2001). *Trends in alcohol-related fatal traffic crashes, United States, 1977–99: Surveillance report #56.* Rockville, MD: U.S. Department of Health and Human Services, Public Health Service, National Institutes of Health, National Institute on Alcohol Abuse and Alcoholism.
160. Wilsnack, S. C. (1996).
161. National Institute on Alcohol Abuse and Alcoholism. (1999).
162. Frieze, I. H., & Schafer, P. C. (1984). Alcohol use and marital violence: Female and male differences in reactions to alcohol. In S. C. Wilsnack & L. J. Beckman (Eds.), *Alcohol problems in women: Antecedents, consequences and intervention* (pp. 260–279). New York: Guilford; Miller,

B. A. (1990). The interrelationships between alcohol and drugs and family violence. In M. De La Rosa, E. Y. Lambert, & B. Gropper (Eds.), *Drugs and violence: Causes, correlates and consequences: NIDA research monograph 103* (DHHS Pub. No. [ADM] 91-1721, pp. 177–207). Rockville, MD: U.S. Department of Health and Human Services, Public Health Service, Alcohol, Drug Abuse, and Mental Health Administration, National Institute on Drug Abuse; Miller, B. A., & Downs, W. R. (1993). The impact of family violence on the use of alcohol by women. *Alcohol Health and Research World, 17*(2), 137–143; Miller, B. A., Downs, W. R., & Gondoli, D. M. (1989). Spousal violence among alcoholic women as compared to a random household sample of women. *Journal of Studies on Alcohol, 50*(6), 533–540; Muehlenhard, C. L., & Linton, M. A. (1987). Date rape and sexual aggression in dating situations: Incidence and risk factors. *Journal of Counseling Psychology, 34*(2), 186–196.

163. CASA. (1999).
164. Collins, J. J., & Messerschmidt, P. M. (1993); Koss, M. P. (1988); Rada, R. T. (1975); Frieze, I. H., & Schafer, P. C. (1984); Groth, A. N. (1978). The older rape victim and her assailant. *Journal of Geriatric Psychiatry, 11*(2), 203–215.
165. Join Together. (2002). *Alcohol more strongly linked to violence than other drugs.* www.jointogether.org (accessed February 26, 2004); CASA. (1999).
166. Malik, S., Sorenson, S. B., & Aneshensel, C. S. (1997). Community and dating violence among adolescents: Perpetration and victimization. *Journal of Adolescent Health, 21*(5), 291–302.
167. CASA. (1999).
168. Frieze, I. H., & Schafer, P. C. (1984); Kantor, G. K., & Straus, M. A. (1989). Substance abuse as a precipitant of wife abuse victimizations. *American Journal of Drug and Alcohol Abuse, 15*(2), 173–189.
169. CASA. (2003). *The formative years.*
170. Task Force of the National Advisory Council on Alcohol Abuse and Alcoholism. (2002). *A call to action: Changing the culture of drinking at U.S. colleges* (NIH Pub. No. 03-5010). Bethesda, MD: U.S. Department of Health and Human Services, National Institutes of Health, National Institute on Alcohol Abuse and Alcoholism.
171. Shafer, M., & Boyer, C. B. (1991). Psychosocial and behavioral factors associated with risk of sexually transmitted diseases, including human immunodeficiency virus infection, among urban high school students. *Journal of Pediatrics, 119*(5), 826–833; CASA. (2003). *The formative years.*
172. Bailey, S. L., Pollock, N. K., Martin, C. S., & Lynch, K. G. (1999). Risky sexual behaviors among adolescents with alcohol use disorders. *Journal of Adolescent Health, 25*(3), 179–181; CASA. (1999).
173. CASA. (1999).
174. Ford, K., & Norris, A. (1994). Urban minority youth: Alcohol and marijuana use and exposure to unprotected intercourse. *Journal of Acquired Immune Deficiency Syndromes, 7*(4), 389–396; Lowry, R., Holtzmann, D., Truman, B. I., Kann, L., Collins, J. L., & Kolbe, L. J. (1994). Substance use and HIV-related sexual activity and alcohol and drug use among U.S.

high school students: Are they related? *American Journal of Public Health, 84*(7), 1116–1120; Mott, F. L., & Haurin, R. J. (1988). Linkages between sexual activity and alcohol and drug use among American adolescents. *Family Planning Perspective, 20*(3), 128–136.

175. CASA. (1999).
176. Avins, A. L., Woods, W. J., Lindan, C. P., Hudes, E. S., Clark, W., & Hulley, S. B. (1994). HIV infection and risk behaviors among heterosexuals in alcohol treatment programs. *JAMA, 251*(7), 515–518.
177. Kruger, T. E., & Jerrells, T. R. (1992). Potential role of alcohol in human immunodeficiency virus infection. *Alcohol Health and Research World, 16*(1), 57–63; MacGregor, R. R. (1988). Alcohol and drugs as co-factors for AIDS. In L. Siegel (Ed.), *AIDS and substance abuse* (pp. 47–71). New York: Harrington Park Press.
178. Bonnie, R. J., & O'Connell, M. E. (Eds.). (2004). *Reducing underage drinking: A collective responsibility.* Washington, DC: National Academy Press.
179. Hommer, D. W., Momenan, R., Kaiser, E., & Rawlings, R. R. (2001). Evidence for a gender-related effect of alcoholism on brain volumes. *American Journal of Psychiatry, 158*(2), 198–204; Mann, K., Batra, A., Günthner, A., & Schroth, G. (1992). Do women develop alcoholic brain damage more readily than men? *Alcoholism: Clinical and Experimental Research, 16*(6), 1052–1056; Tapert, S. F., Brown, G. G., Kindermann, S. S., Cheung, E. H., Frank, L. R., & Brown, S. A. (2001). fMRI measurement of brain dysfunction in alcohol-dependent young women. *Alcoholism: Clinical and Experimental Research, 25*(2), 236–245.
180. Wuethrich, B. (2001, March). Getting stupid. *Discover, 22*(3), 57–63.
181. Swartzwelder, H. S., Wilson, W. A., & Tayyeb, M. I. (1995). Age-dependent inhibition of long-term potentiation by ethanol in immature versus mature hippocampus. *Alcoholism: Clinical and Experimental Research, 19*(6), 1480–1485; Wuethrich, B. (2001, March).
182. Hommer, D. W., Momenan, R., Kaiser, E., & Rawlings, R. R. (2001).
183. Mann, K., Batra, A., Günthner, A., & Schroth, G. (1992).
184. Harrison, P. G. (2001). *Moderate drinking helps preserve women's brains.* www.reuters.com (accessed March 26, 2003).
185. Finlayson, R. E., Hurt, R. D., Davis, L. J., & Morse, R. M. (1988); Oscar-Berman, M., Shagrin, B., Evert, D. L., & Epstein, C. (1997). Impairments of brain and behavior: The neurological effects of alcohol. *Alcohol Health and Research World, 21*(1), 65–75.
186. Finlayson, R. E., Hurt, R. D., Davis, L. J., & Morse, R. M. (1988); Nixon, S. J. (1994). Cognitive deficits in alcoholic women. *Alcohol Health and Research World, 18*(3), 228–232; Oscar-Berman, M., Shagrin, B., Evert, D. L., & Epstein, C. (1997).
187. Nixon, S. J. (1994).
188. Ham, R. J. (1992). Confusion, dementia and delirium. In R. J. Ham & P. D. Sloane (Eds.), *Primary care geriatrics: A case-based approach* (pp. 259–311). St. Louis, MS: Mosby Year Book; Oscar-Berman, M., Shagrin, B., Evert, D. L., & Epstein, C. (1997).
189. Obernier, J. A., Bouldin, T. W., & Crews, F. T. (2002). Binge ethanol exposure in adult rats causes necrotic cell death. *Alcoholism: Clinical and Experimental Research, 26*(4), 547–557.

190. Greenfield, S. F. (2002). Women and alcohol use disorders. *Harvard Review of Psychiatry, 10*(2), 76–85; Ikejima, K., Enomoto, N., Iimuro, Y., Ikejima, A., Fang, D., Xu, J., et al. (1998). Estrogen increases sensitivity of hepatic Kupffer cells to endotoxin. *American Journal of Physiology, 274*(4, Pt. 1), G669-G676.

191. Stranges, S., Freudenheim, J. L., Muti, P., Farinaro, E., Russell, M., Nochajski, T. H., et al. (2004). Differential effects of alcohol drinking pattern on liver enzymes in men and women. *Alcoholism: Clinical and Experimental Research, 28*(6), 949–956.

192. National Institute on Alcohol Abuse and Alcoholism. (2003). *Alcohol.*

193. Bernardy, N. C., King, A. C., & Lovallo, W. R. (2003). Cardiovascular responses to physical and psychological stress in female alcoholics with transitory hypertension after early abstinence. *Alcoholism: Clinical and Experimental Research, 27*(9), 1489–1498; National Institute on Alcohol Abuse and Alcoholism. (2000). *Tenth special report to the U.S. Congress on alcohol and health: Highlights from current research from the Secretary of Health and Human Services* (NIH Pub. No. 00-1583). Rockville, MD: U.S. Department of Health and Human Services, Public Health Service, National Institutes of Health, National Institute on Alcohol Abuse and Alcoholism.

194. Urbano-Marquez, A., Estruch, R., Fernandez-Sola, J., Nicolas, J. M., Pare, J. C., & Rubin, E. (1995). The greater risk of alcoholic cardiomyopathy and myopathy in women compared with men. *JAMA, 274*(2), 149–154.

195. National Institute on Alcohol Abuse and Alcoholism. (2000). *Tenth special report.*

196. Thadhani, R., Camargo, C. A., Stampfer, M. J., Curhan, G. C., Willett, W. C., & Rimm, E. B. (2002). Prospective study of moderate alcohol consumption and risk of hypertension in young women. *Archives of Internal Medicine, 162*(5), 569–574.

197. Mosca, L., Manson, J. E., Sutherland, S. E., Langer, R. D., Manolio, T., & Barrett-Connor, E. (1997). Cardiovascular disease in women: A statement for healthcare professionals from the American Heart Association. *Circulation, 96*(7), 2468–2482.

198. Sempos, C. T., Rehm, J., Crespo, C., & Trevisan, M. (2002). No protective effect of alcohol consumption on coronary heart disease (CHD) in African Americans: Average volume of drinking over the life course and CHD morbidity and mortality in a U.S. national cohort. *Contemporary Drug Problems, 29*(4), 805–820.

199. Honkanen, R., Ertama, L., Kuosmanen, P., Linnoila, M., Alha, A., & Visuri, T. (1983). The role of alcohol in accidental falls. *Journal of Studies on Alcohol, 44*(2), 231–245; Malmivaara, A., Heliovaara, M., Knekt, P., Reunanen, A., & Aromaa, A. (1993). Risk factors for injurious falls leading to hospitalization or death in a cohort of 19,500 adults. *American Journal of Epidemiology, 138*(6), 384–394; O'Loughlin, J. L., Robitaille, Y., Boivin, J. F., & Suissa, S. (1993). Incidence of and risk factors for falls and injurious falls among the community-dwelling elderly. *American Journal of Epidemiology, 137*(3), 342–354; Waller, J. A. (1978). Falls among the elderly: Human and environmental factors. *Accident Analysis and Prevention, 10*(1), 21–33.

200. Centers for Disease Control and Prevention, National Center for Injury Prevention and Control. (2003). *Falls and hip fractures among older adults.* www.cdc.gov/ncipc (accessed October 30, 2003).

201. Ibid.
202. Felson, D. T., Kiel, D. P., Anderson, J. J., & Kannel, W. B. (1988). Alcohol consumption and hip fractures: The Framingham Study. *American Journal of Epidemiology, 128*(5), 1102–1110.
203. Gavaler, J. S. (1995). Alcohol effects on hormone levels in normal postmenopausal women and in postmenopausal women with alcohol-induced cirrhosis. In M. Galanter (Ed.), *Alcoholism and women: Recent developments in alcoholism, volume 12* (pp. 199–208). New York: Plenum; Hankinson, S. E., Willett, W. C., Manson, J. E., Hunter, D. J., Colditz, G. A., Stampfer, M. J., et al. (1995). Alcohol, height, and adiposity in relation to estrogen and prolactin levels in postmenopausal women. *Journal of the National Cancer Institute, 87*(17), 1297–1302; Tivis, L. J., & Galaver, J. S. (1994). Alcohol, hormones and health in postmenopausal women. *Alcohol Health and Research World, 18*(3), 185–188.
204. National Institute on Alcohol Abuse and Alcoholism. (1994).
205. Emanuele, N., & Emanuele, M. A. (1997). The endocrine system: Alcohol alters critical hormonal balance. *Alcohol Health and Research World, 21*(1), 53–64.
206. Sampson, H. W. (1998). Alcohol's harmful effects on bone. *Alcohol Health and Research World, 22*(3), 190–194.
207. National Institute on Alcohol Abuse and Alcoholism. (2003). *Alcohol*; National Institute on Alcohol Abuse and Alcoholism. (2003). *State of the science report on the effects of moderate drinking.* www.niaaa.nih.gov (accessed March 9, 2004).
208. Collaborative Group on Hormonal Factors in Breast Cancer. (2002). Alcohol, tobacco and breast cancer: Collaborative reanalysis of individual data from 53 epidemiological studies, including 58,515 women with breast cancer and 95,067 women without the disease. *British Journal of Cancer, 87*(11), 1234–1245.
209. Vachon, C. M., Cerhan, J. R., Vierkant, R. A., & Sellers, T. A. (2001). Investigation of an interaction of alcohol intake and family history on breast cancer risk in the Minnesota breast cancer family study. *Cancer, 92*(2), 240–248.
210. Chen, W. Y., Colditz, G. A., Rosner, B., Hankinson, S. E., Hunter, D. J., Manson, J. E., et al. (2002). Use of postmenopausal hormones, alcohol, and risk for invasive breast cancer. *Annals of Internal Medicine, 137*(10), 798–804.
211. Baker, L. (2003). *Having more than two alcoholic drinks at a time increases younger women's breast-cancer risk by 80 percent: However, increased risk not found in postmenopausal women.* www.buffalo.edu/reporter (accessed March 1, 2004).
212. Weiss, S. R., Kung, H. C., & Pearson, J. L. (2003). Emerging issues in gender and ethnic differences in substance abuse and treatment. *Current Women's Health Reports, 3*(3), 245–253.
213. Frye, M. A., Altshuler, L. L., McElroy, S. L., Suppes, T., Keck, P. E., Denicoff, K., et al. (2003). Gender differences in prevalence, risk, and clinical correlates of alcoholism comorbidity in bipolar disorder. *American Journal of Psychiatry, 160*(5), 883–889.
214. Stewart, S. H., Agelopoulos, M., Baker, J. M., & Boland, F. J. (2000). Relations between dietary restraint and patterns of alcohol use in young adult women. *Psychology of Addictive Behaviors, 14*(1), 77–82.
215. Wilsnack, S. C. (1996).

216. Brennan, P. L., Moos, R. H., & Kim, J. Y. (1993); Helzer, J. E., & Pryzbeck, T. R. (1988). The co-occurrence of alcoholism with other psychiatric disorders in the general population and its impact on treatment. *Journal of Studies on Alcohol, 49*(3), 219–224.
217. Nolen-Hoeksema, S. (2001). Gender differences in depression. *Current Directions in Psychological Science, 10*(5), 173–176.
218. CASA. (2003). *The formative years.*
219. Grabbe, L., Demi, A., Camann, M. A., & Potter, L. (1997).
220. The National Center on Addiction and Substance Abuse (CASA) at Columbia University. (2003). *Food for thought: Substance abuse and eating disorders.* New York: CASA.
221. CASA. (2003). *The formative years.*
222. Krahn, D., Kurth, C., Demitrack, C., & Drewnowski, A. (1992). The relationship of dieting severity and bulimic behaviors to alcohol and other drug use in young women. *Journal of Substance Abuse, 4*(4), 341–353.
223. CASA. (2003). *Food for thought.*
224. Hughes, J. R., Rose, G. L., & Callas, P. W. (2000). Nicotine is more reinforcing in smokers with a past history of alcoholism than in smokers without this history. *Alcoholism: Clinical and Experimental Research, 24*(11), 1633–1638; CASA. (2003). *The formative years.*
225. Kandel, D. B., Yamaguchi, K., & Chen, K. (1992). Stages of progression in drug involvement from adolescence to adulthood: Further evidence for the gateway theory. *Journal of Studies on Alcohol, 53*(5), 447–457.
226. CASA. (2002).
227. Wilsnack, S. C., & Wilsnack, R. W. (1995).
228. Braude, M. C. (1986). Drugs and drug interactions in elderly women. In B. A. Ray & M. C. Braude (Eds.), *Women and drugs: A new era for research: NIDA research monograph 65* (DHHS Pub. No. [ADM] 86-1447, pp. 58–64). Rockville, MD: U.S. Department of Health and Human Services, Public Health Service, Alcohol, Drug Abuse, and Mental Health Administration, National Institute on Drug Abuse; Galbraith, S. (1991). Women and legal drugs. In P. Roth (Ed.), *Alcohol and drugs are women's issues* (pp. 150–154). Metuchen, NJ: Women's Action Alliance and Scarecrow Press; Trachtenberg, A. I., & Fleming, M. F. (1994). *Diagnosis and treatment of drug abuse in family practice.* Kansas City, MS: American Academy of Family Physicians.
229. Scott, R. B., & Mitchell, M. C. (1988). Aging, alcohol, and the liver. *Journal of the American Geriatrics Society, 36*(3), 255–265.
230. CASA. (1998).
231. Klatsky, A. L. (1999). Moderate drinking and reduced risk of heart disease. *Alcohol Research and Health, 23*(1), 15–23.
232. Britton, A., & Marmot, M. (2004). Different measures of alcohol consumption and risk of coronary heart disease and all-cause mortality: 11-year follow-up of the Whitehall 2 Cohort Study. *Addiction, 99*(1), 109–116; Klatsky, A. L. (1999); Walsh, C. R., Larson, M. G., Evans, J. C., Djousse, L., Ellison, R. C., Vasan, R. C., et al. (2002). Alcohol consumption and risk for

congestive heart failure in the Framingham Heart Study. *Annals of Internal Medicine, 136*(3), 181–191.

233. National Institute on Alcohol Abuse and Alcoholism. (2000). Health risks and benefits of alcohol consumption. *Alcohol Research and Health, 24*(1), 5–11.
234. Sacco, R. L., Elkind, M., Boden-Albada, B., Lin, I. F., Kargman, D. E., Hauser, W. A., et al. (1999). The protective effect of moderate alcohol consumption on ischemic stroke. *JAMA, 281*(1), 53–60.
235. Carlsson, S., Hammar, N., Grill, V., & Kaprio, J. (2003). Alcohol consumption and the incidence of type 2 diabetes: A 20-year follow-up of the Finnish Twin Cohort Study. *Diabetes Care, 26*(20), 2785–2790.
236. Brenner, H., Bode, G., Adler, G., Hoffmeister, A., Koenig, W., & Rothenbacher, D. (2001). Alcohol as a gastric disinfectant? The complex relationship between alcohol consumption and current Helicobacter pylori infection. *Epidemiology, 12*(2), 209–214.
237. Takkacouche, B., Regueira-Mendez, C., Garcia-Closas, R., Figueiras, A., Gestal-Otero, J. J., & Hernan, M. A. (2002). Intake of wine, beer, and spirits and the risk of clinical common cold. *American Journal of Epidemiology, 155*(9), 853–858.
238. National Institute on Alcohol Abuse and Alcoholism. (2003). *State of the science.*
239. Walsh, C. R., Larson, M. G., Evans, J. C., Djousse, L., Ellison, R. C., Vasan, R. C., et al. (2002).
240. National Institute on Alcohol Abuse and Alcoholism. (2003). *Alcohol*; National Institute on Alcohol Abuse and Alcoholism. (2000). Health risks.
241. Fuchs, C. S., Stampfer, M. J., Colditz, G. A., Giovannucci, E. L., Manson, J. E., Kawachi, I., et al. (1995). Alcohol consumption and mortality among women. *New England Journal of Medicine, 332*(19), 1245–1250; National Institute on Alcohol Abuse and Alcoholism. (2003). *State of the science.*
242. Eng, E. T., Ye, J., Williams, D., Phung, S., Moore, R. E., Young, M. K., et al. (2003). Suppression of estrogen biosynthesis by procyanidin dimers in red wine and grape seed. *Cancer Research, 63*(23), 8516–8522; Takkacouche, B., Regueira-Mendez, C., Garcia-Closas, R., Figueiras, A., Gestal-Otero, J. J., & Hernan, M. A. (2002).
243. Barefoot, J. C., Grønbæck, M., Feaganes, J. R., McPherson, R. S., Williams, R. B., & Siegler, I. C. (2002). Alcoholic beverage preference, diet, and health habits in the UNC Alumni Heart Study. *American Journal of Clinical Nutrition, 76*(2), 466–472; National Institute on Alcohol Abuse and Alcoholism. (1999). Alcohol and coronary heart disease. *Alcohol Alert, 45.*
244. National Institute on Alcohol Abuse and Alcoholism. (2000). Health risks.
245. U.S. Department of Agriculture, Center for Nutrition Policy and Promotion. (1997). *Does alcohol have a place in a healthy diet?* www.usda.gov (accessed March 2, 2004).
246. National Institute on Alcohol Abuse and Alcoholism. (2003). *State of the science.*

Chapter 4. Women and Prescription and Illicit Drugs

Epigraph: Murphy, E. F. (1922). *The black candle.* Toronto, Canada: T. Allen.

1. The National Center on Addiction and Substance Abuse (CASA) at Columbia University. (2005). *CASA's analysis of the National Survey on Drug Use and Health (NSDUH), 2003* [Data file]. Rockville, MD: U.S. Department of Health and Human Services, Substance Abuse and Mental Health Services Administration.
2. National Institute on Drug Abuse. (2001). *NIDA research report: Prescription drugs: Abuse and addiction* (NIH Pub. No. 01-4881). Bethesda, MD: U.S. Department of Health and Human Services, National Institutes of Health, National Institute on Drug Abuse.
3. Ibid.
4. Ibid.
5. Substance Abuse and Mental Health Services Administration, Office of Applied Studies. (2002). *Summary of findings from the 2001 National Household Survey on Drug Abuse: Volume 2: Technical appendices and selected data tables* (DHHS Pub. No. [SMA] 02-3759). Rockville, MD: U.S. Department of Health and Human Services.
6. Ibid.
7. National Institute on Drug Abuse. (2000). Gender differences in drug abuse risks and treatment. *NIDA Notes, 15*(4), 6–7.
8. The National Center on Addiction and Substance Abuse (CASA) at Columbia University. (1996). *Substance abuse and the American woman.* New York: CASA.
9. CASA. (2005). *CASA's analysis of NSDUH 2003.*
10. Ibid.
11. Aldrich, M. R. (1994). Historical notes on women addicts. *Journal of Psychoactive Drugs, 26*(1), 61–64; Sandmaier, M. (1992). *The invisible alcoholics: Women and alcohol* (2nd ed.). Blue Ridge Summit, PA: TAB Books; Kandall, S. R. (1998). Women and addiction in the United States: 1850 to 1920. In C. L. Wetherington & A. B. Roman (Eds.), *Drug addiction research and the health of women* (NIH Pub. No. 98 4290, pp. 33–52). Rockville, MD: U.S. Department of Health and Human Services, National Institutes of Health, National Institute on Drug Abuse.
12. Terry, C. E., & Pellons, M. (1970). The extent of chronic opiate use in the United States prior to 1921. In J. C. Ball & C. D. Chambers (Eds.), *The epidemiology of opiate addiction in the United States* (pp. 36–37). Springfield, IL: Thomas.
13. Kandall, S. R. (1998). Women and addiction in the United States: 1850 to 1920.
14. Courtwright, D. T. (2001). *Dark paradise: A history of opiate addiction in America.* Cambridge, MA: Harvard University Press.
15. Brecher, E. M., & Editors of Consumer Reports Magazine. (1972). *Consumers Union report on licit and illicit drugs.* www.druglibrary.org (accessed December 28, 2001).
16. Aldrich, M. R. (1994); Sandmaier, M. (1992).
17. Brecher, E. M., & Editors of Consumer Reports Magazine. (1972); Kandall, S. R. (1996).

Substance and shadow: Women and addiction in the United States. Cambridge, MA: Harvard University Press.

18. University of Buffalo, Addiction Research Unit. (2001). *Before prohibition: Images from the pre-prohibition era when many psychotropic substances were legally available in America and Europe. http://wings.buffalo.edu/aru* (accessed March 4, 2004).
19. Courtwright, D. T. (2001).
20. University of Buffalo, Addiction Research Unit. (2001).
21. Brecher, E. M., & Editors of Consumer Reports Magazine. (1972).
22. Whitebread, C. (1995). *The history of the non-medical use of drugs in the United States.* www.druglibrary.org (accessed June 4, 2004).
23. Ibid.
24. Carlson, P. (1999, May 6). The straight dope: DEA's new museum is a monument to self-destruction. *Washington Post,* C1; Courtwright, D. T. (2001).
25. Clark, D. (2003). *Substance use and misuse: Some historical perspectives.* www.dcresearch.net (accessed November 5, 2004).
26. Quoted in Kandall, S. R. (1996).
27. Brecher, E. M., & Editors of Consumer Reports Magazine. (1972).
28. Kandall, S. R. (1998). Women and addiction in the United States: 1850 to 1920.
29. Brecher, E. M., & Editors of Consumer Reports Magazine. (1972).
30. Ibid.
31. Aldrich, M. R. (1994); Falco, M. (1991). Drug abuse: A national policy perspective. *Bulletin of New York Academy of Medicine, 67*(3), 196–206.
32. Kandall, S. R. (1998). Women and addiction in the United States: 1920 to the present. In C. L. Wetherington & A. B. Roman (Eds.), *Drug addiction research and the health of women* (NIH Pub. No. 98-4290, pp. 53–80). Rockville, MD: U.S. Department of Health and Human Services, National Institutes of Health, National Institute on Drug Abuse.
33. Quoted in Brecher, E. M., & Editors of Consumer Reports Magazine. (1972).
34. Ibid.
35. Courtwright, D. T. (2001).
36. Kandall, S. R. (1998). Women and addiction in the United States: 1920 to the present.
37. Courtwright, D. T. (2001).
38. Winick, C., & Kinsie, P. M. (1971). *The lively commerce: Prostitution in the United States.* Chicago: Quadrangle.
39. Kandall, S. R. (1998). Women and addiction in the United States: 1850 to 1920.
40. Courtwright, D. T. (2001).
41. Metzl, J. (2003). "Mother's little helper": The crisis of psychoanalysis and the Miltown Resolution. *Gender and History, 15*(2), 240–267.
42. Engstrom, F. (1997). Psychotropic drugs: Modern medicine's alternative to purgatives, straitjackets, and asylums. *Postgraduate Medicine, 101*(3), 198–200; Kandall, S. R. (1996).
43. Metzl, J. M., & Angel, J. (2004). Assessing the impact of SSRI antidepressants on popular notions of women's depressive illness. *Social Science and Medicine, 58*(3), 577–584.

44. Kandall, S. R. (1996).
45. Kennedy, B. (1999). *The tranquilizing of America: How mood-altering drugs changed the cultural landscape.* www.cnn.com (accessed April 3, 2003); Koerner, B. I. (1999, December 27). Leo Sternbach: The father of Mother's Little Helper. *U.S. News and World Report, 127*(25), 58.
46. Brecher, E. M., & Editors of Consumer Reports Magazine. (1972).
47. Koerner, B. I. (1999, December 27).
48. Kandall, S. R. (1996).
49. National Commission on Marihuana and Drug Abuse. (1973). *Drug use in America: Problem in perspective: Second report.* Washington, DC: U.S. Government Printing Office. As cited in Kandall, S. R. (1996).
50. Kandall, S. R. (1996).
51. Kennedy, B. (1999).
52. ABC News. (1998). *Mother's little helper: Valium at 35.* www.benzo.org.uk (accessed April 7, 2003).
53. Gordon, B. (1979). *I'm dancing as fast I can.* New York: Harper and Row.
54. Kandall, S. R. (1996).
55. Brecher, E. M., & Editors of Consumer Reports Magazine. (1972).
56. Kandall, S. R. (1996).
57. Substance Abuse and Mental Health Services Administration, Office of Applied Studies. (1997). *Substance use among women in the United States* (DHHS Pub. No. [SMA] 97-3162). Rockville, MD: U.S. Department of Health and Human Services, Substance Abuse and Mental Health Services Administration, Office of Applied Studies.
58. Kendall, S. R. (1996).
59. Ibid.
60. Gfroerer, J. C., Wu, L.-T., & Penne, M. A. (2002). *Initiation of marijuana use. Trends, patterns, and implications.* (Analytic series: A-17, DHHS Pub. No. [SMA] 02-3711). Rockville, MD: Substance Abuse and Mental Health Services Administration, Office of Applied Studies.
61. Kandall, S. R. (1996).
62. Kandall, S. R., & Chavkin, W. (1992). Illicit drugs in America: History, impact on women and infants, and treatment strategies for women. *Hastings Law Journal, 43*(3), 615–643.
63. Kandall, S. R. (1998). The history of drug abuse and women in the United States. In C. L. Wetherington & A. B. Roman (Eds.), *Drug addiction research and the health of women: Executive summary* (NIH Pub. No. 98-4289, pp. 8–16). Rockville, MD: U.S. Department of Health and Human Services, National Institutes of Health, National Institute on Drug Abuse.
64. Kandall, S. R. (1996).
65. CASA. (2005). *CASA's analysis of NSDUH 2003.*
66. Ibid.
67. Substance Abuse and Mental Health Services Administration, Office of Applied Studies. (2002). *Treatment Episode Data Set (TEDS) 1992–2000: National admissions to substance abuse treatment services* (DHHS Pub. No. [SMA] 02-3727). Rockville, MD: U.S. Department of Health and Human Services.

68. National Institute on Drug Abuse. (2003). *NIDA infofacts: Prescription drugs and pain medications.* www.drugabuse.gov (accessed March 5, 2004).
69. The National Center on Addiction and Substance Abuse (CASA) at Columbia University. (2005). *Under the counter: The diversion and abuse of controlled prescription drugs in the United States.* New York: CASA.
70. (CASA). (2005). *CASA's analysis of NSDUH 2003.*
71. Kan, C. C., Breteler, M. H., van der Ven, A. H., Timmermans, M. A., & Zitman, F. G. (2001). Assessment of benzodiazepine dependence in alcohol and drug dependent outpatients: A research report. *Substance Use and Misuse, 36*(8), 1085–1109.
72. The National Center on Addiction and Substance Abuse (CASA) at Columbia University. (2003). *CASA analysis of the National Household Survey on Drug Abuse (NHSDA), 1990–2001* [Data file]. Rockville, MD: U.S. Department of Health and Human Services, Substance Abuse and Mental Health Services Administration.
73. CASA. (2005). *Under the counter.*
74. CASA. (2005). *CASA's analysis of NSDUH 2003.* The National Center on Addiction and Substance Abuse (CASA) at Columbia University. (2004). *CASA analysis of the National Household Survey on Drug Abuse (NHSDA), 1990–2002* [Data file]. Rockville, MD: U.S. Department of Health and Human Services, Substance Abuse and Mental Health Services Administration.
75. CASA. (2005). *CASA's analysis of NSDUH 2003.*
76. Light, H. (1998). Sex differences in adolescent high-risk sexual and drug behaviors. *Psychological Reports, 82*(3, Pt. 2), 1312–1314.
77. National Institute on Drug Abuse. (2001).
78. American Psychiatric Association. (1994). *Diagnostic and statistical manual of mental disorders: DSM-IV.* Washington, DC: American Psychiatric Association.
79. Substance Abuse and Mental Health Services Administration, Office of Applied Studies. (2003). *Overview of findings*; Grunbaum, J. A., Kann, L., Kinchen, S., Ross, J., Hawkins, J., Lowry, R., et al. (2004). Youth Risk Behavior Surveillance: United States, 2003. *Morbidity and Mortality Weekly Report: Surveillance Summaries, 53*(SS-2).
80. Substance Abuse and Mental Health Services Administration, Office of Applied Studies. (2003). *Overview of findings.*
81. The National Center on Addiction and Substance Abuse (CASA) at Columbia University. (2003). *The formative years: Pathways to substance abuse among girls and young women ages 8–22.* New York: CASA.
82. Johnston, L. D., O'Malley, P. M., Bachman, J. G., & Schulenberg, J. E. (2004). *Monitoring the Future: National survey results on drug use, 1975–2003: Volume 2, College students and adults ages 19–45* (NIH Pub. No. 04-5508). Bethesda, MD: U.S. Department of Health and Human Services, National Institutes of Health, National Institute on Drug Abuse.
83. Substance Abuse and Mental Health Services Administration, Office of Applied Studies. (2004).

84. Johnston, L. D., O'Malley, P. M., Bachman, J. G., & Schulenberg, J. E. (2004). *Monitoring the future,* vol. 2.
85. CASA. (2005). *CASA's analysis of NSDUH 2003.*
86. Ibid.
87. Jinks, M. J., & Raschko, R. R. (1990). A profile of alcohol and prescription drug abuse in a high-risk community-based elderly population. *Annals of Pharmacotherapy, 24*(10), 971–975.
88. CASA. (2005). *CASA's analysis of NSDUH 2003.*
89. The National Center on Addiction and Substance Abuse (CASA) at Columbia University. (1998). *Under the rug: Substance abuse and the mature woman.* New York: CASA.
90. Pincus, H. A., Tanielian, T. L., Marcus, S. C., Olfson, M., Zarin, D. A., Thompson, J., et al. (1998). Prescribing trends in psychotropic medications: Primary care, psychiatry, and other medical specialties. *JAMA, 279*(7), 526–531; U.S. General Accounting Office. (1995). *Prescription drugs and the elderly.* Washington, DC: U.S. General Accounting Office; Wysowski, D. K., & Baum, C. (1991). Outpatient use of prescription sedative-hypnotic drugs in the United States, 1970 through 1989. *Archives of Internal Medicine, 151*(9), 1779–1783.
91. U.S. General Accounting Office. (1995).
92. CASA. (1998). *Under the rug.*
93. Ibid.
94. National Institute on Drug Abuse. (2001).
95. Longo, L. P., & Johnson, B. (2000). Addiction: Part 1: Benzodiazepines: Side effects, abuse risk, and alternatives. *American Family Physician, 61*(7), 2121–2128.
96. Miller, N. S., Belkin, B. M., & Gold, M. S. (1991). Alcohol and drug dependence among the elderly: Epidemiology, diagnosis, and treatment. *Comprehensive Psychiatry, 32*(2), 153–165; Ray, W. A., Griffin, M. R., & Downey, W. (1989). Benzodiazepines of long and short elimination half-life and the risk of hip fracture. *JAMA, 262*(23), 3303–3307; Sheahan, S. L., Hendricks, J., & Coons, S. J. (1989). Drug misuse among the elderly: A covert problem. *Health Values, 13*(3), 22–29; Solomon, K., Manepalli, J., Ireland, G. A., & Mahon, G. M. (1993). Alcoholism and prescription drug abuse in the elderly: St. Louis University Grand Rounds. *Journal of the American Geriatric Society, 41*(1), 57–69; Swift, C. G. (1981). Psychotropic drugs and the elderly. In G. Tognoni, C. Bellantuono, & M. Lader (Eds.), *Epidemiological impact of psychotropic drugs: Proceedings of the International Seminar on Impact of Psychotropic Drugs held in Milan, Italy, 24–26 June, 1981* (pp. 325–338). New York: Elsevier/North-Holland Biomedical Press.
97. Cummings, S. R., Nevitt, M. C., Browner, W. S., Stone, K., Fox, K. M., Ensrud, K. E., et al. (1995). Risk factors for hip fracture in white women. *New England Journal of Medicine, 332*(12), 767–773; Lipsitz, L. A., Hirayama, T., Nakajima, I., Kelley, M., Ruthazer, R., Hirayama, T., et al. (1991). Muscle strength, medications and falls in elderly Japanese and American nursing home residents: A cross-cultural study. *Journal of the American Geriatric Society, 39*(8), A10; Ray, W. A., Griffin, M. R., & Downey, W. (1989); Tinetti, M. E., Speechley, M., & Ginter, S. F. (1988). Risk factors for falls among elderly persons living in the community. *New England Journal of Medicine, 319*(26), 1701–1707.

98. Hemmelgarn, B., Suissa, S., Huang, A., Boivin, J.-F., & Pinard, G. (1997). Benzodiazepine use and the risk of motor vehicle crash in the elderly. *JAMA, 278*(1), 27–31; Ray, W. A., Fought, R. L., & Decker, M. D. (1992). Psychoactive drugs and the risk of injurious motor vehicle crashes in elderly drivers. *American Journal of Epidemiology, 136*(7), 873–883.
99. Gomberg, E. S. L. (1994). Risk factors for drinking over a woman's life span. *Alcohol Health and Research World, 18*(3), 220–227.
100. Substance Abuse and Mental Health Services Administration, Office of Applied Studies. (2001). *The NHSDA report: Substance use among older adults.* http://ncadi.samhsa.gov/ (accessed March 11, 2004).
101. Winick, C. (1962). Maturing out of narcotic addiction. *Bulletin on Narcotics, 14,* 1–7.
102. Gfroerer, J., Penne, M., Pemberton, M., & Folsom, R. (2003). Substance abuse treatment need among older adults in 2020: The impact of the aging baby-boom cohort. *Drug and Alcohol Dependence, 69*(2), 127–135; Patterson, T. L., & Jeste, D. V. (1999). The potential impact of the baby-boom generation on substance abuse among elderly persons. *Psychiatric Services, 50*(9), 1184–1188; Substance Abuse and Mental Health Services Administration, Office of Applied Studies. (2001).
103. American Psychiatric Association. (1994).
104. Hanson, G. R. (2002). In drug abuse, gender matters. *NIDA Notes, 17*(2).
105. American Psychiatric Association. (1994).
106. Ibid.
107. National Institute on Drug Abuse. (2002). *NIDA infofacts: Marijuana.* www.nida.nih.gov (accessed October 26, 2001); Kouri, E. M., Pope, H. G., & Lukas, S. E. (1999). Changes in aggressive behavior during withdrawal from long-term marijuana use. *Psychopharmacology, 143*(3), 302–308; Haney, M., Ward, A. S., Comer, S. D., Foltin, R. W., & Fischman, M. W. (1999). Abstinence symptoms following smoked marijuana in humans. *Psychopharmacology, 141*(4), 395–404.
108. American Psychiatric Association. (1994).
109. Kouri, E. M., Pope, H. G., & Lukas, S. E. (1999); Haney, M., Ward, A. S., Comer, S. D., Foltin, R. W., & Fischman, M. W. (1999).
110. Substance Abuse and Mental Health Services Administration, Office of Applied Studies. (2003). *Treatment Episode Data Set (TEDS) 1992–2001: National admissions to substance abuse treatment services* (DHHS Pub. No. 03-3778). Rockville, MD: U.S. Department of Health and Human Services.
111. Brecht, M.-L., O'Brien, A., von Mayrhauser, C., & Anglin, M. D. (2004). Methamphetamine use behaviors and gender differences. *Addictive Behaviors, 29*(1), 89–106.
112. CASA. (2003). *The formative years.*
113. Feigelman, W., Gorman, B. S., & Lee, J. A. (1998). Binge drinkers, illicit drug users and polydrug users: An epidemiological study of American collegians. *Journal of Alcohol and Drug Education, 44*(1), 47–69.
114. Coffin, P. O., Galea, S., Ahern, J., Leon, A. C., Vlahov, D., & Tardiff, K. (2003). Opiates, co-

caine and alcohol combinations in accidental drug overdose deaths in New York City, 1990–98. *Addiction, 98*(6), 739–747.

115. Conway, K. P., Kane, R. J., Ball, S. A., Poling, J. C., & Rounsaville, B. J. (2003). Personality, substance of choice, and polysubstance involvement among substance dependent patients. *Drug and Alcohol Dependence, 71*(1), 65–75.
116. CASA. (2005). *Under the counter.*
117. The National Center on Addiction and Substance Abuse (CASA) at Columbia University. (1999). *CASA analysis of the Youth Risk Behavior Survey (YRBS), 1997* [Data file]. Atlanta, GA: U.S. Department of Health and Human Services, Centers for Disease Control and Prevention, National Center for Chronic Disease Prevention and Health Promotion.
118. Diem, E. C., McKay, L. C., & Jamieson, J. L. (1994). Female adolescent alcohol, cigarette, and marijuana use: Similarities and differences in patterns of use. *International Journal of the Addictions, 29*(8), 987–997; Mott, F. L., & Haurin, R. J. (1988). Linkages between sexual activity and alcohol and drug use among American adolescents. *Family Planning Perspective, 20*(3), 128–136.
119. Logan, T. K., Leukefeld, C., & Farabee, D. (1998). Sexual and drug use behaviors among women crack users: Implications for prevention. *AIDS Education and Prevention, 10*(4), 327–340.
120. National Institute on Drug Abuse. (2000).
121. Centers for Disease Control and Prevention. (1998). U.S. HIV and AIDS cases reported through June, 1998. *HIV/AIDS Surveillance Report, 10*(1).
122. Boston Women's Health Book Collective. (1998). *Our bodies, ourselves for the new century: A book by and for women.* New York: Simon and Schuster.
123. The National Center on Addiction and Substance Abuse (CASA) at Columbia University. (1998). *Behind bars: Substance abuse and America's prison population.* New York: CASA.
124. Ibid.
125. Ericksen, K. P., & Trocki, K. F. (1994). Sex, alcohol and sexually transmitted diseases: A national survey. *Family Planning Perspectives, 26*(6), 257–263.
126. Berenson, A. B., Wilkinson, G. S., & Lopez, L. A. (1995). Substance use during pregnancy and peripartum complications in a triethnic population. *International Journal of the Addictions, 30*(2), 135–145; Battjes, R. J., Sloboda, Z., & Grace, W. C. (Eds.). (1994). *The context of HIV risk among drug users and their sexual partners: NIDA research monograph 143* (NIH Pub. No. 94-3750). Washington, DC: U.S. Department of Health and Human Services, Public Health Service, National Institutes of Health, National Institute on Drug Abuse.
127. The National Center on Addiction and Substance Abuse (CASA) at Columbia University. (2002). *CASA analysis of the Youth Risk Behavior Survey (YRBS), 1999* [Data file]. Atlanta, GA: U.S. Department of Health and Human Services, Centers for Disease Control and Prevention, National Center for Chronic Disease Prevention and Health Promotion.
128. Fullilove, M. T., Fullilove, R. E., Smith, M., Winkler, K., Michael, C., Panzer, P. G., et al. (1993). Violence, trauma, and post-traumatic stress disorder among women drug users.

Journal of Traumatic Stress, 6(4), 533–543; Kantor, G. K., & Straus, M. A. (1989). Substance abuse as a precipitant of wife abuse victimizations. *American Journal of Drug and Alcohol Abuse, 15*(2), 173–189.

129. Miller, B. A. (1998). Partner violence experiences and women's drug use: Exploring the connections. In C. L. Wetherington & A. B. Roman (Eds.), *Drug addiction research and the health of women* (NIH Pub. No. 98-4290, pp. 407–416). Rockville, MD: U.S. Department of Health and Human Services, National Institutes of Health, National Institute on Drug Abuse.
130. Kilpatrick, D. G., Acierno, R., Resnick, H. S., Saunders, B. E., & Best, C. L. (1997). A 2-year longitudinal analysis of the relationships between violent assault and substance use in women. *Journal of Consulting and Clinical Psychology, 65*(5), 834–847.
131. Kilpatrick, D. G., Edmunds, C. N., & Seymour, A. K. (1992). *Rape in America: A report to the nation.* Charleston, SC: Crime Victims' Research and Treatment Center.
132. Courtwright, D. T. (2001).
133. Cohen, E., & Navaline, H. M. D. (1994). High-risk behaviors for HIV: A comparison between crack-abusing and opioid-abusing African-American women. *Journal of Psychoactive Drugs, 26*(2), 233–241; Hunt, D. E. (1990). Drugs and consensual crimes: Drug dealing and prostitution. In M. Tonry & J. Q. Wilson (Eds.), *Drugs and crime* (pp. 159–201). Chicago: University of Chicago Press; Lewis, D. K., & Watters, J. K. (1991). Sexual risk behavior among heterosexual intravenous drug users: Ethnic and gender variations. *AIDS, 5*(1), 77–83; Logan, T. K., Leukefeld, C., & Farabee, D. (1998).
134. Potterat, J. J., Rothenberg, R. B., Muth, S. Q., Darrow, W. W., & Phillips-Plummer, L. (1998). Pathways to prostitution: The chronology of sexual and drug abuse milestones. *Journal of Sex Research, 35*(4), 333–340.
135. Cusick, L., Martin, A., & May, T. (2003). *Vulnerability and involvement in drug use and sex work: Home Office Research Study 268.* London: Home Office Research Development and Statistics Directorate.
136. Hedrich, D. (1990). Prostitution and AIDS risks among female drug users in Frankfurt. In M. A. Plant (Ed.), *AIDS, drugs, and prostitution* (pp. 159–174). New York: Routledge; Ratner, M. S. (1993). *Crack pipe as pimp: An ethnographic investigation of sex-for-crack exchanges.* New York: Lexington Books; Goldstein, P. J. (1979). *Prostitution and drugs.* Lexington, MA: Lexington Books.
137. Cohen, E., & Navaline, H. M. D. (1994); Edlin, B. R., Irwin, K. L., Ludwig, D. D., & McCoy, H. V. (1992). High-risk sex behavior among young street-recruited crack cocaine smokers in three American cities: An interim report. *Journal of Psychoactive Drugs, 24*(4), 363–371; El-Bassel, N., Gilbert, L., Schilling, R. F., Ivanoff, A., & Borne, D. (1996). Correlates of crack abuse among drug-using incarcerated women: Psychological trauma, social support, and coping behavior. *American Journal of Alcohol Abuse, 22*(1), 41–56.
138. Baskin, D. R., & Sommers, I. B. (1998). *Causalities of community disorder: Women's careers in violent crime.* Boulder, CO: Westview Press; Ratner, M. S. (1993).
139. Snyder, H. N. (2002). *Juvenile arrests 2000* (NCJ Pub. No. 191729). Washington, DC: U.S. Department of Justice, Office of Justice Programs, Office of Juvenile Justice and Delinquency Prevention.

140. CASA. (1998). *Behind bars.*

141. Kandall, S. R. (1998). Women and addiction in the United States: 1920 to the present.

142. Snell, T. L., & Morton, D. C. (1994). *Survey of state prison inmates, 1991: Women in prison.* Washington, DC: U.S. Department of Justice, Office of Justice Programs, Bureau of Justice Statistics.

143. Arrestee Drug Abuse Monitoring Program (ADAM). (2002). *Preliminary data on drug use and related matters among adult arrestees and juvenile detainees.* www.adam-nij.net (accessed March 10, 2004).

144. Kassebaum, G., & Chandler, S. M. (1994). Polydrug use and self control among men and women in prisons. *Journal of Drug Education, 24*(4), 333–350; Prendergast, M. L., Wellisch, J., & Falkin, G. P. (1995). Assessment of and services for substance-abusing women offenders in community and correctional settings. *Prison Journal, 75*(2), 240–256.

145. CASA. (1998). *Behind bars.*

146. Inciardi, J. A., Lockwood, D., & Pottieger, A. E. (1993). *Women and crack-cocaine.* New York: Macmillan; Lex, B. W. (1995). Alcohol and other psychoactive substance dependence in women and men. In M. V. Seeman (Ed.), *Gender and psychopathology* (pp. 311–358). Washington, DC: American Psychiatric Press; Maher, L., & Curtis, R. (1992). Women on the edge of crime: Crack cocaine and the changing contexts of street-level sex work in New York City. *Crime, Law and Social Change, 18*(3), 221–258; McCoy, H. V., Inciardi, J. A., Metsch, L. R., Pottieger, A. E., & Saum, C. A. (1995). Women, crack and crime: Gender comparisons of criminal activity among crack cocaine users. *Contemporary Drug Problems, 22*(3), 435–451.

147. Snell, T. L., & Morton, D. C. (1994).

148. Anglin, M. D., & Hser, Y. (1987). Addicted women and crime. *Criminology, 25*(2), 359–397; Erickson, P. G., & Watson, V. A. (1990). Women, illicit drugs and crime. In L. T. Kozlowski, H. M. Annis, H. D. Cappell, F. B. Glaser, M. S. Goodstadt, Y. Israel, et al. (Eds.), *Research advances in alcohol and drug problems, volume 10* (pp. 251–272). New York: Plenum Press; Fagan, J. (1994). Women and drugs revisited: Female participation in the cocaine economy. *Journal of Drug Issues, 24*(2), 179–225; McCoy, H. V., Inciardi, J. A., Metsch, L. R., Pottieger, A. E., & Saum, C. A. (1995).

149. Puzzanchera, C., Stahl, A. L., Finnegan, T. A., Tierney, N., & Snyder, H. N. (2003). *Juvenile court statistics 1999: Celebrating 100 years of the juvenile court, 1899–1999* (NCJ Pub. No. 201241). Pittsburgh, PA: National Center for Juvenile Justice.

150. Prendergast, M. L., Wellisch, J., & Falkin, G. P. (1995); Snell, T. L., & Morton, D. C. (1994); Wellisch, J., Prendergast, M. L., & Anglin, M. D. (1994). Jail: A found opportunity for intervening with drug-abusing pregnant women. *Journal of Correctional Health Care, 1*(1), 17–38.

151. The National Center on Addiction and Substance Abuse (CASA) at Columbia University. (2005). *CASA analysis of the mortality data from the Drug Abuse Warning Network 2002* [Data file]. Rockville, MD: U.S. Department of Health and Human Services, Substance Abuse and Mental Health Services Administration.

152. Miller, N. S., Belkin, B. M., & Gold, M. S. (1991); Montamat, S. C., Cusack, B. J., & Vestal, R. E. (1989). Management of drug therapy in the elderly. *New England Journal of Medicine, 321*(5), 303–309.

153. American Academy of Pediatrics, Committee on Adolescents. (2000). Suicide and suicide attempts in adolescents. *Pediatrics, 105*(4, Pt. 1), 871–874.
154. Litovitz, T. L., Klein-Schwartz, W., Rodgers, G. C., Cobaugh, D. J., Youniss, J., Omslaer, J. C., et al. (2002). 2001 annual report of the American Association of Poison Control Centers Toxic Exposure Surveillance System. *American Journal of Emergency Medicine, 20*(5), 391–452.
155. National Institutes of Health. (2001). *In harm's way: Suicide in America* (NIH Pub. No. 01-4594). Bethesda, MD: U.S. Department of Health and Human Services, National Institutes of Health.
156. Substance Abuse and Mental Health Services Administration, Office of Applied Studies. (2003). *Substance use and risk of suicide among youths.* Rockville, MD: U.S. Department of Health and Human Services, Substance Abuse and Mental Health Services Administration, Office of Applied Studies.
157. CASA. (2002).
158. Substance Abuse and Mental Health Services Administration, Office of Applied Studies. (2003). *Substance use.*
159. Coffin, P. O., Galea, S., Ahern, J., Leon, A. C., Vlahov, D., & Tardiff, K. (2003); Litovitz, T. L., Klein-Schwartz, W., Rodgers, G. C., Cobaugh, D. J., Youniss, J., Omslaer, J. C., et al. (2002).
160. Hagedorn, J., & Omar, H. (2002). Retrospective analysis of youth evaluated for suicide attempt or suicidal ideation in an emergency room setting. *International Journal of Adolescent Medicine and Health, 14*(1), 55–60; Healthyplace.com. (2000). *Frequently asked questions about suicide.* www.healthyplace.com (accessed February 4, 2003).
161. Gauvin, F., Bailey, B., & Bratton, S. L. (2001). Hospitalizations for pediatric intoxication in Washington State, 1987–1997. *Archives of Pediatric and Adolescent Medicine, 155*(10), 1105–1110.
162. Inciardi, J. A., Lockwood, D., & Pottieger, A. E. (1993).
163. Kandall, S. R. (1996).
164. Goode, E. (1999). *Drugs in American society* (5th ed.). Boston: McGraw-Hill College.
165. Johnston, L. D., O'Malley, P. M., & Bachman, J. G. (2003). *Monitoring the future: National survey results on drug use, 1975–2002: Volume 1, secondary school students* (NIH Pub. No. 03-5375). Bethesda, MD: U.S. Department of Health and Human Services, National Institutes of Health, National Institute on Drug Abuse.
166. Jonnes, J. (2002). Hip to be high: Heroin and popular culture in the twentieth century. In D. F. Musto (Ed.), *One hundred years of heroin* (pp. 227–236). Westport, CT: Auburn House.
167. Johnston, L. D., O'Malley, P. M., & Bachman, J. G. (2003).
168. Baker, P. (1997, May 22). Clinton blasts "glorification of heroin" in magazine fashion photo spreads. *Washington Post,* A11.
169. Johnston, L. D., O'Malley, P. M., & Bachman, J. G. (2003).
170. Givhan, R. (2002, October 25). Christian Dior's addict: "Admit" a problem? *Washington Post,* C02.
171. Curley, B. (2003). *Bowing to advocates, Dior agrees to change "addict" marketing campaign.* www.jointogether.org (accessed February 13, 2004).

172. Pinkus, R. L. (2002). From Lydia Pinkham to Bob Dole: What the changing face of direct-to-consumer drug advertising reveals about the professionalism of medicine. *Kennedy Institute of Ethics Journal, 12*(2), 141–158.

173. Rosenthal, M. B., Berndt, E. R., Donohue, J. M., Frank, R. G., & Epstein, A. M. (2002). Promotion of prescription drugs to consumers. *New England Journal of Medicine, 346*(7), 498–505.

174. Ads and prescription pads [Editorial]. (2003). *Canadian Medical Association Journal, 169*(5), 381.

175. Brody, J. E. (1998, December 15). Drug ads lure patients into jargon-strewn territory. *New York Times,* F7.

176. Murray, E., Lo, B., Pollack, L., Donelan, K., & Lee, K. (2003). Direct-to-consumer advertising: Physicians' views of its effects on quality of care and the doctor-patient relationship. *Journal of the American Board of Family Practice, 16*(6), 513–524.

177. National Institute on Drug Abuse. (2001).

178. Ibid.

179. Metzl, J. M., & Angel, J. (2004).

180. Center for Substance Abuse Prevention. (2003). Trouble in the medicine chest (1): Rx drug abuse growing. *Prevention Alert, 6*(4).

181. CASA. (2005). *Under the counter.*

182. National Institute on Drug Abuse. (2001).

183. The National Center on Addiction and Substance Abuse (CASA) at Columbia University. (2004). *You've got drugs!: Prescription drug pushers on the internet.* New York: CASA.

184. Wilford, B. B., Finch, J., Czechowicz, D. J., & Warren, D. (1994). An overview of prescription drug misuse and abuse: Defining the problem and seeking solutions. *Journal of Law, Medicine and Ethics, 22*(3), 197–203; McAuliffe, W. E. (1984). Nontherapeutic opiate addiction in health professionals: A new form of impairment. *American Journal of Drug and Alcohol Abuse, 10*(1), 1–22; O'Connor, P. G., & Spickard, A. (1997). Physician impairment by substance abuse. *Medical Clinics of North America, 81*(4), 1037–1052.

185. Wesson, D. R., & Smith, D. E. (1990). Prescription drug abuse: Patient, physician, and cultural responsibilities. *Western Journal of Medicine, 152*(5), 613–616.

186. National Institute on Drug Abuse. (2001).

187. Ling, W., Wesson, D. R., & Smith, D. E. (2003). Abuse of prescription opioids. In A. W. Graham, T. K. Schultz, M. Mayo-Smith, R, K. Ries, & B. B. Wilford (Eds.), *Principles of Addiction Medicine* (p. 1281). Chevy Chase, MD: American Society of Addiction Medicine.

188. CASA. (2005). *Under the counter.*

Chapter 5. Pregnancy and Substance Abuse

Epigraph: Roberts, L. W., & Dunn, L. B. (2003). Ethical considerations in caring for women with substance use disorders. *Obstetrics and Gynecology Clinics of North America, 30*(3), 559–582.

1. Substance Abuse and Mental Health Services Administration, Office of Applied Studies.

(2004). *Pregnancy and substance use: The NSDUH report.* Rockville, MD: U.S. Department of Health and Human Services, Substance Abuse and Mental Health Services Administration, Office of Applied Studies.

2. American Lung Association. (2000). *Smoking and pregnancy* [Fact sheet]. www.lungusa.org (accessed January 25, 2002); Dwyer, T., Ponsonby, A. L., & Couper, D. (1999). Tobacco smoke exposure at one month of age and subsequent risk of SIDS: A prospective study. *American Journal of Epidemiology, 149*(7), 593–602.
3. Austin, G., & Prendergast, M. (1991). Young children of substance abusers. *Prevention Research Update, 8.*
4. Flynn, H. A., Marcus, S. A., Barry, K. L., & Blow, F. C. (2003). Rates and correlates of alcohol use among pregnant women in obstetrics clinics. *Alcoholism: Clinical and Experimental Research, 27*(1), 81–87.
5. Join Together. (2002). *Most pregnant women don't disclose drug use.* www.jointogether.org (accessed March 2, 2004).
6. Ebrahim, S. H., & Gfroerer, J. (2003). Pregnancy-related substance use in the United States during 1996–1998. *Obstetrics and Gynecology, 101*(2), 374–379.
7. Jos, P. H., Perlmutter, M., & Marshall, M. F. (2003). Substance abuse during pregnancy: Clinical and public health approaches. *Journal of Law, Medicine and Ethics, 31*(3), 340–350.
8. The National Center on Addiction and Substance Abuse (CASA) at Columbia University. (2005). *CASA's analysis of the National Survey on Drug Use and Abuse (NSDUH) 2003* [Data file]. Rockville, MD: U.S. Department of Health and Human Services, Substance Abuse and Mental Health Sources Administration; Ventura, S. J., Martin, J. A., Curtin, S. C., & Mathews, T. J. (1998). Report of final natality statistics, 1996. *Monthly Vital Statistics Report, 46*(Suppl. 11).
9. Hans, S. L. (1999). Demographic and psychosocial characteristics of substance-abusing pregnant women. *Clinics in Perinatology, 26*(1), 55–74.
10. Substance Abuse and Mental Health Services Administration, Office of Applied Studies. (2004).
11. Ebrahim, S. H., & Gfroerer, J. (2003).
12. Brady, J. P., Posner, M., Lang, C., & Rosati, M. J. (1994). *Risk and reality: The implications of prenatal exposure to alcohol and other drugs.* Washington, DC: U.S. Department of Education, Office of Educational Research and Improvement, Educational Resources Information; Richter, L., & Richter, D. M. (2001). Exposure to parental tobacco and alcohol use: Effects on children's health and development. *American Journal of Orthopsychiatry, 71*(2), 182–203; Young, N. K. (1997). Effects of alcohol and other drugs on children. *Journal of Psychoactive Drugs, 29*(1), 23–42.
13. Austin, G., & Prendergast, M. (1991); Richter, L., & Richter, D. M. (2001); Weinberg, N. Z. (1997). Cognitive and behavioral deficits associated with parent alcohol use. *Journal of the American Academy of Child and Adolescent Psychiatry, 36*(9), 1177–1186; Young, N. K. (1997).
14. Famy, C., Streissguth, A. P., & Unis, A. S. (1998). Mental illness in adults with fetal alcohol syndrome or fetal alcohol effects. *American Journal of Psychiatry, 155*(4), 552–554; Streissguth,

A. P., Barr, H. M., Bookstein, F. L., Sampson, P. D., & Olson, H. C. (1999). The long-term neurocognitive consequences of prenatal alcohol exposure: A 14-year study. *Psychological Science, 10*(3), 186–190.

15. Kalotra, C. J. (2002). *Estimated costs related to the birth of a drug and/or alcohol exposed baby.* www.american.edu (accessed February 9, 2004).
16. Hans, S. L. (1999).
17. Leonardson, G. R., & Loudenburg, R. (2003). Risk factors for alcohol use during pregnancy in a multistate area. *Neurotoxicology and Teratology, 25*(6), 651–658; National Institute on Drug Abuse. (1996). *National pregnancy and health survey: Drug use among women delivering livebirths, 1992* (NIH Pub. No. 96-3819). Rockville, MD: U.S. Department of Health and Human Services, National Institutes of Health, National Institute on Drug Abuse.
18. Hans, S. L. (1999).
19. Henry J. Kaiser Family Foundation. (2004). *Racial and ethnic disparities in women's health coverage and access to care: Findings from the 2001 Kaiser Women's Health Survey: Issue brief.* www.kff.org (accessed March 29, 2004); Henry J. Kaiser Family Foundation. (2004). *Health coverage and access challenges for low-income women: Findings from the 2001 Kaiser Women's Health Survey: Issue brief.* www.kff.org (accessed March 29, 2004).
20. National Institute of Child Health and Human Development. (2004). *Contraception and Reproductive Health Branch (NICHD): Report to the NACHHD Council.* www.nichd.nih.gov (accessed February 9, 2004).
21. Henshaw, S. K. (1998). Unintended pregnancy in the United States. *Family Planning Perspectives, 30*(1), 24–29, 46.
22. Centers for Disease Control and Prevention. (2000). National and state-specific pregnancy rates among adolescents: United States, 1995–1997. *Morbidity and Mortality Weekly Report, 49*(27), 605–611.
23. Princeton Survey Research Associates. (1996). *The 1996 Kaiser Family Foundation survey on teens and sex: What they say teens today need to know and who they listen to.* Menlo Park, CA: Henry J. Kaiser Family Foundation.
24. Centers for Disease Control and Prevention. (1997). Alcohol consumption.
25. Streissguth, A. P., Barr, H. M., & Sampson, P. D. (1990). Moderate prenatal alcohol exposure: Effects on child IQ and learning problems at age 7 1/2 years. *Alcoholism: Clinical and Experimental Research, 14*(5), 662–669; Young, N. K. (1997).
26. Hellerstedt, W. L., Pirie, P. L., Lando, H. A., Curry, S. J., McBride, C. M., Grothaus, L. C., et al. (1998). Differences in preconceptional and prenatal behaviors in women with intended and unintended pregnancies. *American Journal of Public Health, 88*(4), 663–666.
27. Hans, S. L. (1999).
28. Haug, N. A. (2003). Motivational enhancement therapy for cigarette-smoking in methadone-maintained pregnant women. *Dissertations Abstracts International, 63*(8-B), 3916.
29. Join Together. (2002). *Depression, alcohol use linked in pregnant women.* www.jointogether.org (accessed April 26, 2004).

30. Hans, S. L. (1999).
31. Lapp, T. (2000). ACOG addresses psychosocial screening in pregnant women. *American Family Physician, 62*(12), 2701–2702.
32. Haller, D. L., & Miles, D. R. (2003). Victimization and perpetration among perinatal substance abusers. *Journal of Interpersonal Violence, 18*(7), 760–780.
33. Martin, S. L., Beaumont, J. L., & Kupper, L. L. (2003). Substance use before and during pregnancy: Links to intimate partner violence. *American Journal of Drug and Alcohol Abuse, 29*(3), 599–617.
34. Haller, D. L., & Miles, D. R. (2003); Tuten, M., Jones, H. E., Tran, G., & Svikis, D. S. (2004). Partner violence impacts the psychosocial and psychiatric status of pregnant, drug-dependent women. *Addictive Behaviors, 29*(9), 1029–1034.
35. Martin, S. L., Clark, K. A., Lynch, S. R., Kupper, L. L., & Cilenti, D. (1999). Violence in the lives of pregnant teenage women: Associations with multiple substance use. *American Journal of Drug and Alcohol Abuse, 25*(3), 425–440.
36. Horrigan, T. J., Schroeder, A. V., & Schaffer, R. M. (2000). The triad of substance abuse, violence, and depression are interrelated in pregnancy. *Journal of Substance Abuse Treatment, 18*(1), 55–58.
37. Tuten, M., Jones, H. E., Tran, G., & Svikis, D. S. (2004).
38. Haller, D. L., & Miles, D. R. (2003); Thompson, M. P., & Kingree, J. B. (1998). The frequency and impact of violent trauma among pregnant substance abusers. *Addictive Behaviors, 23*(2), 257–262.
39. Jasinski, J. L. (2004). Pregnancy and domestic violence: A review of the literature. *Trauma, Violence, and Abuse, 5*(1), 47–64.
40. Kearney, M. H., Munro, B. H., Kelly, U., & Hawkins, J. W. (2004). Health behaviors as mediators for the effect of partner abuse on infant birth weight. *Nursing Research, 53*(1), 36–45.
41. Huth-Bocks, A. C., Levendosky, A. A., Theran, S. A., & Bogat, G. A. (2004). The impact of domestic violence on mothers' prenatal representations of their infants. *Infant Mental Health Journal, 25*(2), 79–98.
42. Miles, D. R., Svikis, D. S., Kulstad, J. L., & Haug, N. A. (2001). Psychopathology in pregnant drug-dependent women with and without comorbid alcohol dependence. *Alcoholism: Clinical and Experimental Research, 25*(7), 1012–1017.
43. Lucas, E. T., Goldschmidt, L., & Day, N. L. (2003). Alcohol use among pregnant African American women: Ecological considerations. *Health and Social Work, 28*(4), 273–283.
44. Webb, D. A., Culhane, J., Metraux, S., Robbins, J. M., & Culhane, D. (2003). Prevalence of episodic homelessness among adult childbearing women in Philadelphia, PA. *American Journal of Public Health, 93*(11), 1895–1896.
45. Kelly, P. J., Blacksin, B., & Mason, E. (2001). Factors affecting substance abuse treatment completion for women. *Issues in Mental Health Nursing, 22*(3), 287–304.
46. Tuten, M., Jones, H. E., & Svikis, D. S. (2003). Comparing homeless and domiciled pregnant substance dependent women on psychosocial characteristics and treatment outcomes. *Drug and Alcohol Dependence, 69*(1), 95–99.

47. Kelly, P. J., Blacksin, B., & Mason, E. (2001); Tuten, M., Jones, H. E., & Svikis, D. S. (2003).
48. Kelly, P. J., Blacksin, B., & Mason, E. (2001).
49. Tuten, M., Jones, H. E., Tran, G., & Svikis, D. S. (2004).
50. Substance Abuse and Mental Health Services Administration, Office of Applied Studies. (2004).
51. Ventura, S. J., Hamilton, B. E., Mathews, B. J., & Chandra, A. (2003). Trends and variations in smoking during pregnancy and low birth weight: Evidence from the birth certificate, 1990–2000. *Pediatrics, 111*(5, Part 2), 1176–1180.
52. Substance Abuse and Mental Health Services Administration, Office of Applied Studies. (2004).
53. Mathews, T. J. (2001). Smoking during pregnancy in the 1990s. *National Vital Statistics Report, 49*(7).
54. Martin, J. A., Hamilton, B. E., Sutton, P. D., Ventura, S. J., Menacker, F., & Munson, M. L. (2003). Births: Final data for 2002. *National Vital Statistics Reports, 52*(10).
55. Mathews, T. J. (2001).
56. Substance Abuse and Mental Health Services Administration, Office of Applied Studies. (2004).
57. Mathews, T. J. (2001).
58. Flynn, H. A., Marcus, S. A., Barry, K. L., & Blow, F. C. (2003).
59. Substance Abuse and Mental Health Services Administration, Office of Applied Studies. (1997). *Substance use among women in the United States* (DHHS Pub. No. [SMA] 97-3162). Rockville, MD: U.S. Department of Health and Human Services, Substance Abuse and Mental Health Services Administration, Office of Applied Studies.
60. Centers for Disease Control and Prevention. (2002). Alcohol use among women of childbearing age: United States, 1991–1999. *Morbidity and Mortality Weekly Report, 51*(13), 273–276.
61. Substance Abuse and Mental Health Services Administration, Office of Applied Studies. (2002). *Substance use among pregnant women during 1999 and 2000.* www.samhsa.gov/oas (accessed February 9, 2004).
62. Substance Abuse and Mental Health Services Administration, Office of Applied Studies. (2004).
63. Substance Abuse and Mental Health Services Administration, Office of Applied Studies. (2002). *Pregnant women in substance abuse treatment: The DASIS report.* Rockville, MD: U.S. Department of Health and Human Services.
64. Substance Abuse and Mental Health Services Administration, Office of Applied Studies. (2004).
65. Join Together. (2002). *Most pregnant women.*
66. Substance Abuse and Mental Health Services Administration, Office of Applied Studies. (2004).
67. Ibid.
68. Ebrahim, S. H., & Gfroerer, J. (2003).

69. National Institute on Drug Abuse. (1996).
70. Substance Abuse and Mental Health Services Administration, Office of Applied Studies. (2002). *Pregnant women.*
71. Public Broadcasting Service. (2001). *American experience: The pill: People and events.* www.pbs.org (accessed April 28, 2004).
72. Kandall, S. R. (1996). *Substance and shadow: Women and addiction in the United States.* Cambridge, MA: Harvard University Press.
73. The smoking report [Editorial]. (1964, January 12). *New York Times,* E12.
74. Schmeck, H. M. (1971, January 12). Surgeon General urges battle to dissuade women smokers. *New York Times,* 17.
75. Sulzberger, A. O. (1981, May 22). Smoking warnings called ineffective: Report to Congress sees need for new caution system for ads and cigarette packages. *New York Times,* A14.
76. Molotsky, I. (1984, May 22). Firmer warnings on cigarettes called likely. *New York Times,* A1, A15; Sulzberger, A. O. (1981, May 22).
77. Sulzberger, A. O. (1981, May 22).
78. Ibid.
79. Roswell Park Cancer Institute. (2004). *The Tobacco Institute: Roots in the Tobacco Industry Research Committee.* http://roswell.tobaccodocuments.org (accessed April 26, 2004).
80. Wall Street Journal Staff Reporter. (1990, January 15). Cigarette labels may need change to alert pregnant women, Surgeon General says. *Wall Street Journal,* 5.
81. United Press International. (1982, March 11). U.S. health officials endorse stronger cigarette warnings. *New York Times,* A15.
82. Schorr, B. (1982, May 11). Should cigarette warnings be even tougher? *Wall Street Journal,* 30.
83. Molotsky, I. (1984, August 11). Tobacco debate: Imports and health. *New York Times,* 6.
84. Lemoine, P., Harousseau, H., Borteyru, J. P., & Menuet, J. C. (1968). Les enfants de parents alcooliques: Anomalies observées à propos de 127 cas. *Ouest Medical, 21,* 476–482.
85. Jones, K. L., & Smith, D. W. (1973). Recognition of the fetal alcohol syndrome in early infancy. *Lancet, 2*(7836), 999–1001.
86. United Press International. (1977, April 24). Advice on alcohol in pregnancy. *New York Times,* 26.
87. Dunning, J. (1977, June 1). Women are warned to give up drinking during pregnancies. *New York Times,* 22.
88. The label on the liquor bottle [Editorial]. (1977, November 26). *New York Times,* 16.
89. Associated Press. (1979, February 9). U.S. asks plan to warn women on alcohol use. *New York Times,* D15.
90. Greenberg, J. (1981, July 18). U.S. advises total abstinence from drinking for pregnant women. *New York Times,* 7.
91. Ibid.
92. Associated Press. (1982, September 23). One in 600 babies affected by fetal alcohol syndrome. *New York Times,* A22.
93. Goodwin, M. (1983, November 16). Council bill warns on drinking during pregnancy. *New York Times,* B5.

94. Hager, P. (1987, August 21). Law on posted alcohol warnings upheld. *Los Angeles Times,* 3.
95. Painter, K. (1988, November 18). Labels to warn pregnant women. *USA Today,* 1D.
96. Molotsky, I. (1984, May 22).
97. Havemann, J. (1989, February 17). Alcohol warning labels may be in small type: Congressionally mandated regulations for beverages issued. *Washington Post,* A03.
98. Glascoff, M. A., & Felts, W. M. (1994). The awareness level of pregnant women of alcoholic beverage health warning labels. *Wellness Perspectives, 10*(2), 24.
99. Painter, K. (1988, November 18).
100. Chicago Tribune Wires. (1990, July 3). FDA widens aspirin warning labels for pregnant women. *Chicago Tribune,* 4.
101. Kandall, S. R. (1996).
102. Office of the Surgeon General. (2001). *Women and smoking: A report of the Surgeon General* (GPO Item No. 0483-L-06). Washington, DC: U.S. Government Printing Office.
103. Pollack, H., Lantz, P. M., & Frohna, J. G. (2000). Maternal smoking and adverse birth outcomes among singletons and twins. *American Journal of Public Health, 90*(3), 395–400; Richter, L., & Richter, D. M. (2001).
104. Office of the Surgeon General. (2001).
105. American Lung Association. (2000).
106. Office of the Surgeon General. (2001).
107. Chung, K. C., Kowalski, C., Kim, H. M., & Buchman, S. R. (2000). Maternal cigarette smoking during pregnancy and the risk of having a child with cleft lip/palate. *Plastic and Reconstructive Surgery, 105*(2), 485–491; Lorente, C., Cordier, S., Goujard, S., Ayme, S., Bianchi, F., Calzolari, E., et al. (2000). Tobacco and alcohol use during pregnancy and risk of oral clefts: Occupational Exposure and Congenital Malformation Working Group. *American Journal of Public Health, 90*(3), 415–419.
108. Lieu, J. E. C., & Feinstein, A. R. (2002). Effect of gestational and passive smoke exposure on ear infections in children. *Archives of Pediatric and Adolescent Medicine, 156*(2), 147–154.
109. Innes, K. E., & Byers, T. E. (2001). Smoking during pregnancy and breast cancer risk in very young women (United States). *Cancer Causes and Control, 12*(2), 179–185.
110. Gilliland, F. D., Berhane, K., McConnell, R., Gauderman, W. J., Vora, H., Rappaport, E. B., et al. (2000). Maternal smoking during pregnancy, environmental tobacco smoke exposure and childhood lung function. *Thorax, 55*(4), 271–276.
111. Montgomery, S. M., & Ekbom, A. (2002). Smoking during pregnancy and diabetes mellitus in a British longitudinal birth cohort. *British Medical Journal, 324*(7328), 26–27.
112. Milunsky, A., Carmella, S. G., Ye, M., & Hecht, S. S. (2000). A tobacco-specific carcinogen in the fetus. *Prenatal Diagnosis, 20*(4), 307–310.
113. Johnson, J. L., & Leff, M. (1999). Children of substance abusers: Overview of research findings. *Pediatrics, 103*(5), 1085–1099; Richter, L., & Richter, D. M. (2001); Young, N. K. (1997).
114. Brook, J. S., Brook, D. W., & Whiteman, M. (2000). The influence of maternal smoking during pregnancy on the toddler's negativity. *Archives of Pediatrics and Adolescent Medicine, 154*(4), 381–385.

115. Brennan, P. A., Brekin, E. R., Mortensen, E. L., & Mednik, S. A. (2002). Relationship of maternal smoking during pregnancy with criminal arrest and hospitalization for substance abuse in male and female adult offspring. *American Journal of Psychiatry, 159*(1), 48–54.
116. Weissman, M. M., Warner, V., Wickramaratne, P. J., & Kandel, D. B. (1999). Maternal smoking during pregnancy and psychopathology in offspring followed to adulthood. *Journal of the American Academy of Child and Adolescent Psychiatry, 38*(7), 892–899.
117. Kandel, D. B., Wu, P., & Davies, M. (1994). Maternal smoking during pregnancy and smoking by adolescent daughters. *American Journal of Public Health, 84*(9), 1407–1413.
118. Becker, A. B., Manfreda, J., Ferguson, A., Dimich-Ward, H., Watson, W. T. A., & Chan-Yeung, M. (1999). Breast-feeding and environmental tobacco smoke exposure. *Archives of Pediatrics and Adolescent Medicine, 153*(7), 689–691; Becker, A. B., Manfreda, J., Ferguson, A., Dimich-Ward, H., Watson, W. T. A., & Chan-Yeung, M. (1999); Mascola, M. A., Van Vunakis, H., Tager, I. B., Speizer, F. E., & Hanrahan, J. P. (1998). Exposure of young infants to environmental tobacco smoke: Breast-feeding among smoking mothers. *American Journal of Public Health, 88*(6), 893–896.
119. Centers for Disease Control and Prevention, National Center for Environmental Health. (2003). *Second national report on human exposure to environmental chemicals.* Atlanta, GA: U.S. Department of Health and Human Services, Centers for Disease Control and Prevention, National Center for Environmental Health.
120. American Lung Association. (2002). *Secondhand smoke* [Fact sheet]. www.lungusa.org (accessed February 24, 2004); Centers for Disease Control and Prevention, National Center for Environmental Health. (2003).
121. American Lung Association. (2002).
122. Join Together. (2002). *Secondhand smoke affects children's learning ability.* www.jointogether.org (accessed March 4, 2004).
123. Aligne, C. A., Moss, M. E., Auinger, P., & Weitzman, M. (2003). Association of pediatric dental caries with passive smoking. *JAMA, 289*(10), 1258–1264.
124. The National Center on Addiction and Substance Abuse (CASA) at Columbia University. (2005). *CASA's analysis of the National Survey on Drug Use and Health (NSDUH), 2003* [Data file]. Rockville, MD: U.S. Department of Health and Human Services, Substance Abuse and Mental Health Services Administration.
125. Schuster, M. A., Franke, T., & Pham, C. B. (2002). Smoking patterns of household members and visitors in homes with children in the United States. *Archives of Pediatrics and Adolescent Medicine, 156*(11), 1094–1100.
126. March of Dimes. (2002). *Drinking alcohol during pregnancy.* www.marchofdimes.com (accessed September 30, 2002).
127. Sood, B., Delaney-Black, V., Covington, C., Nordstrom-Klee, B., Ager, J., Templin, T., et al. (2001). Prenatal alcohol exposure and childhood behavior at age 6 to 7 years: 1. Dose-response effect. *Pediatrics, 108*(2), E34.
128. Willford, J. A., Richardson, G. A., Leech, S. L., & Day, N. L. (2004). Verbal and visuospatial

learning and memory function in children with moderate prenatal alcohol exposure. *Alcoholism: Clinical and Experimental Research, 28*(3), 497–507.

129. Kesmodel, U., Wisborg, K., Olsen, S. F., Henriksen, T. B., & Secher, N. J. (2002). Moderate alcohol intake in pregnancy and the risk of spontaneous abortion. *Alcohol and Alcoholism, 37*(1), 87–92.
130. Willford, J. A., Richardson, G. A., Leech, S. L., & Day, N. L. (2004).
131. Loop, K. Q., & Nettleman, M. D. (2002). Obstetrical textbooks: Recommendations about drinking during pregnancy. *American Journal of Preventive Medicine, 23*(2), 136–138.
132. King James Bible verses. (2003). www.reference-guides.com/king_james_bible/ (accessed March 5, 2004).
133. Sandmaier, M. (1992). *The invisible alcoholics: Women and alcohol* (2nd ed.). Blue Ridge Summit, PA: TAB Books.
134. Day, N. L., Zuo, Y., Richardson, G. A., Goldschmidt, L., Larkby, C. A., & Cornelius, M. D. (1999). Prenatal alcohol use and offspring size at 10 years of age. *Alcoholism: Clinical and Experimental Research, 23*(5), 863–869.
135. March of Dimes. (2002). *Drinking.*
136. Jacobson, S. W. (1999). Assessing the impact of maternal drinking during and after pregnancy. *Alcohol Health and Research World, 21*(3), 199–203; Mattson, S. N., & Riley, E. P. (2000). Parent ratings of behavior in children with heavy prenatal alcohol exposure and IQ-matched controls. *Alcoholism: Clinical and Experimental Research, 24*(2), 226–231; Streissguth, A. P., Barr, H. M., Bookstein, F. L., Sampson, P. D., & Olson, H. C. (1999).
137. Richter, L., & Richter, D. M. (2001).
138. Weinberg, N. Z. (1997); Young, N. K. (1997).
139. Richter, L., & Richter, D. M. (2001).
140. Lupton, C., Burd, L., & Harwood, R. (2004). *Cost of fetal alcohol spectrum disorders.* www.interscience.wiley.com (accessed April 5, 2004); May, P. A., & Gossage, J. P. (2001). Estimating the prevalence of Fetal Alcohol Syndrome: A summary. *Alcohol Research and Health, 25*(3), 159–167.
141. National Association for Children of Alcoholics, & National Clearinghouse for Alcohol and Drug Information. (2002). *Children of alcoholics: Important facts.* www.health.org (accessed September 30, 2002).
142. Jacobson, J. L., & Jacobson, S. W. (2002). Effects of prenatal alcohol exposure on child development. *Alcohol Research and Health, 26*(4), 282–286; May, P. A., & Gossage, J. P. (2001).
143. National Institute on Alcohol Abuse and Alcoholism. (2000). *Tenth special report to the U.S. Congress on alcohol and health from the Secretary of Health and Human Services* (NIH Pub. No. 00-1583). Rockville, MD: U.S. Department of Health and Human Services, Public Health Service, National Institute of Health, National Institute on Alcohol Abuse and Alcoholism; Weinberg, N. Z. (1997).
144. National Association for Children of Alcoholics, & National Clearinghouse for Alcohol and Drug Information. (2002).

145. Lupton, C., Burd, L., & Harwood, R. (2004).
146. Abel, E. L. (1988). Fetal alcohol syndrome in families. *Neurotoxicology and Teratology, 10*(1), 1–2.
147. The National Center on Addiction and Substance Abuse (CASA) at Columbia University. (1996). *Substance abuse and the American woman.* New York: CASA.
148. Prevention of Fetal Alcohol Syndrome (FAS) and Fetal Alcohol Effects (FAE) in Canada. (1997). *Paediatric and Child Health, 2*(2), 143–145.
149. May, P. A., Gossage, J. P., White-Country, M., Goodhart, K., Decoteau, S., Trujillo, P. M., et al. (2004). Alcohol consumption and other maternal risk factors for fetal alcohol syndrome among three distinct samples of women before, during, and after pregnancy: The risk is relative. *American Journal of Medical Genetics Part C: Seminars in Medical Genetics, 127C*(1), 10–20.
150. Day, N. L., & Richardson, G. A. (2004). An analysis of the effects of prenatal alcohol exposure on growth: A teratologic model. *American Journal of Medical Genetics Part C: Seminars in Medical Genetics, 127C*(1), 28–34; Korkman, M., Kettunen, S., & Autti-Rämö, I. (2003). Neurocognitive impairment in early adolescence following prenatal alcohol exposure of varying duration. *Child Neuropsychology, 9*(2), 117–128; May, P. A., Gossage, J. P., White-Country, M., Goodhart, K., Decoteau, S., Trujillo, P. M., et al. (2004).
151. Korkman, M., Kettunen, S., & Autti-Rämö, I. (2003).
152. Thomas, J. D., Leany, B. D., & Riley, E. P. (2003). Differential vulnerability to motor deficits in second replicate HAS and LAS rats following neonatal alcohol exposure. *Pharmacology, Biochemistry and Behavior, 75*(1), 17–24.
153. Baer, J. S., Sampson, P. D., Barr, H. M., Connor, P. D., & Streissguth, A. P. (2003). A 21-year longitudinal analysis of the effects of prenatal alcohol exposure on young adult drinking. *Archives of General Psychiatry, 60*(4), 377–385; Day, N. L., Leech, S. L., Richardson, G. A., Cornelius, M. D., Robles, N., & Larkby, C. (2002). Prenatal alcohol exposure predicts continued deficits in offspring size at 14 years of age. *Alcoholism: Clinical and Experimental Research, 26*(10), 1584–1591; Martínez-Frías, M. L., Bermejo, E., Rodríquez-Pinilla, E., & Frías, J. L. (2004). Risk for congenital anomalies associated with different sporadic and daily doses of alcohol consumption during pregnancy: A case-control study. *Birth Defects Research (Part A): Clinical and Molecular Teratology, 70*(4), 194–200.
154. Centers for Disease Control and Prevention. (2002). *Fetal alcohol syndrome: Frequently asked questions.* www.cdc.gov (accessed September 30, 2002); May, P. A., Gossage, J. P., White-Country, M., Goodhart, K., Decoteau, S., Trujillo, P. M., et al. (2004).
155. Streissguth, A. P., Barr, H. M., & Sampson, P. D. (1990); Young, N. K. (1997).
156. Centers for Disease Control and Prevention. (2002). *Fetal alcohol syndrome.*
157. May, P. A., Gossage, J. P., White-Country, M., Goodhart, K., Decoteau, S., Trujillo, P. M., et al. (2004).
158. Ikonomidou, C., Bittigau, P., Ishimaru, M. J., Wozniak, D. F., Koch, C., Genz, K., et al. (2000). Ethanol-induced apoptotic neurodegeneration and fetal alcohol syndrome. *Science, 287*(5455), 1056–1060.
159. Olney, J. W. (2004). Perinatal drug/alcohol exposure and neuronal suicide: Public health implications. Paper presented at the 2004 Annual Meeting of the American Association for the Advancement of Science. Seattle, WA: American Association for the Advancement of Science.

160. Mennella, J. (2001). Alcohol's effect on lactation. *Alcohol Health and Research World, 25*(3), 230–234.
161. Koletzko, B., & Lehner, F. (2000). Beer and breastfeeding. *Advances in Experimental Medicine and Biology, 478*, 23–28.
162. Mennella, J. A., Pepino, M. Y., & Teff, K. L. (2005). Acute alcohol consumption disrupts the hormonal milieu of lactating women. *Journal of Clinical Endocrinology and Metabolism, 90*(4), 1979–1985.
163. Mennella, J. A., & Garrish, C. J. (1998). Effects of exposure to alcohol in mother's milk on infant sleep. *Pediatrics, 101*(5), E2.
164. Mennella, J. (2001).
165. Little, R. E., Anderson, E. W., Ervin, C. H., Worthington-Roberts, B., & Clarren, S. K. (1989). Maternal alcohol use during breast-feeding and infant mental and motor development at one year. *New England Journal of Medicine, 321*(7), 425–430.
166. Little, R. E., Northstone, K., & Golding, J. (2002). Alcohol, breastfeeding, and development at 18 months. *Pediatrics, 109*(5), e72.
167. Mennella, J. (2001).
168. American Academy of Pediatrics. (2004). *A woman's guide to breastfeeding*. www.aap.org (accessed January 26, 2004).
169. American Medical Association. (2003). *Fact sheet: Effects of alcohol on brains of adolescents*. www.ama-assn.org (accessed March 4, 2004); Bonnie, R. J., & O'Connell, M. E. (Eds.). (2004). *Reducing underage drinking: A collective responsibility*. Washington, DC: National Academy Press.
170. Young, N. K. (1997).
171. Briggs, G. G. (2003). Stimulants, narcotics, hallucinogens. *Ob.Gyn.News, 38*(11), 16–17.
172. Parker, S., Zuckerman, B., Bauchner, H., Frank, D., Vinci, R., & Cabral, H. (1990). Jitteriness in full-term neonates: Prevalence and correlates. *Pediatrics, 85*(1), 17–23.
173. Brady, J. P., Posner, M., Lang, C., & Rosati, M. J. (1994); Ness, R. B., Grisso, J. A., Hirschinger, N., Marcovic, N., Shaw, L. M., Day, N. L., et al. (1999). Cocaine and tobacco use and the risk of spontaneous abortion. *New England Journal of Medicine, 340*(5), 333–339; Richardson, G. A., Hamel, S. C., Goldschmidt, L., & Day, N. L. (1999). Growth of infants prenatally exposed to cocaine/crack: Comparison of a prenatal care and a no prenatal care sample. *Pediatrics, 104*(2), e18.
174. March of Dimes. (2002). *Cocaine use during pregnancy*. www.marchofdimes.com (accessed March 4, 2004); National Institutes of Health. (2002). *Significant deficits in mental skills observed in toddlers exposed to cocaine before birth* [Press release]. www.nih.gov (accessed March 4, 2004).
175. Keller, R. W., & Snyder-Keller, A. (2000). Prenatal cocaine exposure. *Annals of the New York Academy of Sciences, 909*, 217–232; Sherer, D. M., Anyaegbunam, A., & Onyeije, C. (1998). Antepartum fetal intracranial hemorrhage, predisposing factors and prenatal sonography: A review. *American Journal of Perinatology, 15*(7), 431–441.
176. Deren, S. (1986). Children of substance abusers: A review of the literature. *Journal of Sub-*

stance Abuse Treatment, 3(2), 77–94; Potter, S. M., Zelazo, P. R., Stack, D. M., & Papageorgiou, A. N. (2000). Adverse effects of fetal cocaine exposure on neonatal auditory information processing. *Pediatrics, 105*(3), e40; Swanson, M. W., Streissguth, A. P., Sampson, P. D., & Carmichael Olson, H. (1999). Prenatal cocaine and neuromotor outcome at four months: Effect of duration of exposure. *Journal of Developmental and Behavioral Pediatrics, 20*(5), 325–334.

177. Morrow, B. A., Elsworth, J. D., & Roth, R. H. (2002). Male rats exposed to cocaine in utero demonstrate elevated expression of Fos in the prefrontal cortex in response to environment. *Neuropsychopharmacology, 26*(3), 275–285; Morrow, B. A., Elsworth, J. D., & Roth, R. H. (2002). Prenatal cocaine exposure disrupts non-spatial, short-term memory in adolescent and adult male rats. *Behavioural Brain Research, 129*(1–2), 217–223.
178. CASA. (1996).
179. Chavkin, W. (2001). Cocaine and pregnancy: Time to look at the evidence. *JAMA, 285*(12), 1626–1628.
180. Vidaeff, A. C., & Mastrobattista, J. M. (2003). In utero cocaine exposure: A thorny mix of science and mythology. *American Journal of Perinatology, 20*(4), 165–172.
181. Brady, J. P., Posner, M., Lang, C., & Rosati, M. J. (1994); Young, N. K. (1997).
182. Ibid.
183. Kaltenbach, K., Berghella, V., & Finnegan, L. (1998). Opioid dependence during pregnancy: Effects and management. *Substance Abuse in Pregnancy, 25*(1), 139–151; Kaltenbach, K. A., & Finnegan, L. P. (1989). Prenatal narcotic exposure: Perinatal and developmental effects. *NeuroToxicology, 10*(3), 597–604.
184. Kaltenbach, K. A., & Finnegan, L. P. (1989).
185. Kaltenbach, K., Berghella, V., & Finnegan, L. (1998); Kaltenbach, K. A., & Finnegan, L. P. (1989).
186. Chiriboga, C. A. (2003). Fetal alcohol and drug effects. *Neurologist, 9*(6), 267–279.
187. Briggs, G. G. (2003); McElhatton, P. R., Bateman, D. N., Evans, C., Pughe, K. R., & Thomas, S. H. (1999). Congenital anomalies after prenatal ecstasy exposure. *Lancet, 354*(9188), 1441–1442.
188. Briggs, G. G. (2003).
189. World Health Organization. (2000). *Mother-to-child transmission of HIV (MTCT)*. www.who.int (accessed November 1, 2004).
190. Centers for Disease Control and Prevention. (2001). Revised recommendations for HIV screening of pregnant women: Perinatal counseling and guidelines consultation. *Morbidity and Mortality Weekly Report: Recommendations and Reports, 50*(RR19), 59–86.
191. Ibid.
192. Ibid.
193. Ibid.
194. Murphy, S., & Rosenbaum, M. (1999). *Pregnant women on drugs: Combating stereotypes and stigma*. New Brunswick, NJ: Rutgers University Press; Oaks, L. (2001). *Smoking and pregnancy: The politics of fetal protection*. New Brunswick, NJ: Rutgers University Press.

195. Murphy, S., & Rosenbaum, M. (1999).

196. Bolnick, J. M., & Rayburn, W. F. (2003). Substance use disorders in women: Special considerations during pregnancy. *Obstetrics and Gynecology Clinics of North America, 30*(3), 545–558.

197. Murphy, S., & Rosenbaum, M. (1999).

198. Ebrahim, S. H., Floyd, R. L., Merritt, R. K., Decoufle, P., & Holtzman, D. (2000). Trends in pregnancy-related smoking rates in the United States, 1987–1996. *JAMA, 283*(3), 361–366.

199. Office of the Surgeon General. (2001).

200. Ershoff, D. H., Solomon, L. J., & Dolan-Mullen, P. (2000). Predictors of intentions to stop smoking early in prenatal care. *Tobacco Control, 9*(Suppl. 3), iii41–iii45.

201. DiClemente, C. C., Dolan-Mullen, P., & Windsor, R. A. (2000). The process of pregnancy smoking cessation: Implications for interventions. *Tobacco Control, 9*(Suppl. 3), iii16–iii21.

202. DiClemente, C. C., Dolan-Mullen, P., & Windsor, R. A. (2000); Mullen, P. D., Richardson, M. A., Quinn, V. P., & Ershoff, D. H. (1997). Postpartum return to smoking: Who is at risk and when. *American Journal of Health Promotion, 11*(5), 323–330.

203. Ershoff, D. H., Solomon, L. J., & Dolan-Mullen, P. (2000).

204. National Cancer Institute, & California Environmental Protection Agency. (1999). *Health effects of exposure to environmental tobacco smoke: The report of the California Environmental Protection Agency* (NIH Pub. No. 99-4645). Bethesda, MD: U.S. Department of Health and Human Services, Public Health Service, National Institutes of Health, National Cancer Institute.

205. Centers for Disease Control and Prevention. (1997). *Smoking and pregnancy* [Fact sheet]. Atlanta, GA: Centers for Disease Control and Prevention, Office of Smoking and Health, Division of Media Relations.

206. Lindley, A. A., Becker, S., Gray, R. H., & Herman, A. A. (2000). Effect of continuing or stopping smoking during pregnancy on infant birth weight, crown-heel length, head circumference, ponderal index, and brain:body weight ratio. *American Journal of Epidemiology, 152*(3), 219–225.

207. Association of Maternal and Child Health Programs. (1999). *Smoking cessation makes cents: The cost-effectiveness of tobacco interventions* [Fact sheet]. www.amchp.org (accessed February 9, 2004).

208. Moran, S., Thorndike, A. N., Armstrong, K., & Rigotti, N. A. (2003). Physicians' missed opportunities to address tobacco use during prenatal care. *Nicotine and Tobacco Research, 5*(3), 363–368.

209. National Association for Children of Alcoholics, & National Clearinghouse for Alcohol and Drug Information. (2002).

210. Haller, D. L., Miles, D. R., & Dawson, K. S. (2003). Factors influencing treatment enrollment by pregnant substance abusers. *American Journal of Drug and Alcohol Abuse, 29*(1), 117–131.

211. Center for Substance Abuse Treatment. (2001). *Benefits of residential substance abuse treatment for pregnant and parenting women: Highlights from a study of 50 demonstration programs of the Center for Substance Abuse Treatment.* www.samhsa.gov (accessed February 11, 2004).

212. Office of the Surgeon General. (2001).
213. Van't Hof, S. M., Wall, M. A., Dowler, D. W., & Stark, M. J. (2000). Randomised controlled trial of a postpartum relapse prevention intervention. *Tobacco Control, 9*(Suppl. 3), III64–III66.
214. Office of the Surgeon General. (2001).
215. Hymowitz, N., Schwab, M., McNerny, C., Schwab, J., Eckholdt, H., & Haddock, K. (2003). Postpartum relapse to cigarette smoking in inner city women. *Journal of the National Medical Association, 95*(6), 461–474; Perkins, K. A. (2001). Smoking cessation in women: Special considerations. *CNS Drugs, 15*(5), 391–411.
216. The National Center on Addiction and Substance Abuse (CASA) at Columbia University. (2003). *Food for thought: Substance abuse and eating disorders.* New York: CASA.
217. McBride, C. M., & Pirie, P. L. (1990). Postpartum smoking relapse. *Addictive Behaviors, 15*(2), 165–168.
218. O'Campo, P., Faden, R. R., Brown, H., & Gielen, A. C. (1992). The impact of pregnancy on women's prenatal and postpartum smoking behavior. *American Journal of Preventive Medicine, 8*(1), 8–13.
219. Bolnick, J. M., & Rayburn, W. F. (2003); Dailard, C., & Nash, E. (2000). State responses to substance abuse among pregnant women. *Guttmacher Report on Public Policy, 3*(6), 3–6; Jos, P. H., Perlmutter, M., & Marshall, M. F. (2003).
220. Dailard, C., & Nash, E. (2000).
221. Alan Guttmacher Institute. (2004). *State policies in brief: Substance abuse during pregnancy.* www.guttmacher.org (accessed March 4, 2004).
222. Hankin, J., McCaul, M. E., & Heussner, J. (2000). Pregnant, alcohol-abusing women. *Alcoholism: Clinical and Experimental Research, 24*(8), 1276–1286.
223. Dailard, C., & Nash, E. (2000); Marshall, M. F., Menikoff, J., & Paltrow, L. M. (2003). Perinatal substance abuse and human subjects research: Are privacy protections adequate? *Mental Retardation and Developmental Disabilities Research Reviews, 9*(1), 54–59.
224. Alan Guttmacher Institute. (2004).
225. Marshall, M. F., Menikoff, J., & Paltrow, L. M. (2003).
226. Alan Guttmacher Institute. (2004).
227. Jos, P. H., Perlmutter, M., & Marshall, M. F. (2003).
228. The National Center on Addiction and Substance Abuse (CASA) at Columbia University. (2003). *Shoveling up: The impact of substance abuse on state budgets.* Washington, DC: CASA.
229. Eckenwiler, L. (2004). Why not retribution? The particularized imagination and justice for pregnant addicts. *Journal of Law, Medicine and Ethics, 32*(1), 89–99; Roberts, L. W., & Dunn, L. B. (2003).
230. Jos, P. H., Perlmutter, M., & Marshall, M. F. (2003).
231. Dailard, C., & Nash, E. (2000).
232. Jos, P. H., Perlmutter, M., & Marshall, M. F. (2003).
233. Thompson, M. P., & Kingree, J. B. (1998).
234. Roberts, L. W., & Dunn, L. B. (2003).

235. NARAL Foundation. (2001). *Limitations on the rights of pregnant women.* www.naral.org.nal (accessed October 4, 2004).

Chapter 6. Getting Over the Influence

Epigraph: National Clearinghouse for Alcohol and Drug Information. (1995). *Making the link: Alcohol, tobacco, and other drugs and pregnancy and parenthood.* www.health.org (accessed October 12, 2002).

1. Substance Abuse and Mental Health Services Administration, Office of Applied Studies. (2002). *Treatment Episode Data Set (TEDS) 1992–2000: National admissions to substance abuse treatment services* (DHHS Pub. No. [SMA] 02-3727). Rockville, MD: U.S. Department of Health and Human Services.
2. Office of the Surgeon General. (2001). *Women and smoking: A report of the Surgeon General* (GPO Item No. 0483-L-06). Washington, DC: U.S. Government Printing Office.
3. The National Center on Addiction and Substance Abuse (CASA) at Columbia University. (2005). *CASA's analysis of the National Survey on Drug Use and Health (NSDUH), 2003* [Data file]. Rockville, MD: U.S. Department of Health and Human Services, Substance Abuse and Mental Health Services Administration.
4. Substance Abuse and Mental Health Services Administration, Office of Applied Studies. (2001). *Women in substance abuse treatment: The DASIS report.* Rockville, MD: U.S. Department of Health and Human Services.
5. CASA. (2005). *CASA's analysis of NSDUH 2003.*
6. Substance Abuse and Mental Health Services Administration, Office of Applied Studies. (2003). *National Survey of Substance Abuse Treatment Services (N-SSATS): 2002: Data on substance abuse treatment facilities* (DHHS Pub. No. [SMA] 03-3777). Rockville, MD: U.S. Department of Health and Human Services.
7. Kandall, S. R. (1998). The history of drug abuse and women in the United States. In C. L. Wetherington & A. B. Roman (Eds.), *Drug addiction research and the health of women: Executive summary* (NIH Pub. No. 98-4289, pp. 8–16). Rockville, MD: U.S. Department of Health and Human Services, National Institutes of Health, National Institute on Drug Abuse.
8. Ibid.; National Institute on Drug Abuse. (2002). *Overview of NIDA research on women's health and gender differences.* www.drugabuse.gov (accessed March 17, 2002).
9. Lynch, W. J., Roth, M. E., & Carroll, M. E. (2002). Biological basis of sex differences in drug abuse: Preclinical and clinical studies. *Psychopharmacology, 164*(2), 121–137.
10. The National Center on Addiction and Substance Abuse (CASA) at Columbia University. (2003). *The formative years: Pathways to substance abuse among girls and young women ages 8–22.* New York: CASA.
11. CASA. (2005). *CASA's analysis of NSDUH 2003.*
12. Substance Abuse and Mental Health Services Administration, Office of Applied Studies. (2001). *Coerced treatment among youths: 1993 to 1998: The DASIS report.* www.samhsa.gov (accessed 2002).

13. Ibid.; Substance Abuse and Mental Health Services Administration, Office of Applied Studies. (2002). *Treatment Episode Data Set.*
14. The National Center on Addiction and Substance Abuse (CASA) at Columbia University. (2004). *Criminal neglect: Substance abuse, juvenile justice and the children left behind.* New York: CASA.
15. Shillington, A. M., & Clapp, J. D. (2003). Adolescents in public substance abuse treatment programs: The impacts of sex and race on referrals and outcomes. *Journal of Child and Adolescent Substance Abuse, 12*(4), 69–91.
16. Substance Abuse and Mental Health Services Administration, Office of Applied Studies. (2001). *Coerced treatment;* Substance Abuse and Mental Health Services Administration, Office of Applied Studies. (2002). *Treatment Episode Data Set.*
17. Rounds-Bryant, J. L., Kristiansen, P. L., Fairbank, J. A., & Hubbard, R. L. (1998). Substance use, mental disorders, abuse, and crime: Gender comparisons among a national sample of adolescent drug treatment clients. *Journal of Child and Adolescent Substance Abuse, 7*(4), 19–34.
18. Harrison, P. A., Hoffman, N. G., & Edwall, G. E. (1989). Differential drug use patterns among sexually abused adolescent girls in treatment for chemical dependency. *International Journal of the Addictions, 24*(6), 499–514.
19. Substance Abuse and Mental Health Services Administration, Office of Applied Studies. (2001). *How men and women enter substance abuse treatment: The DASIS report.* Rockville, MD: U.S. Department of Health and Human Services, Substance Abuse and Mental Health Services Administration, Office of Applied Studies.
20. Substance Abuse and Mental Health Services Administration, Office of Applied Studies. (2001). *Women.*
21. Wechsberg, W. M., Craddock, S. G., & Hubbard, R. L. (1998). How are women who enter substance abuse treatment different than men? A gender comparison from the Drug Abuse Treatment Outcome Study (DATOS). *Drugs and Society, 13*(1–2), 97–115.
22. National Institute on Drug Abuse. (2000). Gender differences in drug abuse risks and treatment. *NIDA Notes, 15*(4), 6–7.
23. Substance Abuse and Mental Health Services Administration, Office of Applied Studies. (2001). *Women.*
24. The National Center on Addiction and Substance Abuse (CASA) at Columbia University. (2005). *CASA's analysis of the Treatment Episode Data Set (TEDS), 2002* [Data file]. Rockville, MD: U.S. Department of Health and Human Services, Substance Abuse and Mental Health Services Administration.
25. Hanson, G. R. (2002). In drug abuse, gender matters. *NIDA Notes, 17*(2).
26. Fiorentine, R., Anglin, M. D., Gil-Rivas, V., & Taylor, E. (1997). Drug treatment: Explaining the gender paradox. *Substance Use and Misuse, 32*(6), 653–678.
27. Lynch, W. J., Roth, M. E., & Carroll, M. E. (2002).
28. Substance Abuse and Mental Health Services Administration, Office of Applied Studies. (2002). *Pregnant women in substance abuse treatment: The DASIS report.* Rockville, MD: U.S. Department of Health and Human Services, Substance Abuse and Mental Health Services Administration, Office of Applied Studies.

29. Ibid.
30. Haller, D. L., Miles, D. R., & Dawson, K. S. (2003). Factors influencing treatment enrollment by pregnant substance abusers. *American Journal of Drug and Alcohol Abuse, 29*(1), 117–131.
31. The National Center on Addiction and Substance Abuse (CASA) at Columbia University. (1998). *Under the rug: Substance abuse and the mature woman.* New York: CASA.
32. Substance Abuse and Mental Health Services Administration, Office of Applied Studies. (2001). *Older adults in substance abuse treatment: The DASIS report.* www.samhsa.gov (accessed March 23, 2004).
33. Ibid.
34. White, W. L. (1998). *Slaying the dragon: The history of addiction treatment and recovery in America.* Bloomington, IL: Chestnut Health Systems/Lighthouse Institute.
35. Kandall, S. R. (1996). *Substance and shadow: Women and addiction in the United States.* Cambridge, MA: Harvard University Press.
36. Ibid.
37. White, W. L. (1998).
38. Straussner, S. L. A., & Attia, P. R. (2002). Women's addiction and treatment through a historical lens. In S. L. A. Straussner & S. Brown (Eds.), *The handbook of addiction treatment for women* (pp. 3–25). San Francisco: Jossey-Bass.
39. White, W. L. (1998).
40. Kandall, S. R. (1996).
41. White, W. L. (1998); Morgan, H. W. (1981). *Drugs in America: A social history, 1800–1980.* Syracuse, NY: Syracuse University Press; Caron, J. (2002). *Keeley Institute: Fargo, ND.* www.fargohistory.com (accessed March 24, 2004).
42. White, W. L. (1998).
43. Edwards, G. (2003). *Alcohol: The world's favorite drug.* New York: Thomas Dunne Books.
44. Kandall, S. R. (1996).
45. Kandall, S. R. (1998). Women and addiction in the United States: 1850 to 1920. In C. L. Wetherington & A. B. Roman (Eds.), *Drug addiction research and the health of women* (NIH Pub. No. 98-4290, pp. 33–52). Rockville, MD: U.S. Department of Health and Human Services, National Institutes of Health, National Institute on Drug Abuse.
46. Kandall, S. R. (1996).
47. Ibid.
48. Ibid.
49. Ibid.
50. Ibid.
51. Ibid.; White, W. L. (2003). The history of "medicinal specifics" as addiction cures in the United States. *Addiction, 98*(3), 261–267.
52. Kandall, S. R. (1996).
53. Ibid.
54. Ibid.

55. The National Center on Addiction and Substance Abuse (CASA) at Columbia University. (2000). *Missed opportunity: National survey of primary care physicians and patients on substance abuse.* New York: CASA.
56. Koenig, H. G., George, L. K., & Meador, K. G. (1997). Use of antidepressants by nonpsychiatrists in the treatment of medically ill hospitalized depressed elderly patients. *American Journal of Psychiatry, 154*(10), 1369–1375; Pincus, H. A., Tanielian, T. L., Marcus, S. C., Olfson, M., Zarin, D. A., Thompson, J., et al. (1998). Prescribing trends in psychotropic medications: Primary care, psychiatry, and other medical specialties. *JAMA, 279*(7), 526–531.
57. Sarigiani, P. A., Ryan, L., & Petersen, A. C. (1999). Prevention of high-risk behaviors in adolescent women. *Journal of Adolescent Health, 25*(2), 109–119.
58. Most doctors don't counsel teens about smoking. (1999). *Alcoholism and Drug Abuse Weekly, 11*(44), 8.
59. Sarigiani, P. A., Ryan, L., & Petersen, A. C. (1999).
60. Ellen, J. M., Franzgrote, M., Irwin, C. E., & Millstein, S. G. (1998). Primary care physicians' screening of adolescent patients: A survey of California physicians. *Journal of Adolescent Health, 22*(6), 433–438.
61. CASA. (2000).
62. CASA. (1998).
63. Hallfors, D., & Van Dorn, R. A. (2002). Strengthening the role of two key institutions in the prevention of adolescent substance abuse. *Journal of Adolescent Health, 30*(1), 17–28.
64. CASA. (2003). *The formative years.*
65. CASA. (1998).
66. Trachtenberg, A. I., & Fleming, M. F. (1994). *Diagnosis and treatment of drug abuse in family practice.* Kansas City, MS: American Academy of Family Physicians.
67. Stewart, D., Gossop, M., Marsden, J., Kidd, T., & Treacy, S. (2003). Similarities in outcomes for men and women after drug misuse treatment: Results from the National Treatment Outcome Research Study (NTORS). *Drug and Alcohol Review, 22*(1), 35–41.
68. Ashley, O. S., Marsden, M. E., & Brady, T. M. (2003). Effectiveness of substance abuse treatment programming for women: A review. *American Journal of Drug and Alcohol Abuse, 29*(1), 19–53.
69. Wechsberg, W. M., Craddock, S. G., & Hubbard, R. L. (1998).
70. Comfort, M., Sockloff, A., Loverro, J., & Kaltenbach, K. (2003). Multiple predictors of substance-abusing women's treatment and life outcomes: A prospective longitudinal study. *Addictive Behaviors, 28*(2), 199–224.
71. Simpson, T. L. (2002). Women's treatment utilization and its relationship to childhood sexual abuse history and lifetime PTSD. *Substance Abuse, 23*(1), 17–30.
72. Jessup, M. A., Humphreys, J. C., Brindis, C. D., & Lee, K. A. (2003). Extrinsic barriers to substance abuse treatment among pregnant drug dependent women. *Journal of Drug Issues, 33*(2), 285–304.
73. The National Center on Addiction and Substance Abuse (CASA) at Columbia University. (2004). *CASA's analysis of the Drug Evaluation Network System (DENS).* [Data file]. www.tre-

search.org/tx_systems/dcns.htm (accessed January 2, 2004); Carise, D., McLellan, A. T., Gifford, L., & Kleber, H. D. (1999). Developing a national addiction treatment information system: An introduction to the Drug Evaluation Network System. *Journal of Substance Abuse Treatment, 17*(1–2), 67–77.

74. CASA. (1998).
75. Substance Abuse and Mental Health Services Administration, Office of Applied Studies. (2002). *Facilities offering special programs or services for women.* Rockville, MD: U.S. Department of Health and Human Services, Substance Abuse and Mental Health Services Administration, Office of Applied Studies.
76. CASA. (2005). *CASA's analysis of NSDUH 2003.*
77. Centers for Disease Control and Prevention. (2002). Cigarette smoking among adults: United States, 2000. *Morbidity and Mortality Weekly Report, 51*(29), 642–645.
78. Gillespie, M. (1999). *Majority of smokers want to quit, consider themselves addicted.* www.gallup.com (accessed January 29, 2002).
79. Centers for Disease Control and Prevention, Grunbaum, J. A., Kann, L., Kinchen, S. A., Williams, B., Ross, J. G., et al. (2002). Youth risk behavior surveillance: United States, 2001. *Morbidity and Mortality Weekly Report: Surveillance Summaries, 51*(SS-4).
80. Office of the Surgeon General. (2001).
81. Ibid.; Perkins, K. A. (2001). Smoking cessation in women: Special considerations. *CNS Drugs, 15*(5), 391–411.
82. Centers for Disease Control and Prevention. (2002).
83. Sarna, L., & Bialous, S. A. (2004). Why tobacco is a women's health issue. *Nursing Clinics of North America, 39*(Pt. 1), 165–180.
84. Samet, J. M., & Yoon, S.-Y. (Eds.). (2001). *Women and the tobacco epidemic: Challenges for the 21st century.* Geneva, Switzerland: World Health Organization, Johns Hopkins School of Health, Institute for Global Tobacco Control.
85. Perkins, K. A. (2001).
86. Office of the Surgeon General. (2001).
87. Perkins, K. A. (1995). Individual variability in responses to nicotine. *Behavior Genetics, 25*(2), 119–132.
88. Office of the Surgeon General. (2001).
89. Taylor, D. H., Hasselblad, V., Henley, S. J., Thun, M. J., & Sloan, F. A. (2002). Benefits of smoking cessation for longevity. *American Journal of Public Health, 92*(6), 990–996.
90. Rich-Edwards, J. W., Manson, J. E., Hennekens, C. H., & Buring, J. E. (1995). The primary prevention of coronary heart disease in women. *New England Journal of Medicine, 332*(26), 1758–1766; Willett, W. C., Green, A., Stampfer, M. J., Speizer, F. E., Colditz, G. A., Rosner, B., et al. (1987). Relative and absolute excess risks of coronary heart disease among women who smoke cigarettes. *New England Journal of Medicine, 317*(21), 1303–1309.
91. Hermanson, B., Omenn, G. S., Kronmal, R. A., & Gersh, B. J. (1988). Beneficial six-year outcome of smoking cessation in older men and women with coronary artery disease. *New England Journal of Medicine, 319*(21), 1365–1369; LaCroix, A. Z., Lang, J., Scherr, P., Wallace,

R. B., Cornoni-Huntley, J., Berkman, L., et al. (1991). Smoking and mortality among older men and women in three communities. *New England Journal of Medicine, 324*(23), 1619–1625; Office of the Surgeon General. (1990). *Health benefits of smoking cessation: A report of the Surgeon General 1990* (GPO Item No. 483-L–6). Washington, DC: U.S. Government Printing Office; Vogt, M. T., Cauley, J. A., Scott, J. C., Kuller, L. H., & Browner, W. S. (1996). Smoking and mortality among older women. *Archives of Internal Medicine, 156*(6), 630–636.

92. Office of the Surgeon General. (2001).
93. Ibid.
94. Hunter, S. M. (2001). Quitting. In J. M. Samet & S.-Y. Yoon (Eds.), *Women and the tobacco epidemic: Challenges for the 21st century* (pp. 121–146). Geneva, Switzerland: World Health Organization.
95. Office of the Surgeon General. (2001).
96. Perkins, K. A., Marcus, M. D., Levine, M. D., D'Amico, D., Miller, A., Broge, M., et al. (2001). Cognitive-behavioral therapy to reduce weight concerns improves smoking cessation outcome in weight-concerned women. *Journal of Consulting and Clinical Psychology, 69*(4), 604–613.
97. Hall, S. M., Tunstall, C. D., Vila, K. L., & Duffy, J. (1992). Weight gain prevention and smoking cessation: Cautionary findings. *American Journal of Public Health, 82*(6), 799–803; Perkins, K. A. (2001).
98. Hunter, S. M. (2001); Perkins, K. A. (2001); Perkins, K. A., Marcus, M. D., Levine, M. D., D'Amico, D., Miller, A., Broge, M., et al. (2001).
99. Fiore, M. C., Bailey, W. C., Cohen, S. J., Dorfman, S. F., Goldstein, M. G., Gritz, E. R., et al. (2000). *Treating tobacco use and dependence: Clinical practice guideline* (GPO Item No. 0491-B–17). Washington, DC: U.S. Government Printing Office.
100. Sarna, L., & Bialous, S. A. (2004).
101. CASA. (2003). *The formative years.*
102. National Institute on Drug Abuse. (2001). *Quitting smoking harder for women than for men: Review of research finds variety of reasons for why it is harder for women to break free of nicotine addiction* [Press release]. http://165.112.78.61 (accessed June 13, 2001).
103. Office of the Surgeon General. (2001).
104. Fiore, M. C., Bailey, W. C., Cohen, S. J., Dorfman, S. F., Goldstein, M. G., Gritz, E. R., et al. (2000).
105. Slotkin, T. A. (1998). Fetal nicotine or cocaine exposure: Which one is worse? *Journal of Pharmacology and Experimental Therapeutics, 285*(3), 931–945.
106. Dunner, D. L., Zisook, S., Billow, A. A., Batey, S. R., Johnston, A., & Ascher, J. A. (1998). A prospective safety surveillance study for bupropion sustained-release in the treatment of depression. *Journal of Clinical Psychiatry, 59*(7), 366–373.
107. U.S. Public Health Service. (2000). *Treating tobacco use and dependence: Summary.* www.surgeongeneral.gov/tobacco/smokesum.htm (accessed April 21, 2005).
108. National Institute on Drug Abuse. (1999). *Principles of drug addiction treatment: A research based guide* (NIH Pub. No. 99-4180). Rockville, MD: U.S. Department of Health and Human Services, National Institutes of Health, National Institute on Drug Abuse.

109. Ashley, O. S., Marsden, M. E., & Brady, T. M. (2003).

110. Copeland, J., & Hall, W. (1992). A comparison of women seeking drug and alcohol treatment in a specialist women's and two traditional mixed-sex treatment services. *British Journal of Addiction, 87*(9), 1293–1302, 1361, 1365.

111. Howell, E. M., Heiser, N., & Harrington, M. (1999). A review of recent findings on substance abuse treatment for pregnant women. *Journal of Substance Abuse Treatment, 16*(3), 195–219.

112. Ibid.; Roberts, L. W., & Dunn, L. B. (2003). Ethical considerations in caring for women with substance use disorders. *Obstetrics and Gynecology Clinics of North America, 30*(3), 559–582.

113. Substance Abuse and Mental Health Services Administration, Office of Applied Studies. (2000). *Uniform Facility Data Set (UFDS) 1998: Data on substance abuse treatment facilities* (DHHS Pub. No. [SMA] 99-3463). Rockville, MD: U.S. Department of Health and Human Services.

114. Ashley, O. S., Marsden, M. E., & Brady, T. M. (2003).

115. Bride, B. E. (2001). Single-gender treatment of substance abuse: Effect on treatment retention and completion. *Social Work Research, 25*(4), 223–231; Kandall, S. R. (1998).

116. Guthrie, B. J., Rotheram, M. J., Genero, N., Amaro, H., Chesney-Lind, M., Flinchbaugh, L. J., et al. (2001). *A guide to understanding female adolescents' substance abuse: Gender and ethnic considerations for prevention and treatment policy* (DHHS Pub. No. [SMA] 00-3309). Rockville, MD: U.S. Department of Health and Human Services, Substance Abuse and Mental Health Services Administration, Center for Substance Abuse Prevention; National Institute on Drug Abuse. (2002). *Advances in research on women's health and gender differences.* www.drugabuse.gov (accessed March 15, 2002).

117. Ellis, R. A., O'Hara, M., & Sowers, K. M. (2000). Profile-based intervention: Developing gender-sensitive treatment for adolescent substance abusers. *Research on Social Work Practice, 10*(3), 327–347.

118. Center for Substance Abuse Treatment. (2000). *Substance abuse in brief: Successful treatment for adolescents: Multiple needs require diverse and special services* [Pamphlet]. Rockville, MD: U.S. Department of Health and Human Services, Substance Abuse and Mental Health Services Administration.

119. CASA. (2003). *The formative years.*

120. Schultz, S. K., Arndt, S., & Liesveld, J. (2003). Locations of facilities with special programs for older substance abuse clients in the US. *International Journal of Geriatric Psychiatry, 18*(9), 839–843.

121. Zimberg, S. (1984). Diagnosis and management of the elderly alcoholic. In R. M. Atkinson (Ed.), *Alcohol and drug abuse in old age* (pp. 23–34). Washington, DC: American Psychiatric Press.

122. Brennan, P. L., & Moos, R. H. (1996). Late-life drinking behavior: The influence of personal characteristics, life context and treatment. *Alcohol Health and Research World, 20*(3), 197–204; Kofoed, L. L., Tolson, R. L., Atkinson, R. M., Toth, R. L., & Turner, J. A. (1987). Treatment compliance of older alcoholics: An elder specific approach is superior to "mainstreaming."

Journal of Studies on Alcohol, 48(1), 47–51; Schonfeld, L., & Dupree, L. W. (1995). Treatment approaches for older problem drinkers. *International Journal of the Addictions, 30*(13–14), 1819–1842; Zimberg, S. (1984).

123. Blow, F. C. (1998). *Substance abuse among older adults: Treatment Improvement Protocol (TIP) Series 26* (DHHS Pub. No. [SMA] 98-3179). Rockville, MD: U.S. Department of Health and Human Services, Public Health Service, Substance Abuse and Mental Health Services Administration, Center for Substance Abuse Treatment.
124. Mitchell, J. L. (1995). *Pregnant, substance-using women: Treatment Improvement Protocol (TIP) Series 2* (DHHS Pub. no. [SMA] 95-3056). Rockville, MD: U.S. Department of Health and Human Services, Public Health Service, Substance Abuse and Mental Health Services Administration, Center for Substance Abuse Treatment.
125. Mitchell, J. L. (1995).
126. Kaltenbach, K., Berghella, V., & Finnegan, L. (1998). Opioid dependence during pregnancy: Effects and management. *Substance Abuse in Pregnancy, 25*(1), 139–151; Kaltenbach, K. A., & Finnegan, L. P. (1989). Prenatal narcotic exposure: Perinatal and developmental effects. *NeuroToxicology, 10*(3), 597–604; National Institute on Drug Abuse. (2000). *NIDA research report: Heroin abuse and addiction.* Bethesda, MD: U.S. Department of Health and Human Services, National Institutes of Health, National Institute on Drug Abuse.
127. Kaltenbach, K., Berghella, V., & Finnegan, L. (1998); Kaltenbach, K. A., & Finnegan, L. P. (1989).
128. Mitchell, J. L. (1995).
129. Clark, H. W. (2001). Residential substance abuse treatment for pregnant and postpartum women and their children: Treatment and policy implications. *Child Welfare, 80*(2), 179–198; Comfort, M., & Kaltenbach, K. A. (2000). Predictors of treatment outcomes for substance-abusing women: A retrospective study. *Substance Abuse, 21*(1), 33–45.
130. The National Center on Addiction and Substance Abuse (CASA) at Columbia University. (2003). *Shoveling up: The impact of substance abuse on state budgets.* New York: CASA.
131. Ibid.
132. National Women's Law Center, & Oregon Health and Science University. (2003). *Women and smoking: A national and state-by-state report card.* Washington, DC: National Women's Law Center, Oregon Health and Science University.

Chapter 7. Prevention and Policy Opportunities across the Life Span

1. The National Center on Addiction and Substance Abuse (CASA) at Columbia University. (2003). *The formative years: Pathways to substance abuse among girls and young women ages 8–22.* New York: CASA.
2. Simons-Morton, B. (2004). Prospective association of peer influence, school engagement, drinking expectancies, and parent expectations with drinking initiation among sixth graders. *Addictive Behaviors, 29*(2), 299–309.
3. CASA. (2003). *The formative years.*

4. Fleming, M. F., Barry, K. L., Manwell, L. B., Johnson, K., & London, R. (1997). Brief physician advice for problem alcohol drinkers: A randomized controlled trial in community-based primary care practices. *JAMA, 277*(13), 1039–1045.

5. Johnston, L. D., O'Malley, P. M., & Bachman, J. G. (2003). *Monitoring the Future: National survey results on drug use, 1975–2002: Volume 2, college students and adults ages 19–40* (NIH Pub. No. 03-5376). Bethesda, MD: U.S. Department of Health and Human Services, National Institutes of Health, National Institute on Drug Abuse.

6. CASA. (2003). *The formative years.*

7. Johnston, L. D., O'Malley, P. M., & Bachman, J. G. (2003).

8. Arnett, J. J. (2000). Emerging adulthood: A theory of development from the late teens through the twenties. *American Psychologist, 55*(5), 469–480.

9. U.S. Census Bureau, Population Division. (2003). *Marital status of people 15 years and over, by age, sex, personal earnings, race, and Hispanic origin: 1, March 2002.* www.census.gov (accessed March 18, 2004).

10. Arnett, J. J. (1998). Risk behavior and family role transitions during the twenties. *Journal of Youth and Adolescence, 27*(3), 301–320; Brook, J. S., Richter, L., Whiteman, M., & Cohen, P. (1999). Consequences of adolescent marijuana use: Incompatibility with the assumption of adult roles. *Genetic, Social, and General Psychology Monographs, 125*(2), 193–207.

11. The National Center on Addiction and Substance Abuse (CASA) at Columbia University. (1996). *Substance abuse and the American woman.* New York: CASA.

12. Schoenbaum, M. (1997). Do smokers understand the mortality effects of smoking? Evidence from the health and retirement survey. *American Journal of Public Health, 87*(5), 755–759.

13. Johnson, P. B., & Johnson, H. L. (2000). Reaffirming the power of parental influence on adolescent smoking and drinking decisions. *Adolescent and Family Health, 1*(1), 37–43; The National Center on Addiction and Substance Abuse (CASA) at Columbia University. (2001). *National survey of American attitudes on substance abuse VI: Teens.* New York: CASA.

14. CASA. (2003). *The formative years.*

15. CASA. (2001). *National survey.*

16. Partnership for a Drug-Free America. (2000). *Partnership Attitude Tracking Study 1999: Parents.* www.drugfreeamerica.org (accessed April 15, 2002).

17. CASA. (2003). *The formative years.*

18. Ibid.

19. The National Center on Addiction and Substance Abuse (CASA) at Columbia University. (2003). *National survey of American attitudes on substance abuse VIII: Teens and parents.* New York: CASA.

20. Brody, G. H., Flor, D. L., Hollet-Wright, N., McCoy, J. K., & Donovan, J. (1999). Parent-child relationships, child temperament profiles and children's alcohol use norms. *Journal of Studies on Alcohol, Suppl. 13,* 45–51.

21. Noller, P. (1995). Parent-adolescent relationships. In M. A. Fitzpatrick & A. L. Vangelisti (Eds.), *Explaining family interactions* (pp. 77–111). Thousand Oaks, CA: Sage.

22. Anderson, A. R., & Henry, C. S. (1994). Family system characteristics and parental behaviors as predictors of adolescent substance use. *Adolescence, 29*(114), 405–420; Wills, T. A., Vaccaro, D., & McNamara, G. (1992). The role of life events, family support, and competence in adolescent substance use: A test of vulnerability and protective factors. *American Journal of Community Psychology, 20*(3), 349–374.
23. The National Center on Addiction and Substance Abuse (CASA) at Columbia University. (2002). *CASA analysis of the National Household Survey on Drug Abuse (NHSDA), 1999* [Data file]. Rockville, MD: U.S. Department of Health and Human Services, Substance Abuse and Mental Health Services Administration.
24. Andrews, J. A., Hops, H., Ary, D., Tildesley, E., & Harris, J. (1993). Parental influence on early adolescent substance use: Specific and non-specific effects. *Journal of Early Adolescence, 13*(3), 285–310; Barnes, G. M., & Farrell, A. D. (1992). Parental support and control as predictors of adolescent drinking, delinquency, and related behavior problems. *Journal of Marriage and the Family, 54*(4), 763–776; Peterson, P. L., Hawkins, J. D., Abbott, R. D., & Catalano, R. F. (1994). Disentangling the effects of parental drinking, family management, and parental alcohol norms on current drinking by black and white adolescents. *Journal of Research on Adolescence, 4*(2), 203–227; CASA. (2003). *The formative years;* Andersen, M. R., Leroux, B. G., Marek, P. M., Peterson Jr., A. V., Kealey, K. A., Bricker, J., et al. (2002). Mothers' attitudes and concerns about their children smoking: Do they influence kids? *Preventive Medicine, 34*(2), 198–206; Sargent, J. D., & Dalton, M. (2001). Does parental disapproval of smoking prevent adolescents from becoming established smokers? *Pediatrics, 108*(6), 1256–1262.
25. The National Center on Addiction and Substance Abuse (CASA) at Columbia University. (2005). *CASA's analysis of the National Survey on Drug Use and Health (NSDUH), 2003* [Data file]. Rockville, MD: U.S. Department of Health and Human Services, Substance Abuse and Mental Health Services Administration.
26. CASA. (2003). *The formative years.*
27. Fletcher, A. C., & Jefferies, B. C. (1999). Parental mediators of associations between perceived authoritative parenting and early adolescent substance use. *Journal of Early Adolescence, 19*(4), 465–487.
28. Catalano, R. F., Morrison, D. M., Wells, E. A., Gillmore, M. R., Iritani, B., & Hawkins, J. D. (1992). Ethnic differences in family factors related to early drug initiation. *Journal of Studies on Alcohol, 53*(3), 208–217.
29. CASA. (2003). *The formative years.*
30. Richter, L., & Richter, D. M. (2001). Exposure to parental tobacco and alcohol use: Effects on children's health and development. *American Journal of Orthopsychiatry, 71*(2), 182–203.
31. Brody, G. H., Flor, D. L., Hollet-Wright, N., McCoy, J. K., & Donovan, J. (1999).
32. CASA. (2003). *National survey.*
33. Ibid.
34. The National Center on Addiction and Substance Abuse (CASA) at Columbia University. (2003). *The importance of family dinners.* New York: CASA.

35. Griffin, K. W., Botvin, G. J., Scheier, L. M., Diaz, T., & Miller, N. L. (2000). Parenting practices as predictors of substance use, delinquency, and aggression among urban minority youth: Moderating effects of family structure and gender. *Psychology of Addictive Behaviors, 14*(2), 174–184.
36. The National Center on Addiction and Substance Abuse (CASA) at Columbia University. (2003). *Food for thought: Substance abuse and eating disorders.* New York: CASA.
37. Turrisi, R., Jaccard, J., Taki, R., Dunnam, H., & Grimes, J. (2001). Examination of the short-term efficacy of a parent intervention to reduce college student drinking tendencies. *Psychology of Addictive Behaviors, 15*(4), 366–372.
38. The National Center on Addiction and Substance Abuse (CASA) at Columbia University. (2005). *Substance abuse, mental health and engaged learning: Summary of findings from CASA's focus groups and national survey.* New York: CASA.
39. Turrisi, R., Wiersma, K. A., & Hughes, K. K. (2000). Binge-drinking-related consequences in college students: Role of drinking beliefs and mother-teen communications. *Psychology of Addictive Behaviors, 14*(4), 342–355.
40. CASA. (2003). *The formative years.*
41. Gomberg, E. (1982). Alcohol use and problems among the elderly. In National Institute on Alcohol Abuse and Alcoholism (Ed.), *Special population issues: Alcohol and health monograph no. 4* (DHHS Pub. No. [ADM] 82-1193, pp. 263–290). Washington, DC: U.S. Government Printing Office.
42. Blake, S. M., Amaro, H., Schwartz, P., & Flinchbaugh, L. J. (2001). A review of substance abuse prevention interventions for young adolescent girls. *Journal of Early Adolescence, 21*(3), 294–324.
43. CASA. (2003). *The formative years.*
44. The National Center on Addiction and Substance Abuse (CASA) at Columbia University. (2001). *Malignant neglect: Substance abuse and America's schools.* New York: CASA.
45. Acoca, L. (1998). Outside/inside: The violation of American girls at home, on the streets, and in the juvenile justice system. *Crime and Delinquency, 44*(4), 561–589.
46. CASA. (2003). *The formative years.*
47. The National Center on Addiction and Substance Abuse (CASA) at Columbia University. (2003). *Depression, substance abuse and college student engagement: A review of the literature.* New York: CASA.
48. Task Force of the National Advisory Council on Alcohol Abuse and Alcoholism. (2002). *A call to action: Changing the culture of drinking at U.S. colleges* (NIH Pub. No. 03-5010). Bethesda, MD: U.S. Department of Health and Human Services, National Institutes of Health, National Institute on Alcohol Abuse and Alcoholism.
49. Task Force of the National Advisory Council on Alcohol Abuse and Alcoholism. (2002); The National Center on Addiction and Substance Abuse (CASA) at Columbia University. (2003). *Alcohol abuse on college campuses: A reconnaissance mission: Report to funders.* New York: CASA.
50. Fleming, M. F., Barry, K. L., Manwell, L. B., Johnson, K., & London, R. (1997).
51. The National Center on Addiction and Substance Abuse (CASA) at Columbia University.

(2000). *Missed opportunity: National survey of primary care physicians and patients on substance abuse.* New York: CASA.

52. CASA. (2003). *The formative years.*
53. Centers for Disease Control and Prevention, National Center for Health Statistics. (2001). *Healthy people 2000 final review: National health promotion and disease prevention objectives* (DHHS Pub. No. 01-0256). Hyattsville, MD: U.S. Department of Health and Human Services, Centers for Disease Control and Prevention, National Center for Health Statistics.
54. Hallfors, D., & Van Dorn, R. A. (2002). Strengthening the role of two key institutions in the prevention of adolescent substance abuse. *Journal of Adolescent Health, 30*(1), 17–28; Most doctors don't counsel teens about smoking. (1999). *Alcoholism and Drug Abuse Weekly, 11*(44), 8.
55. Hallfors, D., & Van Dorn, R. A. (2002).
56. Brener, N. D., McMahon, P. M., Warren, C. W., & Douglas, K. A. (1999). Forced sexual intercourse and associated health-risk behaviors among female college students in the United States. *Journal of Consulting and Clinical Psychology, 67*(2), 252–259.
57. CASA. (2003). *Depression.*
58. Bergen-Cico, D., Barretto, C., & Vermette, J. (2003). *The impact of alcohol and other drug policies on gender and referrals to substance abuse counseling.* Unpublished manuscript.
59. Abel, E. L. (1988). Fetal alcohol syndrome in families. *Neurotoxicology and Teratology, 10*(1), 1–2; Abel, E. L., & Sokol, R. J. (1987). Incidence of fetal alcohol syndrome and economic impact of FAS-related anomalies. *Drug and Alcohol Dependence, 19*(1), 51–70.
60. CASA. (2000).
61. Brown, E. R., Wyn, R., Cumberland, W. G., Yu, H., Abel, E., Gelberg, L., et al. (1995). *Women's health-related behaviors and use of clinical preventive services: A report to the Commonwealth Fund.* Los Angeles: UCLA Center for Health Policy Research.
62. Bernstein, L. R., Folkman, S., & Lazarus, R. S. (1989). Characterization of the use and misuse of medications by an elderly, ambulatory population. *Medical Care, 27*(6), 654–663.
63. The National Center on Addiction and Substance Abuse (CASA) at Columbia University. (1998). *Under the rug: Substance abuse and the mature woman.* New York: CASA.
64. Burns, B. J., Wagner, H. R., Taube, J. E., Magaziner, J., Permutt, T., & Landerman, L. R. (1993). Mental health service use by the elderly in nursing homes. *American Journal of Public Health, 83*(3), 331–337; Goldstrom, I. D., Burns, B. J., Kessler, L. G., Feuerberg, M. A., Larson, D. B., Miller, N. E., et al. (1987). Mental health services use by elderly adults in a primary care setting. *Journal of Gerontology, 42*(2), 147–153.
65. Beardsley, R. S., Gardocki, G. J., Larson, D. B., & Hidalgo, J. (1988). Prescribing of psychotropic medication by primary care physicians and psychiatrists. *Archives of General Psychiatry, 45*(12), 1117–1119.
66. Ascione, F. J., & Shimp, L. A. (1988). Helping patients to reduce medication: Misuse and error. *Generations, 12*(4), 52–55.
67. National Institute on Drug Abuse. (2001). *NIDA research report: Prescription drugs: Abuse and addiction* (NIH Pub. No. 01-4881). Bethesda, MD: U.S. Department of Health and Human Services, National Institutes of Health, National Institute on Drug Abuse.

68. CASA. (2000).
69. CASA. (1998).
70. U.S. General Accounting Office. (1995). *Prescription drugs and the elderly.* Washington, DC: U.S. General Accounting Office.
71. Sheahan, S. L., Hendricks, J., & Coons, S. J. (1989). Drug misuse among the elderly: A covert problem. *Health Values, 13*(3), 22–29.
72. Blow, F. C. (1998). *Substance abuse among older adults: Treatment Improvement Protocol (TIP) Series 26* (DHHS Pub. No. [SMA] 98-3179). Rockville, MD: U.S. Department of Health and Human Services, Public Health Service, Substance Abuse and Mental Health Services Administration, Center for Substance Abuse Treatment; Ives, T. J. (1992). Pharmacotherapeutics. In R. J. Ham & P. D. Sloane (Eds.), *Primary care geriatrics: A case-based approach* (pp. 194–208). St. Louis, MO: Mosby Year Book.
73. Ascione, F. J., & Shimp, L. A. (1988).
74. CASA. (2003). *Alcohol abuse.*
75. Farrell, E. F. (2005, March 18). The battle for hearts and lungs. *Chronicle of Higher Education.*
76. Office of National Drug Control Policy. (2002). *Ad gallery: Jessica Simpson.* www.mediacampaign.org (accessed October 12, 2004).
77. Partnership for a Drug-Free America. (2002). *Campaign viewer: Cause of death: Ecstasy.* www.drugfreeamerica.org (accessed October 12, 2004).
78. TheTruth.com. (2004). www.thetruth.com (accessed October 12, 2004).
79. CASA. (2003). *The formative years.*
80. Hystert, P. E., Mirand, A. L., Giovino, G. A., Cummings, K. M., & Kuo, C. L. (2003). "At Face Value": Age progression software provides personalised demonstration of the effects of smoking on appearance. *Tobacco Control, 12*(2), 238.
81. Farrelly, M. C., Healton, C. G., Davis, K. C., Messeri, P., Hersey, J. C., & Haviland, M. L. (2002). Getting to the truth: Evaluating national tobacco countermarketing campaigns. *American Journal of Public Health, 92*(6), 901–907; Join Together. (2002). *Walters says anti-drug ad campaign a failure.* www.jointogether.org (accessed June 11, 2002); Office of National Drug Control Policy, & National Youth Anti-Drug Media Campaign. (2002). *Investing in our nation's youth: The National Youth Anti-Drug Media Campaign surpasses expectations in phase II* [Press release]. www.mediacampaign.org (accessed June 11, 2002).
82. Straus, R. (1986). Alcohol problems among the elderly: The need for a biobehavioral perspective. In G. Maddox, L. N. Robins, & N. Rosenberg (Eds.), *Nature and extent of alcohol problems among the elderly* (pp. 9–28). New York: Springer.
83. Centers for Disease Control and Prevention, National Center for Chronic Disease Prevention and Health Promotion. (2004). *Tobacco industry marketing: Fact sheet.* www.cdc.gov (accessed May 18, 2004).
84. Center on Alcohol Marketing and Youth. (2004). *Summary: Youth exposure to alcohol advertising.* http://camy.org (accessed May 18, 2004).
85. Tobacco ads retreat [Editorial]. (1999, November 17). *Christian Science Monitor,* 10.

86. Center on Alcohol Marketing and Youth. *Alcohol advertising on sports television 2001 and 2002.* http://camy.org (accessed June 1, 2004).

87. Center for Science in the Public Interest. (2003). *Coaching legends help launch "alcohol-free sports TV" effort: 71 percent want colleges to dump beer ads.* www.cspinet.org (accessed May 18, 2004).

88. Foster, S. E., Vaughan, R. D., Foster, W. H., & Califano, J. A. (2003). Alcohol consumption and expenditures for underage drinking and adult excessive drinking. *JAMA, 289*(8), 989–995.

89. U.S. Food and Drug Administration. (2001). *Buying medicines and medical products online: General FAQs.* www.fda.gov (accessed March 5, 2004).

90. The National Center on Addiction and Substance Abuse (CASA) at Columbia University. (2004). *You've got drugs!: Prescription drug pushers on the internet.* New York: CASA.

91. National Drug Intelligence Center. (2001). *Drugs and the internet: An overview of the threat to America's youth.* www.gpo.gov (accessed March 5, 2004).

92. Greenspan, R. (2003). *Surfing with seniors and boomers.* www.clickz.com (accessed March 5, 2004).

93. CASA. (2004).

94. Ribisl, K. M., Williams, R. S., & Kim, A. E. (2003). Internet sales of cigarettes to minors. *JAMA, 290*(10), 1356–1359.

95. Pacific Institute for Research and Evaluation, Mosher, J. F., & Stewart, K. (1999). *Regulatory strategies for preventing youth access to alcohol: Best practices.* Calverton, MD: Pacific Institute for Research and Evaluation.

96. Ibid.

97. Grossman, M., Sindelar, J. L., Mullahy, J., & Anderson, R. (1993). Policy watch: Alcohol and cigarette taxes. *Journal of Economic Perspectives, 7*(4), 211–222; National Institute on Alcohol Abuse and Alcoholism. (2000). *Tenth special report to Congress on alcohol and health: Highlights from current research* (NIH Pub. No. 00-1583). Rockville, MD: U.S. Department of Health and Human Services, National Institute on Alcohol Abuse and Alcoholism.

98. Ringel, J. S., & Evans, W. N. (2001). Cigarette taxes and smoking during pregnancy. *American Journal of Public Health, 91*(11), 1851–1856.

99. The National Center on Addiction and Substance Abuse (CASA) at Columbia University. (2002). *Teen tipplers: America's underage drinking epidemic.* New York: CASA.

100. Sargent, R. P., Shepard, R. M., & Glantz, S. A. (2004). Reduced incidence of admissions for myocardial infarction associated with public smoking ban: Before and after study. *British Medical Journal, 328*(7446), 977–980; Of smoking bans and heart attacks [Editorial]. (2004, April 27). *New York Times,* A24.

101. New York City Department of Health and Mental Hygiene, Office of Communications. (2004). *New York City's smoking rate declines rapidly from 2002 to 2003, the most significant one-year drop ever recorded* [Press release]. www.nyc.gov.1993.

102. CASA. (2002). *Teen tipplers.*

103. Pacific Institute for Research and Evaluation. Mosher, J. F., & Stewart, K. (1999).

104. Abt Associates. (2002). *8th Abt tobacco report: Independent evaluation of the Massachusetts Tobacco Control Program eighth annual report: January 1994 to June 2001.* www.mass.gov (accessed June 7, 2004); Centers for Disease Control and Prevention, National Center for Chronic Disease Prevention and Health Promotion. (2003). *What is needed to reduce smoking among women* [Fact sheet]. www.cdc.gov (accessed June 7, 2004).

105. Centers for Disease Control and Prevention. (2003).

106. Centers for Disease Control and Prevention. (2000). Declines in lung cancer rates: California, 1988–1997. *Morbidity and Mortality Weekly Report, 49*(47), 1066–1069.

107. Pacific Institute for Research and Evaluation, Mosher, J. F., & Stewart, K. (1999).

108. Grover, P. L. (Ed.). (1999). *Preventing problems related to alcohol availability: Environmental approaches: Reference guide* (DHHS Pub. No. [SMA] 99-3298). Rockville, MD: U.S. Department of Health and Human Services, Substance Abuse and Mental Health Services Administration, Center for Substance Abuse Prevention, Division of State and Community Systems Development; Grube, J. W. (1997). Preventing sales of alcohol to minors: Results from a community trial. *Addiction, 92*(Suppl. 2), S251-S260.

109. National Women's Law Center, & Oregon Health and Science University. (2003). *Women and smoking: A national and state-by-state report card.* Washington, DC: National Women's Law Center, Oregon Health and Science University.

110. Ibid.; Richter, L., Vaughan, R. D., & Foster, S. E. (2004). Public attitudes about underage drinking policies: Results from a national survey. *Journal of Public Health Policy, 25*(1), 58–77; CASA. (2002). *Teen tipplers.*

111. CASA. (2005). *CASA's analysis of NSDUH 2003.*

indexindexindexindex

5 14 44 (258) 51?

6 17

40 63

53

55